Deep Nutrition

Why Your Genes Need Traditional Food

Every effort has been made to ensure that the information contained in the book is complete and accurate. However, neither the author nor the publisher is engaged in rendering advice to the individual reader.

Deep Nutrition

Why Your Genes Need Traditional Food

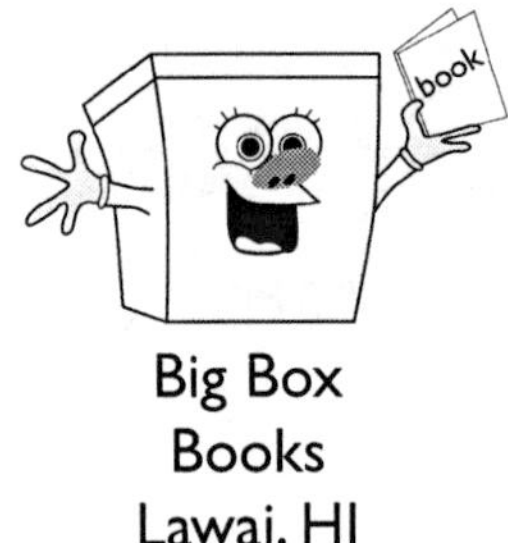

Big Box
Books
Lawai, HI

Cover and Book Design: Catherine & Luke Shanahan
Nautilus Pompilus photo by Ethan Hern
Amarna Tablet clay replica by Luke Shanahan
Interior cartoons by Catherine Shanahan

Library of Congress Cataloging-in-Publication Data

Shanahan, Catherine MD
Deep Nutrition: Why Your Genes Need Traditional Food
Catherine Shanahan, MD; Luke Shanahan, MFA

Includes bibliographical references and index

Library of Congress Control Number: 200890981

To order, visit www.DrCate.com

ISBN-10: 0-615-22838-0
ISBN-13 13:978-0-615-22838-9

Photo And Image Credits

Nautilus Pompilus graphic, courtesy of John N. Harris 37
Persian girl, by Hamed Saber CC 3.0..38
Clark Gable, from *Gone With The Wind* trailer, uncopyrighted 38
Tyson Beckford, by Jesse Gross CC 2.5..38
Tom Cruise, by Alan Light CC 2.0..38
Halle Berry, by Alexander Horn CC 2.5..38
Blonde Student, by Yuri Arcurs..........38
Dick Cheney, Karen Ballard White House staff 42
Marquardt Mask and overlays, © Stephen Marquardt, Marquardt Beauty Analysis, courtesy of Dr. Marquardt, www.beautyanalysis.com.................44
Cerebellum, photomicrograph courtesy of Jhodie Duncan 46
Ingrid Bergman, from *Dr. Jekyll & Mr. Hyde* trailer, uncopyrighted..............50
Christopher Reeve and Jane Seymour, from *Somewhere In Time*, publicity photo 52
Oprah Winfrey, by Alan Light CC 2.0..53
Narrow Marquardt Mask, © Stephen Marquardt, MD 56
Maasai woman, © Price Pottenger Nutrition Foundation, PPNF.org 62
Marquardt Mask, © Stephen Marquardt,www.beautyanalysis.com62
Thai woman, photo courtesy of David Miller 64
Girl from Hamar tribe, photo courtesy of Terry Buxton 64
Children milking goat, photo courtesy of Iman MP Heijboer........................66
Kevin Dillon, photo courtesy of Allistair McMannis.......................................78
Matt Dillon, photo courtesy of Devin Hyde 78
Nicky Hilton, by Eduardo Sciammarella, CC2.0........................81
Paris Hilton, by Paul Schäfermeier, CC2.5 81
Prince William and Prince Harry, Getty Images...82
Three Turlington sisters, by Sharon Wohlmuth..84
Ralph Fiennes, promotional photo....90
Martha, Magnus, Sophie, and Joseph Fiennes, Getty Images 90
Jacob Fiennes, *Madam* magazine 90
Fetal Alcohol Syndrome, photo by Teresa Kellerman, wwwlfasstar.com .95
Petroglyph, by Andras Zboray, Fliegel Jerniczy Expeditions, gourd portion of petroglyph was digitally modified for better viewing in black and white ..120
Tiger Woods, by Molly A Burgess, US Navy Petty Officer 2nd Class..........266
Maasai Man, photo courtesy of John Hanley 277
Dean Ornish, by Pierre Omidyar....277
Saccade tracings, by Alfred Yarbus..281
Petroglyph at Anasazi Ridge, courtesy of Don Austin.................................288

Key

CC 2.0 **Creative Commons Attribution 2.0 Generic http://creativecommons.org/licenses/by/2.0/**

CC 2.5 **Creative Commons Attribution Share Alike 2.5 Generic http://creativecommons.org/licenses/by-sa/2.5/**

CC 3.0 **Creative Commons Attribution Unported http://creativecommons.org/licenses/by/3.0/**

To Buddy

Of all the souls we have met, he was the most human.

Special Thanks

To dozens of physicians at UCLA and UCSF for interviews and opinions. To Dr. Stephen Marquardt for insights into his groundbreaking research. To Jo Robinson for her story of the discovery of omega-3 fatty acids. To the Price-Pottenger Nutrition Foundation for making the extensive works of Weston A. Price and Dr. Francis Pottenger publicly available. To Yvette Bambas for questions from healthcare consumers. To George Brown for design. To my brother Dan Shanahan for cartoons. To Sandra Yue for countless hours of editing.To Matt Olds for last-minute editing. To Jeff Tucker and Rob Kvidt of Techspokes.com for social media marketing. To Carol Pimental, Leona Soares, Lizelle Hernandez, and the staff of West Kauai Clinic Kalaheo for being so caring to my patients through the years. And to all the scientists and researchers who still believe in the scientific method.

Blending Cultures, Bridging Time

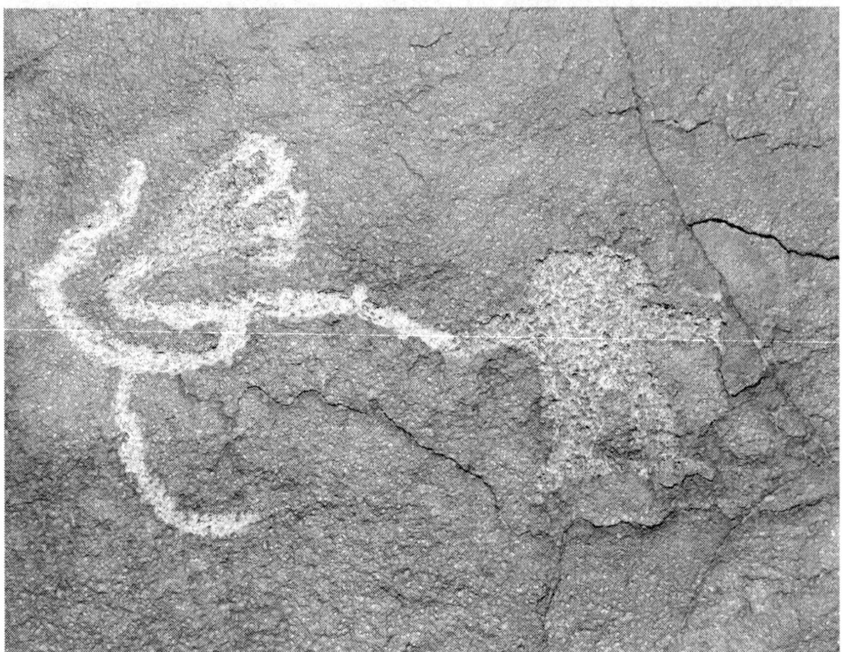

Petroglyph Found on Anasazi Ridge, New Mexico. The childlike glyph on the right is probably Anasazi, agrarians who lived between 400 and 1000 AD. The left is possibly Numic, hunter gatherers who displaced the Anasazi after 1200 AD. No one knows for certain what story it tells. What most attracted me to this particular petroglyph, however, is how the meaning of the original has been modified in a wonderful way, by a younger artist who attached his own symbol to it, in much the same way that our own, ancient genetic code has been modified over time by everyone who has carried it.

Table Of Contents

Introduction..i

1. Reclaiming Your Health..1

   The Origins of Deep Nutrition

2. The Intelligent Gene..22

   Epigenetics and the Language of DNA

3. Dynamic Symmetry..36

   Nature's Desire for Beauty

4. The Greatest Gift..58

   The Creation and Preservation of Genetic Wealth

5. A Mother's Wisdom..76

   Letting Your Body Create a Perfect Baby

6. The Great Nutrition Migration..103

   From the Culinary Garden of Eden to Outer Space

7. The Four Pillars of World Cuisine..121

   Foods that Program Your Body for Beauty, Brains, and Health

8. Good Fats and Bad..166

   How the Cholesterol Theory Created a Sickness Epidemic

9. Sickly Sweet..201

   How Carbohydrate-Rich Diets Block Metabolic Function

10. Beyond Calories..234

    Using Food as a Language to Achieve Ideal Body Weight

11. Forever Young..261

    Collagen Health and Life Span

12. Epilogue..285
Health Without Healthcare

Appendices..288

Tests to Measure Your Health..289

Steps for Including The Four Pillars in Your Diet...................................292

Our Four Pillar Menu..294

Selected Recipes..297

Shopping, Reading, and Resources..299

Index...302

References 307..313

Introduction

This book describes the diet to end all diets.

That's easy to say, of course. All kinds of nutrition books claim to describe the one and only, best-of-all diet—the last one you'll ever need. The truth is, there really are a lot of good diets out there. You're already familiar with some of them: the Okinawan, the Mediterranean, and the French—who "paradoxically" live long, healthy lives though their foods are so heavy and rich.

As a physician, I've often wondered—as have many of my patients—what it is, exactly, that makes all these good diets so special. If the people in Japan, eating lots of fish and fresh vegetables, and the people of the Mediterranean, eating dairy and foods drenched in olive oil, can enjoy superior health, and attribute their good health to the foods they eat, then how is it that—enjoying apparently different foods—they can both lay claim to the number one, best diet on Earth? Could it be that many cultures hold equal claim to a fantastically successful nutritional program? Might it be that people all over the world are doing things right, acquiring the nutrients their bodies need to stay healthy and feel young by eating what appear to be different foods but which are, in reality, nutritionally equivalent?

This book comprehensively describes what could be called *The Human Diet*. It is the first to identify and describe the commonalities between all the most successful nutritional programs people the world over have depended on for millennia to protect their health and encourage the birth of healthy children so that the heritage of optimum health can be gifted to the next generation, and the generations that follow.

We like to talk about leaving a sustainable, healthy environment for our children. The latest science fuses the environmental discussion with the genetic one; when we talk environmental sustainability, we are necessarily talking about our genomic sustainability.

This is also the first book to discuss health across generations. Because of a new science called *epigenetics*, it will no longer make sense to consider our health purely on the personal level. When we think of our health, we think of our own bodies, as in "I feel good," "I like my weight," "I'm doing fine." Epigenetics is teaching us that our genes can be healthy or sick, just like we can. And if our genes are healthy when we have children, that health is imparted to them. If our genes are ailing, then that illness can be inherited as well. Because epigenetics allows us to consider health in the context of a longer timeline, we are now able to understand how what we eat as parents can change everything about our children, even the way they look. We'll talk about how, with the right foods, we can get our genome into shape to give our kids a fighting chance.

One of the most important new concepts of *Deep Nutrition* is this idea that the foods parents eat can change the way their children look. Actually, it's not entirely new. Most of us are familiar with fetal alcohol syndrome, a developmental impairment characterized by a set of facial abnormalities caused by alcohol consumption during pregnancy. Those very same developmental impairments can be caused by malnutrition. I see this every day in my clinic. You'll learn why following the standard dietary recommendations currently promoted by nutritionists and dietitians means running the risk that your child's development will be similarly affected—something I call *second sibling syndrome*.

There's been a reluctance to equate good looks with good health—even, for that matter, to broach the subject. But with the healthcare infrastructure creaking under the bloat of chronically ill children and adults, it's time to get real. We're not talking about abstract aesthetic concepts of beauty. If you're planning on having a child, and you want them to have every opportunity in life, you want them to be physically attractive. How do we know what's attractive? We met with the world's leading expert in the science of beauty to find out for ourselves what exactly makes a person pretty or plain. His name is Dr. Stephen Marquardt. He's a highly sought-after plastic surgeon living outside LA, and his "Marquardt Mask" shows how the perfect human face is the inevitable result of a person's body growing in accordance with the mathematical rules of nature.

You're going to meet another maverick, a man who should be considered the father of modern nutrition. Like Marquardt, the plastic surgeon, this modest dentist refused to accept the idea that it was natural for children's teeth to crowd and shift as haphazardly as tombstones on frost-heaved ground. Teeth should fit, he insisted. He traveled the world to determine if remaining on traditional foods would ensure the proper growth of children so that their teeth, their eyes, and every organ in their body would match one another in perfect proportion, ensuring optimum function and extraordinary health. He discovered that human health depends on traditional foods. Epigenetics proves that this is so because our genes expect the nutrients traditional foods provide.

When you have finished reading this book, you will have completely revised the way you think about food. We're going to do away with calorie counting and struggling to find the perfect ratio of carbs to protein to fat. These terms aren't useful because they say nothing about what really matters about your food. Food is like a language, an unbroken information stream that connects every cell in your body to an aspect of the natural world. The better the source and the more undamaged the message when it arrives to your cells, the better your health will be. If you eat a properly cooked steak from an open-range, grass-fed cow, then you are receiving information not only about the health of that cow's body, but about the health of the grasses from which it ate, and the soil from which those grasses grew. If you want to know whether or not a steak, or a fish, or a carrot is good for you, ask yourself what portions of the natural world it represents, and whether or not the bulk of that information remains intact. This requires traveling backwards down the food chain, step by step, until you reach the ground or the sea.

In the following chapters, you will learn that the secret to health—the big secret, the one no one's talking about—is that there is no secret. Getting healthy, really healthy, and staying healthy can be easy. Avoiding cancer and dependence on medications, staving off heart disease, keeping a razor sharp mind well into advanced years, and even having healthy, beautiful children are all aspects of the human experience that can be, and should be, under your control. You *can* live better, and it doesn't have to be that difficult. You just have to be armed with the right information.

No matter what you already believe about diet, medicine, or health—including the limits of your own health—the book you're about to read will enable you to make better sense of what you already know. To answer what is for many people a nagging question: *Who's right?* What's the simple, complete picture that ties all the best information together, so that I can know, once and for all, which foods my family is supposed to eat and which ones we need to avoid? How can I be sure that what I'm preparing for my children will give them a better chance to grow normally, succeed in school, and live long, happy lives?

What am I supposed to make for dinner?

This book will give you the answer.

One

Reclaiming Your Health

The Origins of Deep Nutrition

Ask ten people what the healthiest diet in the world is and you'll get ten different answers. Some people swear by the Okinawa diet. Others like the Mediterranean or the French. But have you ever thought to wonder what it is about all these traditional diets that makes the people eating them so healthy? This book will describe the common rules that link all successful diets. We call them the Four Pillars of World Cuisine. Throughout history, people have used them to protect their own health, and grow healthy, beautiful children.

In other words, they used diet to engineer their bodies. Most of us probably have something we'd want to change about the way we look, or about our health. What if you could use food to change your body at the genetic level?

Think about it: What if you could re-engineer your genes to your liking? Want to be like Mike? How about Tiger Woods? Halle Berry? George Clooney? Or maybe you want to change your genes so that you can still be you, only better. Just a modest upgrade—a sexier body, better health, greater athleticism, and a better attitude. When you start to consider what you might be willing to pay for all this, you realize that the greatest gift on Earth is a set of healthy genes. The lucky few who do inherit pristinely healthy genes are recognized as "genetic lottery winners" and spend their lives enjoying the many benefits of beauty, brains, and brawn. Being a genetic marvel doesn't mean you automatically get everything you want. But if you have the genes and the desire, you can have the world at your feet.

Back in the mid 1980s, a handful of biotech millionaires thought they had the technology to bring daydreams like these to life. They organized the Human Genome Project, which, we were told, was going to revolutionize how medicine was practiced and how babies were conceived and born.

At the time, conventional medical wisdom held that some of us turn out beautiful and talented while others don't because, at some point, Mother Nature made a mistake or two while reproducing DNA. These mistakes lead to random *mutations* and, obviously, you can't be a genetic marvel if your genes are scabbed with mutations. The biotech wiz kids got the idea that if they could get into our genes and fix the mutations—with genetic vaccines or patches—they could effectively rig the lottery. On June 26, 2000, they reached the first milestone in this ambitious scheme and announced they'd cracked the code.

"This is the outstanding achievement not only of our lifetime but in terms of human history," Dr. Michael Dexter, the project's administrator, declared.[1] Many were counting on new technology such as this to magically address disease at its source. Investors and geneticists promised the mutations responsible for hypertension, depression, cancer, male pattern baldness—potentially whatever we wanted—would soon be neutralized and corrected. In the weeks that followed, I listened to scientists on talk shows stirring up publicity by claiming the next big thing would be made-to-order babies, fashioned using so-called *designer genes*. But I was skeptical. Actually, more than skeptical—I knew it to be hype. I knew this because a decade earlier, in 1989, while at Cornell University, I learned from leaders in the field that a layer of biologic complexity existed which would undermine such bullish predictions. It was an inconvenient reality these scientists kept tucked under their hats.

While the project's supporters described our chromosomes as static chunks of information that could be easily (and safely) manipulated, a new field of science, called *epigenetics*, had already proved this fundamental as-

Do These Men Look Tough to You?

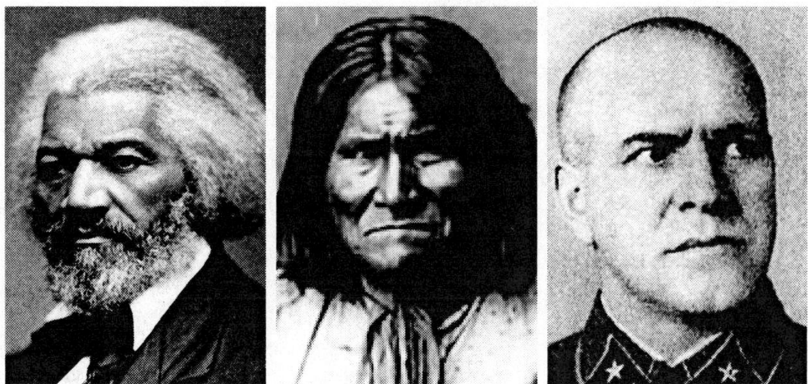

Figure 1. What Healthy Genes Can Do. Left to right: American abolitionist and statesman, Frederick Douglass; Apache leader, Geronimo; Russian war hero, Georgy Zhukov. These men look tough because they are tough. Like other historical figures, they were not raised on Pop Tarts and power drinks, but on The Four Pillars of Traditional Cuisine.

sumption wrong. Epigenetics helps us understand that the genome is more like a dynamic, living being—growing, learning, and adapting constantly. You may have heard that most disease is due to random mutations, or "bad" genes. But epigenetics tells us otherwise. If you need glasses or get cancer or age faster than you should, you very well may have perfectly normal genes. What's gone wrong is how they function, what scientists call *genetic expression*. Just as we can get sick when we don't take care of ourselves, it turns out, so can our genes.

Your Diet Changes How Your Genes Work

In the old model of genetic medicine, diseases arise from permanent damage to DNA, called mutations, portions of the genetic code where crucial data has been distorted by a biological typo. Mutations were thought to arise from mistakes DNA makes while generating copies of itself, and therefore, the health of your genes (and Darwinian evolution) was dependent on random rolling of the dice. Mutations were, for many decades, presumed to be the root cause of everything from knock-knees to short stature to high blood pressure and depression. This model of inheritance is the reason doctors tell people with family histories of cancer, diabetes, and so on that they've inherited genetic time bombs ready to go off at any moment. It's also the reason we call the genetic lottery a lottery. The underlying principle is that we have little or no control. But epigenetics has identified a ghost in the machine, giving us a different vision of Mother Nature's most fantastic molecule.

Epigenetic translates to *upon the gene.* Epigenetic researchers study how our own genes react to our behavior, and they've found that just about everything we eat, think, breathe, or do can, directly or indirectly, trickle down to touch the gene and affect its performance in some way. These effects are carried forward into the next generation where they can be magnified. In laboratory experiments researchers have shown that, simply by feeding mice with different blends of vitamins, they can change the next generation's adult weight and susceptibility to disease, and these new developments can then be passed on again, to grandchildren.[2] It's looking as though we've grossly underestimated the dictum *You are what you eat.* Not only does what we eat affect us down to the level of our genes, our physiques have been sculpted, in part, by the foods our parents and grandparents ate (or didn't eat) generations ago.

The body of evidence compiled by thousands of epigenetic researchers working all over the world suggests that the majority of people's medical problems do not come from mutations, as previously thought, but rather from harmful environmental factors that force good genes to behave badly, by switching them on and off at the wrong time. And so, genes that were once healthy can, at any point in our lives, start acting sick.

The environmental factors controlling how well our genes are working will vary from minute to minute, and each one of your cells reacts differently. So you can imagine how complex the system is. It's this complexity which makes it impossible to predict whether a given smoker will develop lung cancer, colon cancer, or no cancer at all. The epigenetic modulation is so elaborate and so dynamic that it's unlikely we'll ever develop a technologic fix for most of what ails us. So far, it may sound like epigenetics is all bad news. But ultimately, epigenetics is showing us that the genetic lottery is anything but random. Though some details may forever elude science, the bottom line is clear: *We* control the health of our genes.

The concept of gene health is simple. Genes work fine until disturbed. External forces that disturb the normal ebb and flow of genetic function can be broken into two broad categories: toxins and nutrient imbalances. Toxins are harmful compounds we may eat, drink, or breathe into our bodies, or even manufacture internally when we experience undue stress. Nutrient imbalances are usually due to deficiencies, missing vitamins, minerals, fatty acids, or other raw materials required to run our cells. You may not have control over the quality of the air you breathe or be able to quit your job in order to reduce stress. But you do have control over what may be the most powerful class of gene regulating factors: food.

A Holistic Perspective of Food

Believe it or not, designer babies aren't a new idea. People "designed" babies in ancient times. No, they didn't aim for a particular eye or hair color; their goal was more practical—to give birth to healthy, bright, and happy babies. Their tools were not high technology in the typical sense of the word, of course. Their tool was biology, combined with their own common sense wisdom and careful observation. Reproduction was not entered into casually, as it too often is today, because the production of healthy babies was necessary to the community's long-term survival. Through trial and error people learned that, when certain foods were missing from a couple's diet, their children came out with problems. They learned which foods helped to ease delivery, which encouraged the production of calmer, more intelligent children who grew rapidly and rarely fell sick, and then passed this information on. Without this nurturing wisdom, we—as *we* are presently defined—never would have made it this far.

Widely scattered evidence indicates that all successful cultures accumulated vast collections of nutritional guidelines anthologized over the course of many generations and placed into a growing body of wisdom. This library of knowledge was not a tertiary aspect of these cultures. It was ensconced safely within the vaults of religious doctrine and ceremony to ensure its unending revival. The following excerpt offers one example of what the locals living in Yukon Territory (in Canada) knew about scurvy, a disease of vitamin C deficiency, which at the time (in 1930), still killed European explorers to the region:

> *When I asked an old Indian [...]why he did not tell the white man how [to prevent scurvy], his reply was that the white man knew too much to ask the Indian anything. I then asked him if he would tell me. He said he would if the chief said he might. He returned in an hour, saying that the chief said he could tell me because I was a friend of the Indians....He then described how when the Indian kills a moose he opens it up and at the back of the moose just above the kidney there are what he described as two small balls in the fat [the adrenal glands]. These he said the Indian would take and cut up into as many pieces as there were little and big Indians in the family and each one would eat his piece.*[3]

When I first encountered this passage, it was immediately obvious just how sophisticated the accumulated knowledge once was—far better than my medical school training in nutrition. My textbooks said that vitamin C only comes from fruits and vegetables. In the text, the chief makes specific reference to his appreciation of the interviewer's advice to avoid the food in the trading posts, demonstrating how, in indigenous culture, advice regarding food and nutrition is held in high esteem, even treated as a valuable object that can serve as consideration in a formal exchange. We've become accustomed to using the word "share" these days, as in, *Let me share a story with you.* But this was sharing in the truest sense, as in offering a gift of novel weaponry or a fire-starting device—items not to be given up lightly. In fact, the book's author admitted consistent difficulty extracting nutrition-related information for this very reason. There is an old African saying, *When an elder dies, a library burns to the ground.* And so, unfortunately, this particular human instinct—an understandable apprehension of sharing with outsiders —has allowed much of what used to be known to die away.

Today we are raised to think of food as a kind of enriched fuel, a source of calories and a carrier for vitamins, which help prevent disease. In contrast, ancient peoples understood food to be a holy thing, and eating was a sanctified act. Their songs and prayers reflected the belief that, in consuming food, each of us comes in contact with the great, interconnected web of life. Epigentics proves that intuitive idea to be essentially true. Our genes make their day-to-day decisions based on chemical information they receive from the food we eat, information encoded in our food and carried from that food item's original source, a microenvironment of land or sea. In that sense, food is less like a fuel and more like a language conveying information from the outside world. That information programs your genes, for better or for worse. Today's genetic lottery winners are those people who inherited well-programmed, healthy genes by virtue of their ancestor's abilities to properly plug into that chemical information stream. If you want to help your genes get healthy, you need to plug in too—and this is the book that can help.

For ten years, I have studied how food programs genes and how that programming affects physiology. I've learned that food can tame unruly genetic behavior far more reliably than biotechnolgy. By simply replenishing your body with the nourishment that facilitates optimal gene expression, it's possible to eliminate genetic malfunction and, with it, pretty much all known disease. No matter what kind of genes you were born with, I know that eating right can help reprogram them, immunizing you against cancer, premature aging and dementia, enabling you to control your metabolism, your moods, your weight—and much, much more. And if you start planning early enough, and your genetic momentum is strong enough, you can give your children a shot at reaching for the stars.

Who Am I?

In many ways, it was my own unhealthy genes that inspired me to go to medical school and, later, to write this book. I'd had more than my fair share of problems from the beginning of my sports career. In high school track, I suffered with Achilles tendonitis, then calcaneal bursitis, then iliotibial band syndrome, and it seemed to me that I was constantly fitting corrective inserts into my shoes or adding new therapeutic exercises to my routine. In college I developed a whole new crop of soft tissue problems, including a case of shin splints so severe it almost cost me my athletic scholarship.

When my shin splints got bad enough that I had to start skipping practice, I paid another visit to the team physician. Dr. Scotty, a stubby, mustached man with thick black hair and a high-pitched voice, told me that this time he couldn't help me. All I could do was cut back my training and wait. But I was sure there was something else I needed to do. Perhaps I had some kind of dietary deficiency? Applying my newly acquired mastery of biology 101, I suggested that, perhaps, my connective tissue cells couldn't make normal tendons. Like many of my own patients insist today, I pushed Dr. Scotty to get to the bottom of my problem. I even had a plan, simply take some kind of biopsy of the tendon in my leg and compare the material to a healthy tendon. My ideas went nowhere, as I imagine such suggestions often do. Dr. Scotty furrowed his bushy eyebrows and said he'd never heard of any such test. I'd read stories in *Newsweek* and *Time* about the powerful diagnostics being brought to us by molecular biology. In my naiveté, I couldn't believe Dr. Scotty didn't know how to use any of that science to help me. I was so confounded by the unwillingness to consider what seemed to me to be the obvious course of action, and so enamored with the idea of getting to the molecular root of physical problems—and so enthralled by the promise of the whole burgeoning biotech field—that I scrapped my plans to be a chemical engineer and enrolled in every course I could to study genetics. I went to graduate school at Cornell, where I learned about gene regulation and epigenetics from Nobel Prize-winning researchers, then straight to Robert Wood Johnson Medical School in New Jersey, in hopes of putting my knowledge of the fundamentals of genetics to practical use.

I then found out why Dr. Scotty had been dumfounded by my questions years before. Medical school doesn't teach doctors to address the root of the problem. It teaches doctors to treat the problem. It's a practical science with practical aims. In this way, medicine differs quite drastically from other natural sciences. Take, for instance, physics, which has built a body of deep knowledge by always digging down to get to the roots of a problem. Physicists have now dug so deep that they are grappling with one of the most fundamental questions of all: How did the universe begin? But medicine is different from other sciences because, more than being a science, it is first and foremost a business. This is why, when people taking a heart pill called Loniten started growing unwanted hair on their arms, researchers didn't ask why. Instead, they looked for customers. And Loniten the heart pill became Rogaine, the spray for balding men. Medicine is full of examples like this, one the most lucrative being the discovery of Sildafenil, originally for blood pressure until found to have the happy side effect of prolonging erections and repackaged into Viagra. Since medicine is a business, medical research must ultimately generate some kind of saleable product. And that is why we still don't know what leads to common problems like shin splints.

I didn't go to medical school to become a businesswoman. My dreams had sprouted from a seed planted in my psyche when I was five, during an incident with a baby robin. Sitting on the street curb in front of my house one spring morning, the plump little fledgling flew down from the maple tree to land on the street in front of me. Looking directly at me, he chirped and flapped his wings as if to say "Look what I can do!"—and then I saw the front tire of a station wagon roll up behind him. In a blink, the most adorable creature I'd ever seen was smashed into a feather pancake, a lifeless stain on the asphalt. Dead. I was outraged. Overwhelmed with guilt. Whoever was driving that car had no idea of the trauma he'd just inflicted on two young lives. This was my first experience with the finality of death, and it awoke a protective instinct that has driven my career decisions ever since: Prevent harm. It was why I'd wanted to be a chemical engineer (to invent nontoxic baby diapers) and why I had gone to medical school. I was all about prevention, and that meant I needed to understand what makes us tick and what makes us sick.

Unfortunately, soon after enrolling in medical school, I found that the gap between my childhood dream and the reality of limited medical knowledge was enormous. So enormous that, I concluded, it wasn't yet possible to breach. To pursue my dream of preventing harm, the best I could do was practice "preventive medicine," and the best place to do this was within the specialty of primary care. To tell the truth, I kind of forgot about the whole idea of getting to the bottom of what makes people sick, and for many years after graduation I went on with ordinary life. Until something drew me back in.

Respecting Our Ancient Wisdom

It was those malfunctioning genes of mine, again. Shortly after moving to Hawaii, I developed another musculoskeletal problem. But this one was different from all the others. This time no doctor, not even five different specialists, could tell me what it was. And it didn't go away. A year after I developed the first unusual stinging pain around my right knee, I could no longer walk more than a few feet without getting feverish. It was unlike anything I'd ever heard of. I'd had exploratory surgery, injections, physical therapy, and I'd even seen a Hawaiian *kahuna*. But everything I tried seemed to make the problem worse. Just as I was giving up hope, Luke came up with an idea: Try studying nutrition. As an excellent chef and an aficionado of all things relating to cuisine, he'd been impressed by the variety and flavors he encountered at the local Filipino buffets. Like many professional chefs I've spoken with since, he suspected there might be other opinions out there on what healthy food might actually be. Having fought his own battles against malnutrition while growing up on the wrong side of the tracks in small-town USA, he recognized that there were nutritional haves and have-nots, as there is with everything else. And he suspected that my high-sugar, convenience-food diet put me in the have-not category and might even be impairing my ability to heal.

Sure, I thought, everyone has an opinion. I—on the other hand—went to medical school. Hel-l-l-lo-o-o…I took a course on nu-tri-tion. I learned bi-o-chem-is-try. I already knew to eat low-fat, low-cholesterol and count my calories. What more did I need to know? The next day, Luke brought home a book. Had I not been literally immobilized, I may never have bothered opening Andrew Weil's book *Spontaneous Healing* and started reading.

Medical school teaches us to believe that we're living longer now, and so today's diet must beat the diets of the past, hands down. This argument had me so convinced that I never considered questioning the dietary dogma I'd absorbed throughout my schooling. But realize that today's eighty-year-olds grew up on an entirely different, more natural diet. They were also the first generation to benefit from antibiotics, and many have been kept alive thanks only to technology. Today's generation has yet to prove its longevity, but given that many forty-year-olds already have joint and cardiovascular problems that their parents didn't get until much later in life (as is true in my practice), I don't think we can assume they have the same life expectancy. And the Millennium Generation's lifespan may be 10 to 20 years shorter.[4] I was going to get my first inkling of this reality very soon.

Once I cracked the book open, it didn't take much reading to bump into something I'd never heard of before, omega-3 fatty acids. According to Weil, these are fats we need to eat, just like vitamins. These days, our diets are so deficient that we need to supplement. This blew my mind. First of all, I'd thought fats were bad. Secondly, we were supposed to be eating better today than at any point in human history. Either he was off base, or my medical education had failed to provide some basic information. Like a kid who gets into the bathtub kicking and screaming and then doesn't want to get out, I soon couldn't get enough of these "alternative" books. Inside them wasn't just new information, but hope that I might walk normally again.

In another publication, I came across an intriguing article entitled *Guts and Grease: The Diet of Native Americans* which suggested that Native

Hygieia: The Goddess of Nutrition in the Hippocratic Oath

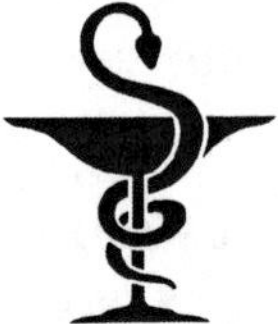

Figure 2. Hygieia's Bowl. In Greek mythologic emblems, Hygieia is depicted holding a bowl, from which she feeds the serpent, a symbol of medical learning.

In ancient Greece the philosophy of wellness was balanced by two complementary ideas. The female, Hygieia, the goddess of health, personified the first. Hygieia was all about building healthy bodies with sound nutrition from the start—prenatally and throughout the formative years of childhood—and maintaining health for the rest of a person's life. In other words, she embodied the most effective form of preventative medicine there is. When that first line of defense failed, and people succumbed to infections or the inevitable accident, Aesculapius, the god of medicine, acted as a kind of Johnny-on-the-spot. He provided knowledge of healing surgical procedures and therapeutic potions. The Hippocratic oath I took on graduation day invokes the wisdom of Aesculapius, Hygieia, and Panacea (the god of potions or cure-alls). But like hundreds of other fresh-faced MDs standing beside me in the lecture hall, hands raised, I had no idea who she was or what she stood for.

Over the last 3000 years of civilization, the male aspect of medical science has completely taken over. Hygiene, which was once a highly scientific and advanced compendium of nutritional information, has been reduced to simplistic notions of cleanliness, like washing your hands and brushing your teeth. It's time to bring Hygieia back.

Americans were healthier than their European counterparts because they ate the entire animal. Not just muscle, but all the "guts and grease."

> *According to John (Fire) Lame Deer, the eating of guts had evolved into a contest. "In the old days we used to eat the guts of the buffalo, making a contest of it, two fellows getting hold of a long piece of intestines from opposite ends, starting chewing toward the middle, seeing who can get there first; that's eating. Those buffalo guts, full of half-fermented, half-digested grass and herbs, you didn't need any pills and vitamins when you swallowed those.*[5]

I liked the voice of authority this Native American assumed, as if he were drawing from a secret well of knowledge. I also liked that the article's authors offered healthy people as evidence instead of statistics of lab simulations. At the time, the approach struck me as novel—focusing on health rather than disease. Early European explorers Cabeza de Vaca, Francisco Vaquez de Coronado, and Lewis and Clark described Native Americans as superhuman warriors, able to run down buffalo on foot and, in battle, continue fighting after being shot through with an arrow. Photographs taken two hundred years later, in the 1800s, capture the Native American's imposing visage and broad, balanced bone structure. Presenting a people's stamina and strength as evidence of a healthy diet seemed reasonable, and it rang true with my own clinical experience in Hawaii: The healthiest family members are, in many cases, the oldest, raised on foods vastly different from those being fed to their great grand children. I began to doubt my presumption that today's definition of a healthy diet was nutritionally superior to diets of years past.

Still, the dietary program of Native Americans seemed bizarre. Reading the passage about two grown men chewing their way through an animal's unwashed, fat-encased intestine forever changed the way I remember the spaghetti scene from *Lady and the Tramp*. It also brought up some serious questions. For one thing, wouldn't eating buffalo poo make the men ill? And isn't animal fat supposed to be unhealthy? The first issue—eating unwashed intestine—was too much for me to tackle (though later I would). So I sunk my teeth into the matter of the health effects of animal fat.

Two things I learned about nutrition in medical school were that saturated fat raises cholesterol levels, and cholesterol is a known killer. Who was right, the American Medical Association, or John (Fire) Lame Deer?

This was how I began to close the knowledge gap that, years ago, had derailed me from pursuing further studies of the fundamentals of disease. To determine the best dietary stance, I would look at all the necessary basic science data (on free radicals, fatty acid oxidation, eicosanoid signaling, gene regulation, and the famous Framingham studies), which, fortunately, I had the training to decipher. It took six months of research to get to the bottom of this one nutritional question, but I ultimately came to understand that the nutrition science I'd learned in medical school was full of contradictions, and resting on assumptions proved false by researchers in other, related scientific fields. The available evidence failed to support the AMA's position, and overwhelmingly sided with that of John (Fire) Lame Deer.

This was a big deal. Contrary to the opinion of medical leaders today, saturated fat and cholesterol appeared to be beneficial nutrients. (Chapter 8 explains how heart disease really develops.) Fifty years of removing foods containing these nutrients from our diets—foods like eggs, fresh cream, and liver—to replace them with low-fat or outright artificial chemicals—like trans-rich margarine—would have starved our genes of the chemical information on which they've come to depend. Simply by cutting eggs and sausage (originally made with lactic acid starter culture instead of nitrates, and containing chunks of white cartilage) from our breakfasts to replace them with cold cereals would mean that generations of children have been fed fewer fats, B vitamins, and collagenous proteins than required for optimal growth.

Here's why. The yolk of an egg is full of brain-building fats, including lecithin, phospholipids, and, (only if from free-range chickens), essential fatty acids and vitamins A and D. Meanwhile, low-fat diets have been shown to reduce intelligence in animals.[6] B vitamins play key roles in the development of every organ system, and women with vitamin B deficiencies give birth to children prone to developing weak bones, diabetes, and more.[7,8] Chunks of cartilage supply us with collagen and glycosaminoglycans,factors that help facilitate the growth of robust connective tissues, which would help to prevent later-life tendon and ligament problems—including shin splints![9]

By righting the wrong assumptions that mushroomed from this one piece of nutritional misinformation, I had already gained a greater understanding of the root causes of disease than I'd thought possible—at least since attending medical school. A single item of medical misinformation, that cholesterol-rich foods are dangerous, had drastically changed our eating habits and with that our access to nutrients. The effect on my personal physiology was to weaken my connective tissues, an epigenetic response that had already managed to change the course of my life in ways that I can't begin to calculate. After reading every old-fashioned cookbook I could get my hands on, and enough biochemistry to understand the essential character of traditional cuisine, I changed everything about the way I eat. For me, eating in closer accordance with historical human nutrition corrected some of my damaged epigenetic programming. I got fewer colds, less heartburn, improved my moods, lost my belly fat, had fewer headaches, and increased my mental energy. And eventually my swollen knee got better.

What Our Ancestors Knew That Your Doctor Doesn't

It seems like every day another study comes out showing the benefits of some vitamin or mineral or antioxidant supplement in the prevention of a given disease. All these studies taken together send the strong message that doctors still underestimate the power of nutrition to fortify and to heal. Of course, people know this intuitively, which is why dietary supplements and nutraceuticals sell so well. Unfortunately, in all this research there is also something that's not talked about very often: Artificial vitamins and powdered, encapsulated antioxidant products are not as effective as the real thing—not even close. They can even be harmful. A far better option is to eat more nutritious *food.*

To identify the most nutritious food Luke and I have studied traditions from all over the world. The goal was not to identify the "best" tradition, but to understand what all traditions have in common. We identified four universal elements, each of which represent a distinct set of ingredients along with the cooking (or other preparation technique) that maximize the nutrition delivered to our cells. For the bulk of human history, these techniques and materials have proved indispensable. The reason that so many of us have health problems today is that we no longer eat in accordance with any culinary tradition. In the worst cases of recurring illnesses and chronic diseases that I see, more often than not, the victims parents and grandparents haven't either. This means that most Americans are carrying around very sick genes. But by returning to the same four categories of nourishing foods our ancestors ate—the "Four Pillars"—our personal genetic health will be regained.

Genetic Health and Wealth

The health of your genes represents a kind of inheritance. Two ways of thinking about this inheritance, *genetic wealth* and *genetic momentum*, help explain why some people can abuse this inheritance and, for a time, get away with it. Just as a lazy student born into a prominent family can be assured he'll get into Yale no matter his grades, healthy genes don't have to be attended to very diligently in order for their owner's bodies to look beautiful. The next generation, however, will pay the price.

We've all seen the twenty-year-old supermodel who abuses her body with cigarettes and Twinkies. For years, her beautiful skeletal architecture will still shine though. Beneath the surface, poor nutrition will deprive those bones of what they need, thinning them prematurely. The connective tissue supporting her skin will begin to break down, stealing away her beauty. Most importantly, deep inside her ovaries, inside each egg, her genes will be affected. Those deleterious genetic alterations mean that her child will have lost *genetic momentum* and will not have the same potential for health or beauty as she did. He or she may benefit from mom's sizable financial portfolio—*à la* Danielynn Nichole Smith—but junior's genetic wealth will, unfortunately, have been drawn down.

That's a real loss. Over the millennia, our genes developed under the influence of a steady stream of nourishing foods gleaned from the most nutritionally potent corners of the natural world. Today's supermodels have benefited not just from their parents and grandparents' healthy eating habits, but from hundreds, even thousands, of generations of ancestors who, by eating the right foods, maintained—and even improved upon—the genetic heirloom that would ultimately construct a beautiful face in the womb. All of this accumulated wealth can be disposed of as easily and as mindlessly as the twenty-year-old supermodel would flick away a cigarette.

Such squandering of *genetic wealth*—a measure of the intactness of epigenetic programming—has affected many of us. My own father grew up drinking powdered milk and ate margarine on Wonderbread every day at lunch. My mother spent much of her childhood in postwar Europe, where dairy products were scarce. Because they had inherited genetic wealth from their parents, my parents never had significant soft tissue problems in spite of these shortcomings. But those suboptimal diets did take a toll on their genes. Much of the genetic wealth of my family line had been squandered by the time I was born. Unlike my parents and grandparents, I had to struggle to keep my joints from falling apart. Fortunately for me, my story is not over—and neither is yours. Thanks to the plasticity of genetic response we can all improve the health of our genes and rebuild our genetic wealth.

Anyone who has chronically neglected a plant and watched its leaves curl and its color fade knows that proper care and feeding can have dramatic, restorative effects. The same applies to our genes—and our epigenetic programming. Not only will you personally benefit from this during your lifetime with improved health, normalization of fat distribution, remission of chronic disease, and resistance to the effects of age, your children will benefit as well. If you think saving money for college or moving to a neighborhood with a good school system is important, then consider the importance of ensuring that your children are as healthy and beautiful as they can be. If you start early enough, the fruits of your efforts will be clearly visible in the bones of your child's face, the face they may one day be presenting to the one person who can give them the opportunity—over all the other candidates—to inaugurate the career of their dreams. It all depends on you—what you eat and how you choose to live. I am not a specialist in stress reduction (though stress reduction is vital), and I won't be talking that much about exercise other than to describe how different types of exercise will help you lose weight and build healthy tissue. However, by virtue of my training and subsequent studies I am an expert at predicting the physiologic effects of eating different types of food. And my basic philosophy is simple.

Deep Nutrition

I subscribe to the school of nutritional thought that counsels us to eat the same foods people ate in the past because, after all, that's how we got here. It's how we're designed to eat. Epigenetics supplies the scientific support for the idea by giving molecular evidence that we are who we are, in large part, because of the foods our ancestors ate. But because healthy genes, like healthy people, can perform well under difficult conditions for a finite amount of time there is, in effect, a delay in the system. Since nutritional researchers don't ask study participants what their parents ate, the conclusions drawn from those studies are based on incomplete data. A poor diet can seem healthy if studied for a 24-hour period. A slightly better diet can seem successful for months or even years. Only the most complete diets, however, can provide health generation after generation.

Diet books that adopt this long-term philosophy such as *Paleodiet, Evolution Diet,* and *Health Secrets of The Stone Age* have been incredibly successful partly by virtue of the philosophy itself, which has intuitive appeal. Fleshing out the bare bones of the nutritional philosophy with specifics, real ingredients, and real recipes, is another matter. Authors of previously published books are still working on the old random mutation model, and so, they don't realize how fast genetic change can occur. In going all the way back to the prehistoric era, they take the idea too far to be practical. Their evidence is so limited it's literally skeletal—gleaned from campfire debris, chips of bone, and the cleanings of mummified stomachs. These books do give us fascinating glimpses of life in the distant past. And I'm impressed by how the authors use modern physiologic science to expand tiny tidbits of data into a complete dietary regime. But each of these books, often citing the same information, leaves us with contradicting advice. Why? The data they have is simply too fragmented, too old, and too short on detail to give us meaningful guidance. How can we reproduce the flavors and nutrients found in our Paleolitic predecessors' dinners when the only instructions they left behind come in the form of such artifacts as "the 125,000-year-old spear crafted from a yew tree found embedded between the ribs of an extinct straight-tusked elephant in Germany" and "cut marks that have been found on the bones of fossilized animals."[10] The authors do their best to make educated guesses, but clearly, a creative mind could follow this ancient trail of evidence to end up wherever they like.

Fortunately, we don't have to rely on prehistory or educated guesses. There is a much richer, living source of information available to us. It's called *cuisine*. Specifically, authentic cuisine. By "authentic," I'm not talking about the Americanized salad-and-seafood translation of Mediterranean or Okinawan or Chinese diets. I'm not talking about modern molecular gastronomy or functional food or fast food. The authentic cuisine I'm referring to is what fondest memories are made of. It's the combination of ingredients and skills that enable families in even the poorest farming communities around the world to create fantastic meals, meals that would be fit for a king and that would satisfy even the snarkiest of New Yorkers—even, say, a food connoisseur whose glance has been known to weaken many a *Top Chef* contender's knees. I am of course referring to former punk rock chef turned world-trotting celebrity, Anthony Bourdain.

As evidence that there's plenty of detailed information surviving to inform us exactly how people used to eat (and still should), I submit Bourdain's travel TV show *No Reservations*. If you haven't seen it already, it's your chance to have the colorful, vastly inventive, and diverse world of culinary arts served to you for an hour each week in your living room. Bourdain gets right to the heart of his host country's distinct food culture, beginning each show by casting a historical light on the local food. Guided by foodwise natives—be they a busty former Miss Russia or a perpetually sweaty sometime-chef named Zamir, he ends up at the right spots to sample food that captures each geographical region's soul. More often than not, these spots end up being the mom-and-pop holes in the wall where people cook the way food has been cooked in that country for as long as anyone can remember. Shows like Bourdain's have helped to convince me that growing up in America is growing up—culinarily speaking—in an underdeveloped country.

While Americans have hot dogs and apple pie, Happy Meals, meatloaf, casseroles, and variations on the theme of salad, citizens of other countries seem to have so much more. In one region of China, a visitor could experience pit-roasted boar, rooster, or rabbit, with a side of any number of different kind of pickle or fermented beans, hand-crafted noodles, or fruiting vegetation of every shape, color, size, and texture. In burgeoning, ultramodern cities, at the base of towering glass buildings around the world, farmers' markets still sell the quality, local ingredients pulled from the earth or fished from the rivers and lakes that morning. My point is not to suggest that America isn't a wonderful country with our own rich history of cuisine. My point is that we're out of touch with our roots. That disconnection is the biggest reason why we have bookshelves full of conflicting nutritional advice. It's also why, though many of us still have good genes, we have not maintained them very well. Like plump grapes left to bake on a French hillside, American chromosomes are wilting on the vine. They can be revitalized simply by enjoying the delightful products of traditional cuisine.

The messy amalgamation of vastly different dishes comprising every authentic cuisine can be cleaved into four neat categories, which I call the Four Pillars of Authentic Cuisine. We need to eat them as often as we can, preferably daily. They are as follows: I: meat cooked on the bone; II: organs and offal (what Bourdain calls "the nasty bits"); III: fresh (raw) plant and animal products; and IV: better than fresh—fermented and sprouted. These categories have proved to be *essential* by virtue of their ubiquitousness. In almost every country other than ours people eat them every day. They've proved to be *successful* by virtue of their practitioners health and survival. Like cream rising in a glass, these traditions have percolated upwards from the past, buoyed by their intrinsic value. They have endured the test of time simply by being delicious and nutritious, and in celebrating them we can reconnect with our roots and with each other, and bring our lives towards their full potential.

Tending the Sacred Flame

Not too long ago, and without understanding genetics, stem cell biology, or biochemistry, cultures everywhere survived based on living in accordance with the cause and effect realities of their daily experience. Their successes are now memorialized in our existence and in the healthy genetic material we have managed to retain. Solutions to the all-important omnivore's dilemma—the question of what we *should* be eating—are all around us, encapsulated in traditions still practiced by foodies, culinary artists, devoted grandmothers, and chefs throughout the world, some in your very own neighborhood. Unfortunately, this wisdom has gone unappreciated, thanks to the cholesterol theory of heart disease and other byproducts of what Michael Pollan calls "scientific reductionism" (a decidedly unscientific exercise, as Pollan explains in his recent book *In Defense of Food*).[11] Fortunately, those who love—really love—good cooking and good food have kept culinary traditions alive. In doing so, not only have their own families benefitted, they also serve as the modern emissaries of our distant relatives, carriers of an ancient secret once intended to be shared only with members of the tribe. Today, we are that tribe. And that message—how to use food to stay healthy and beautiful—is the most precious gift we could possibly receive.

Throughout the book we are going to be highlighting the power of food to shape your daily life. In fact, every bite you eat changes your genes a little bit. Just as the genetic lottery follows a set of predictable rules, so do the small changes that occur after every meal. If the machinery of physiologic change is not random, and is instead guided by rules, then who—or what—keeps track of them? In the next chapter, we'll see how the gene responds to nourishment with what can best be described as intelligence, and why this built-in ability makes me certain that many of us have untapped genetic potential waiting to be released.

Two

The Intelligent Gene

Epigenetics and the Language of DNA

I remember getting caught up in the nostalgia when Halle Berry took the stage at the 2002 Oscars, how she stood before the audience and tearfully thanked God for her blessings. "Thank you. I'm so honored. I'm so honored. And I thank the Academy for choosing me to be the vessel for which His blessing might flow. Thank you." A laudable Hollywood milestone, she had become the first woman of African American descent to be awarded the Oscar for a leading role. While so much focus was placed on what made this actor, and that evening, unique in the history of Hollywood movies, I couldn't avoid the nagging feeling that there was something familiar about the woman in the stunning Elie Saab gown, something about her face that reminded me of every other woman who had, over the years, clutched the little golden statue in her hands. What was the link between Ms. Berry and all her Academy-honored sisters like Charlize Theron, Nicole Kidman, Cate Blanchett, Angelina Jolie, Julia Roberts, Kim Basinger, Jessica Lange, Elizabeth Taylor, Ingrid Bergman, and the rest? Yes, they are all talented masters of their craft. But there was something else about them, something more obvious, maybe so obvious that it was one of those things you just learn to take for granted.

Then it occurred to me: They are *all* breathtakingly gorgeous.

Like Halle Berry, we are all vessels—not necessarily designed to win Oscars, but to eat, survive, and reproduce genetic material. So if you happen to win an Oscar, you could make history by extending one last note of gratitude to your extraordinary DNA. When your PR agent chastises you the next morning, just explain to her that we are all active participants in one of the oldest and most profound relationships on our planet—between our bodies, our DNA, and the food that connects both to the outside world. Halle Berry's perfectly proportioned, fit, healthy body is evidence of a happy relationship between her genes and the natural environment, one that has remained so for several generations. As this chapter will explain, if you hope to create a more fruitful relationship with your own genes, to get healthier and improve the way you look, you need to learn to work with the intelligence within your DNA.

DNA's Giant "Brain"

Every cell of your body contains a nucleus, floating within the cytoplasm like the yolk inside an egg. The nucleus holds your chromosomes, 46 super-coiled molecules, and each one of those contains up to 300 million pairs of genetic letters, called *nucleic acids*. These colorless, gelatinous chemicals (visible to the naked eye only when billions of copies are reproduced artificially in the lab) constitute the genetic materials that make you who you are. If you stretched out the DNA in one of your cells, its 2.8 billion base pairs would end up totaling two to three meters long. The DNA from all your cells strung end to end would reach to the moon and back at least 5000 times.[12] That's a lot of chemical information. But your genes take up only two percent of it. The rest of the sequence—the other 98 percent—is what scientists used to call "junk." Not that they thought this remaining DNA was useless; they just didn't know what any of it was for. In the last two decades, scientists have discovered this material has some amazing abilities.

Epigenetic researchers exploring this expansive genetic territory are finding a hidden world of ornate complexity. Unlike genes, which function as a relatively static repository of encoded data, the so-called "Junk DNA" seems designed for change, both over the short term—within our lifetimes—and over periods of several generations, and longer. It appears that

Junk DNA assists biology in making key decisions, like turning one stem cell into part of an eye, and another stem cell with identical DNA into, say, part of your liver. These decisions seem to be made based on environmental influences. We know this because when you take a stem cell and place it into an animal's liver, it becomes a liver cell. If you took that same stem cell and placed it into an animal's brain, it would become a nerve cell.[13] Junk DNA does all this by using the chemical information floating around it to determine which genes should get turned on when, and in what quantity.

One of the most fascinating, and unexpected, lessons of the Human Genome Project is the discovery that our genes are very similar to mouse genes, which are very much like other mammalian genes, which in turn are surprisingly similar to fish. It appears that the proteins humans produce are not particularly unique in the animal kingdom. What makes us uniquely human are the regulatory segments of our genetic material, the same regulatory segments that direct stem cell development during in-utero growth and throughout the rest of our lives. Could it be that the same mechanisms facilitating cell maturation also function over generations, enabling species to evolve? According to Arturas Petronis, head of the Krembil Family Epigenetics Laboratory at the Centre for Addiction and Mental Health in Toronto, "We really need some radical revision of key principles of the traditional genetic research program." Another epigeneticist puts our misapprehension of evolution in perspective. Mutation- and selection-driven evolutionary change is just the tip of the iceberg. "The bottom of the iceberg is epigenetics." [14]

The more we study this mysterious 98 percent, the more we find it seems to function as a massively complicated regulatory system which serves to control our cellular activities as if it were a huge, molecular brain. A genetic lottery winner's every cell carries DNA that regulates cell growth and activity better than your average Joe's. Not because they're just dumb-lucky, but because their regulatory DNA—their chromosomal "brain"—functions better. Just like your brain, to function properly, DNA needs to be able to remember what it's learned.

How Chromosomes Learn

To understand the genetic brain, how it works, and why it might sometimes forget how to function as perfectly as we may wish, let's get a closer look at chromosomes.

Each of your 46 chromosomes is actually one very long DNA molecule containing up to 300 million pairs of genetic letters, called *nucleic acids*. The genetic alphabet only has four "letters," A,G,T, and C. All of our *genetic* data is encrypted in the patterns of these four letters. Change a letter and you change the pattern, and with it the meaning. Change the meaning, and you very well may change an organism's growth.

Biologists had long assumed that letter substitution was the only way to generate such physiologic change. Epigenetics has taught us that, more often, the reason different individuals develop different physiology stems not from permanent letter substitutions but from temporary markers—or *epigenetic tags*—that attach themselves to the double helix and change how genes are expressed. Some of these markers are in place at birth, but throughout a person's life, many of them detach while others accumulate. Researchers needed to know what this tagging meant. Is it just a matter of DNA aging, or is something else—something more exciting—going on? If everyone developed the same tags during their lives, then it was simple aging. But if the tagging occurred differentially, then it suggests different life experiences can lead to different genetic function. It also means that, in a sense, our genes can *learn*.

In 2005, scientists in Spain found a way to solve the mystery. They prepared chromosomes from two sets of identical twins, one set aged three and the other aged 50. Using fluorescent green and red molecules that bind, respectively, to epigenetically modified and unmodified segments of DNA, they examined the two sets of genes. The children's genes looked very similar, indicating that, as one would expect, twins start life with essentially identical genetic tags. In contrast, the 50-year-old chromosomes lit up green and red like two Christmas trees with different decorations. Their life experiences had tagged their genes in ways that meant these identical twins were, in terms of their genetic function, no longer identical.[15] This means the tagging is not just due to aging. It is a direct result of how we live our lives. Other studies since have shown that epigenetic tagging occurs in response to chemicals that form as a result of everything we eat, drink, breathe, think, and do. It seems our genes are always listening, always on the ready to respond and change. In photographing the different patterns in red and green on the two 50-year-old chromosomes, scientists were capturing the two different "personalities" the women's genes had developed.

This differential genetic tagging would help explain why twins with identical DNA might develop completely different medical problems. If one twin smokes, drinks and eats nothing but junk food while the other takes care of her body, the two sets of DNA are getting entirely different chemical "lessons"—one is getting a balanced education when the other is getting schooled in the dirty streets of chemical chaos.

In a sense, our lifestyles teach our genes how to behave. In choosing between healthy or unhealthy foods and habits, we are programming our genes for either good or bad conduct. Scientists are identifying numerous techniques by which two sets of identical DNA can be coerced into functioning dissimilarly. So far, the processes identified include bookmarking, imprinting, gene silencing, X chromosome inactivation, position effect, reprogramming, transvection, maternal effects, histone modification, and paramutation. Many of these epigenetic regulatory processes involve tagging sections of DNA with markers that govern how often a gene uncoils and unzips. Once exposed, a gene is receptive to enzymes that translate it into protein. If *un*exposed, it remains dormant and the protein it codes for doesn't get expressed.

If one twin sister drinks a lot of milk and moves to Hawaii (where her skin can make vitamin D in response to the sun), while the other avoids dairy and moves to Minnesota, then one will predictably develop weaker bones than the other and will likely suffer from more hip, spine, and other osteoporosis-related fractures.[16] The epigenetic twin study tells us that it's not only their X-rays that will look different, their genes will too. Scientists are becoming convinced that failure to attend to the proper care and feeding of our bodies doesn't just affect us, it affects our genes—and that means it may affect our offspring. Research shows that when one sibling has osteoporosis and the other doesn't, you'll find the genes encoding for bone growth in the osteoporotic member have gone to sleep, having been tagged, temporarily, to stay unexposed and dormant.[17] Fortunately, they'll wake up from their slumber if we change our habits. Unfortunately, the twin who smoked (in our previous example) may have lost too much bone to ever catch up to her milk-drinking, vitamin-D fortified sister. What is worse, any epigenetic markings she developed before conceiving children can be transmitted to her offspring—so that her avoidance of bone-building nutrients has consequences for them. Her children will inherit relatively sleepy bone-growth genes and be born epigenetically prone to osteoporosis. You could say that when it comes to remembering how to build bone, the epigenetic brain had grown a wee bit forgetful. Marcus Pembry, professor of clinical genetics at the Institute of Child Health in London, believes that "we are all guardians of our genome. The way people live and their lifestyle no longer just affects them, but may have a knockoff effect for their children and grandchildren."[18]

What fascinates me most is the intelligence of the system. It seems our genes have found ways to take notes, to remind themselves what to do with the various nutrients they are fed. Here's how. Let's say a gene for building bone is tagged with two epigenetic markers, one that binds to vitamin D and another that binds to calcium. And let's say that when vitamin D and calcium are both bound to their respective markers at the same time, the gene uncoils and can be expressed. If there is no calcium and no vitamin D, then the gene remains dormant and less bone is built. The epigenetic regulatory tags are effectively serving as a kind of Post-it note: *When there's lots of vitamin D and calcium around, make a bunch of the protein encoded for right here.* When they do, *voilà!* You're building bone! It's truly an elegant design.

Of course, DNA doesn't "know" what a given gene actually does. It doesn't even know what the various nutrients it contacts are good for. Through mechanisms not fully understood, DNA has been programmed at some point in the past by epigenetic markers that can turn certain DNA portions on or off in response to certain nutrients. The entire programming system is designed for change; these markers can, apparently, fall off, causing the genetic brain to forget, at least temporarily, previously programed information.

This forgotten information can be recalled, given the right environment. This is why I believe we all have the potential to be—or at least give birth to—genetic lottery winners, because a forgetful genome can be retrained.

You can see evidence of this retraining in laboratory animals. Dr. Randy Jirtle at Duke University studied the effects of nutrient fortification on a breed of mice, called *agouti,* known for their yellow color and predisposition for developing severe obesity and subsequent diabetes. Starting with a female agouti raised on ordinary mouse chow, he fed her super-fortified pellets enriched with vitamin B_{12}, folic acid, choline, and betaine and mated her to another agouti male. Instead of the usual overweight, unhealthy yellow-coat babies she'd normally give birth to, she instead bore brown mice that developed normally.[19] You could interpret this study as follows: The agouti breed has regulatory DNA that's essentially been brain damaged by some past traumas in the history of the lineage. As a result, agouti chromosomes, unlike other mice, are typically incapable of building healthy, normal offspring. In this study, researchers were able to rehabilitate the agouti's genome by blasting the sleepy genes with enough nutrients to wake them up, reprogramming their genes for better function.

This has enormous implications for us, as researchers are finding abnormal regulatory scars all over our genes, records of our ancestors' experiences—even with the weather. Toward the end of WWII, an unusually harsh winter combined with a German-imposed food embargo led to death by starvation of some 30,000 people. Those who survived suffered from a range of developmental and adult disorders, including low birth weight, diabetes, obesity, coronary heart disease, breast and other cancers. A group of Dutch researchers has associated this exposure with the birth of smaller-than-normal *grandchildren*.[20] This finding is remarkable as it suggests the effects of a pregnant woman's diet can ripple, at the least, into the next two generations. Unlike the agouti mice, which required massive doses of vitamins, these people would possibly respond well to normal or only slightly above normal levels of nutrients as their genes have been affected only for a short while—just a generation or two (unlike the mice)—meaning it might not take quite so much extra nutrition to wake them up.

Some epigenetic reactions are not merely passed on but magnified. In a study of the effects of maternal smoking on a child's risk of developing asthma, doctors at the Keck School of Medicine in Los Angeles discovered that children whose mothers smoked while pregnant were 1.5 times more likely to develop asthma than those born to non-smoking mothers. If grandma smoked, the child was 1.8 times more likely to develop asthma—even if mom never touched a cigarette! Those children whose mother and grandmother both smoked while pregnant had their risk elevated by 2.6

Figure 1. The Nucleus: Where Food Programs Genes

Here we see one loop of the DNA double helix wrapped around nuclear regulatory proteins, shown as smaller coils. The tightness or looseness of the association helps determine how often a given gene gets expressed. When tightly coiled, genes are isolated from enzymes that transcribe their information, and protein production is turned off. When a tightly coiled gene segment loosens enough for enzymes to bind to it, the gene is now effectively turned on again. But epigenetics is showing that these binary designations of "off" and "on" aren't the whole story, and that we have all kinds of in-between settings. This means that the chromosomal data is stored and expressed in analog terms rather than digital, enabling our DNA to compute more information than we imagined.

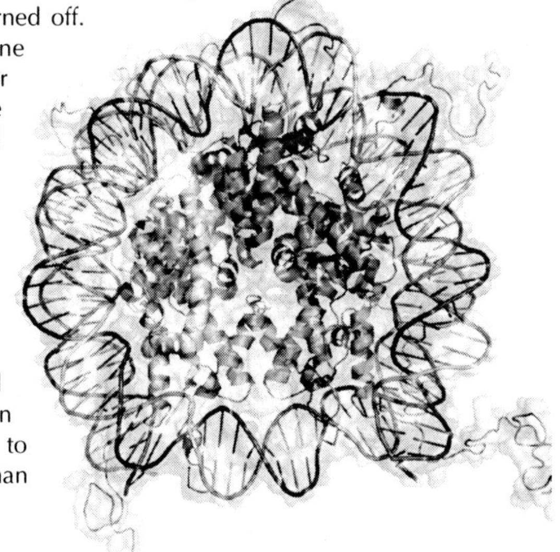

times.[21] Why would DNA react this way? If you look for the logic in this decision, you might see it like this: By smoking during pregnancy, you are telling the embryo that the air is full of toxins and that breathing is sometimes dangerous. The developing lungs would do well to be able to react quickly to any inhaled irritants. Asthmatic lungs are *over*-reactive. They cough and spit at the slightest whiff of foreign aerosols. Still, I believe even a genome as abused as this can be reminded of normal function.

Why do I have so much faith in the restorative power of good epigenetic care? Because contrary to the old ways of thinking we now know it is rarely anything as permanent as a mutation that causes most disease. As we've seen, environmentally derived chemicals mark the long molecule with tags that change its behavior. Such a system, according to Randy Jirtle, seems to be to provide a "rapid mechanism by which [an organism] can respond to the environment without having to change its hardware."[22] This way, any physiologic tweak or modification can be recalled based on its apparent success or failure. Call it test marketing for a proposed "mutation." That may seem a rather sophisticated operation for a molecule to pull off, but remember we're talking about a molecule that has been in development ever since life on Earth began. With this new understanding of how DNA works, we can now appreciate how easily nutrient deficiencies or exposure to toxins might lead to chronic disease—and how readily these diseases might respond to eliminating toxins and improving nutrition.

At Yale's Center for Excellence in Genomic Science, Dr. Dov S. Greenbaum shares my faith in the intellect behind the design of our genetic apparatus. In describing how Junk DNA functions to guide evolution, he writes, "The movement of transposable Junk results in a dynamic system of gene activation, which allows for the organism to adapt to its environment...."[23] He describes the function very much like Jirtle, adding that this transposition system "allows for the organism to adapt to its environment without redesigning its hardware...."[24] To further the analogy, it's conceivable that genetic modifications are introduced under a protocol similar to that used by software designers: test for bugs, then run concurrent with other software on a provisional basis (the beta version of the program), then integrate into the operating system, and finally—when proved to be indispensable—build it into the hardware.

This might have been exactly what happened with the human gene for making vitamin C. After generations of non-use (due to abundance of vitamin C in our food), the gene would have grown very "sleepy." Eventually, when epigenetic test marketing had demonstrated that we could live without being able to make our own vitamin C, a mutation within the gene permanently deactivated it. How, exactly, might this test marketing work? Certain markers increase the error rate during reproduction, and thus a temporary epigenetic change can set up the gene to be permanently altered by a base pair mutation.[25] Genes are like tiny protein-producing machines that create different products. If a factory worker (epigenetic tagging) shuts off one machine and everything in the cell continues to run smoothly over the ensuing generations, then that particular machine (gene) can be refashioned to produce something else, or turned off altogether. The more we learn about epigenetics, the more it seems that genetic change—both the development of disease and even evolution itself—is as tightly controlled and subject to feedback as every other biologic process from cell development to breathing to reproduction, and, therefore, isn't so random after all.

What helps regulate all these cellular events? Food, mostly. After all, food is the primary way we interact with our environment. But here's what's really remarkable: Those tags that get placed on the genes to control how they work and help drive the course of evolution are made out of simple nutrients, like minerals, vitamins, and fatty acids, or are influenced by the presence of these nutrients. In other words, there's essentially no middleman between the food you eat and what your genes are being told to do, enacting changes that can ultimately become permanent and inheritable. If food can alter genetic information in the space of a single generation, then this powerful and immediate relationship between diet and DNA should place nutritional shifts at the front of the stage in the continuing drama of human evolution.

Evidence for Language in DNA

We have no clear idea how nature keeps track of which programming codes work best for what, or how the many environmental inputs—minerals, vitamins, toxins, and so on—might be translated into a new epigenetic strategy, but recent research offers intriguing support to the idea that DNA can indeed take notes.

In 1994, mathematicians observed that Junk contained patterns reminiscent of natural language, since it follows, among other things, Zipf's law (a hierarchical word distribution pattern found in all natural languages).[26,27,28,29] Some geneticists disagree with this assessment, while others think this added layer of complexity might eventually help explain many of DNA's hidden mysteries. But everyone agrees there's plenty of space in Junk DNA for all kinds of data storage. Junk DNA is a large enough repository of information to function as a kind of chemical software programmed to, for want of a better term, *recognize* something about the dietary conditions provided it and then include this updated information when it reproduces itself. Some molecular biologists feel that this capability to orchestrate a measured response to environmental change demands that we consider the language encoded in Junk DNA as an "independent mechanism for the gradual regulation of gene expression in [higher organisms]."[30] "Independent" meaning something other than the previously accepted mechanisms of selection and random mutation.

One example of the logic underlying DNA's behavior can be found by observing the effects of vitamin A deficiency. In the late 1930s, Professor Fred Hale of the Texas Agricultural Experiment Station at College Station was able to deprive pigs of vitamin A before conception so that the mother would produce a litter without any eyeballs.[31] When the mother was re-fed vitamin A, her next litter of babies developed normal eyeballs, suggesting that eyeball growth was not switched off due to (permanent) mutation, but to a temporary epigenetic modification. Vitamin A is derived from retinoids, which come from plants, which in turn depend on sunlight. So in responding to the absence of vitamin A by turning off the genes to grow eyes, it is as if DNA interpreted the lack of vitamin A as a lack of light, or a lightless environment in which eyes would be of no use. The eyeless pigs had lids, very much like blind cave salamanders. It's possible that these and other blind cave dwellers have undergone a similar epigenetic modification of the genes controlling eye growth in response to low levels of vitamin A in a lightless, plantless cave environment.

Taken together, epigenetic evidence paints DNA as a far more dynamic and intelligent mechanism of adaptation than has been generally appreciated. In effect, DNA seems capable of collecting information—through the language of food—about changing conditions in the outside world, enacting alteration based on that information, and documenting both the collected data and its response for the benefit of subsequent generations. Junk DNA is full of genetic treasure. It may function as a kind of ever-expanding library, complete with its own insightful librarian capable of researching previously written volumes of successful and unsuccessful genetic adaptation strategies. It follows that more complex organisms, with larger cells—whose genomes represent a more complex evolutionary history—would carry relatively more substantial libraries filled with more Junk DNA. And we do.[32]

The intelligent library stands in direct opposition to the placement of selection and random mutation as the sole mechanisms of genetic change and the development of new species. Given the highly competitive world of survival, it seems obvious that those genetic codes capable of listening to the outside world and using that information to guide decisions would enjoy a marked advantage compared with those stumbling in the dark, dependent completely on luck. This understanding may give rise to an entirely new perspective on how we came to be, placing a new spin on "intelligent design." DNA's ability to respond intelligently to changes in its nutritional environment enables it to take advantage of the shifting cornucopia, exploiting rich nutritional contexts like the way an interior decorator would make use of a surprise shipment of high-quality silk upholstery. Our genes may help us survive periods of famine and stress by way of experiment, and take advantage of any nutritional glut to experiment further—not blindly, not with random mutations, but with memory and purpose, guided by past experiences encoded within its own structure.

How does this matter to you?

The chemical intelligence encoded in your DNA and the intelligence of our distant ancestors shared the same ultimate goal: survive. Inside your ancestors' bodies, their genomes shuffled themselves to match nutrient supply with physiologic demands while the people who carried them shared tool-making tips and rumors of food sources which—propelled by this synergy of purpose—would catapult a small group of primates from a nook of the African continent to a state of world domination.

Under the watchful eye of grandmothers and midwives, special foods and preparations proved themselves effective at creating children who could learn faster and grow stronger than the generation before. Children who, naturally, would grow to become parents themselves, able to form their own sets of observations and conclusions about the way the world works and how best to guarantee survival. One of the things that makes human beings (and their ancestors) unique is the sophistication of tool use that enabled consumption of a greater proportion of the edible world than the competition, furthering the agenda of our perpetually reincarnating, self-revising, constantly upgrading, ruthlessly selfish genes. We have managed to shepherd our own genomes through millennia, roaming from one ocean to another, over mountains and across whole continents, and into the modern age.

Those hoping to maintain the product of that achievement—a beautiful, healthy human body—will want to acquaint themselves with the foods and preparation techniques that allowed us to get this far in the first place. By eating the foods described later in this book, you will be talking directly to your genes. Your foods will tell your epigenome to make your body stronger, more energized, healthier, and more beautiful. And your epigenome will listen.

Unblocking Your Genetic Potential

Whether you believe in the idea of genetic intelligence or not, the one thing I hope I've made clear in this chapter is that our genes are not written in stone. They are exquisitely sensitive to how we treat them. Like a fine painting passed down through generations, conditions that either harm or preserve are permanently recorded in the provenance of a family's DNA. When the DNA is mistreated, like a Monet thrown into the corner of a damp musty basement, the inheritance loses its value. And the losses may be devastating. Between Halle Berry and the person who cleans her bathrooms, and between all the tall, trim, and beautiful people strutting the red carpets in Hollywood or the tennis courts in the Hamptons and the rest of us who can only watch are untold stories of nutritional starvation, of lost or distorted genetic information. This variability in our ancestors' ability to safeguard their genetic wealth is the reason why, today, we have so many people wishing for better health, better looks, greater athleticism, and all the manifold benefits of healthy genes.

In Chapter 1, I introduced the idea that the genetic lottery is not random, and in this chapter we saw how genes make what seem to be intelligent decisions guided in part by chemical information in the food we eat. In the next chapter, we'll see that when we've eaten right—when our chromosomes have marinated long enough in the chemical soup that enables them to do their utmost best—*Homo sapiens* genes can produce extraordinary beauty. In fact, no matter what race you are talking about, our genetic minds seem to dream of the same ideal. This is why beautiful people of every race share the same basic skeletal geometry, and why for the bulk of human history, Hollywood beauties were as plentiful as the stars.

Three

Dynamic Symmetry

Nature's Desire for Beauty

Few people can make sense when they talk about beauty. The subject is either too profound or too emotionally charged to describe objectively. Even talent agents who make their living in the beauty trade characterize it using imprecise euphemisms: *a glow, that certain something*. Press a publisher, judge, or news reporter hard enough and you might get them to confess, privately, that good looks matter more to them than they'd rather admit. On the other hand, feminists, including author Camile Paglia, have suggested that beauty may all be a big put-on, and that without cover girls, movie stars, and other models saturating the media, we'd be immune to its effects. Controversial and enigmatic as the subject of beauty may seem, in reality, beauty is simply another natural phenomenon which, like gravity or the speed of light, can be quantified, analyzed, and understood. Though poets and songwriters might object, significant benefits can be derived from deconstructing human beauty using the same tools we would bring to any other scientific question. For starters, beauty can tell us quite a lot about our genetic histories, our bodies, and our health.

Ancient people, by comparison, may have been far more rational in their consideration of beauty. Their emblems, art, and artifacts of worship consistently feature geometric forms, and many today believe the Inca, Maya, Athenians, Romans, Druids, and ancient Egyptians recognized that beauty and health were related.

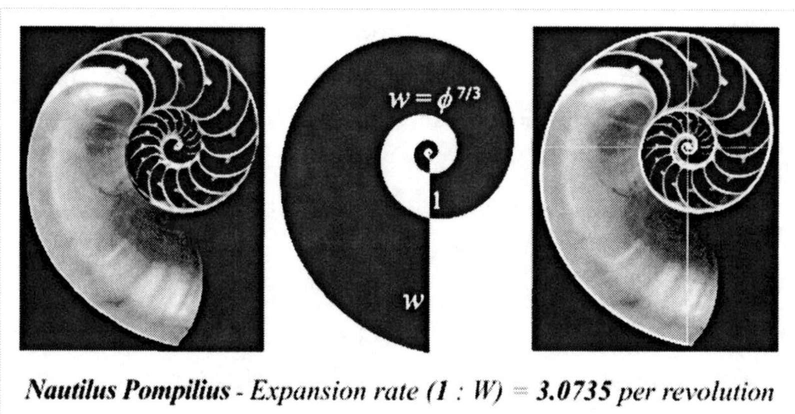

Nautilus Pompilius* - *Expansion rate (1 : W) = 3.0735 per revolution

Figure 1. What Is Beauty? The nautilus has been a symbol of balanced form since ancient times. Its entire body pattern can be described by the simple formula written above. As it turns out, the ideal human face can also be mathematically described as a formula.

Even today, outside of the field of medicine, many life-science professionals apply their ability to judge physical attractiveness without hesitation. When a farmer or a racehorse breeder or a rare orchid grower sees obvious disruptions in healthy growth, they naturally consider the nutritional context in which the specimen was raised. If a prize-winning mare gives birth to a foal with abnormally bowed legs, the veterinarian recognizes that something went wrong and, often, asks the logical question, *What was the mother eating?* But physicians rarely do that, even when life-threatening problems show up right at birth. And we continue to neglect the nutrition-development equation when our patients develop scoliosis, joint malformations, aneurysms, autism, schizophrenia, and so on later in life. If doctors and nutritionists were as willing to use their basic senses as other professionals, every child would have a better chance to grow up healthy.

The way we look speaks volumes about our health because of the fact that form implies function, and this means our desire for beauty is no simple matter of vanity. Less attractive facial forms are less functional. Children with suboptimal skull architecture may need glasses, braces, or oral surgery, whereas children with more ideal architecture won't.[33] Such a child may have narrow airways, leading to nasal irritation and allergies.[34, 35] Or even sleep apnea, which starves the brain of oxygen needed to develop normal intelligence.[36,37] One of the few instances in which doctors do use visual assessments to screen for health disorders is with a condition known loosely as "minor anomalies" also known, much less formally, as the "funny looking kid." It's common enough that it even has an acronym, FLK. This diagnosis is one of the primary reasons for genetic testing. Children with growth anomalies are the group most often found to have genetic disease and internal organ malformations, and they frequently develop learning disorders, socialization disorders, and cancer.[38] And let's not pretend a person's physi-

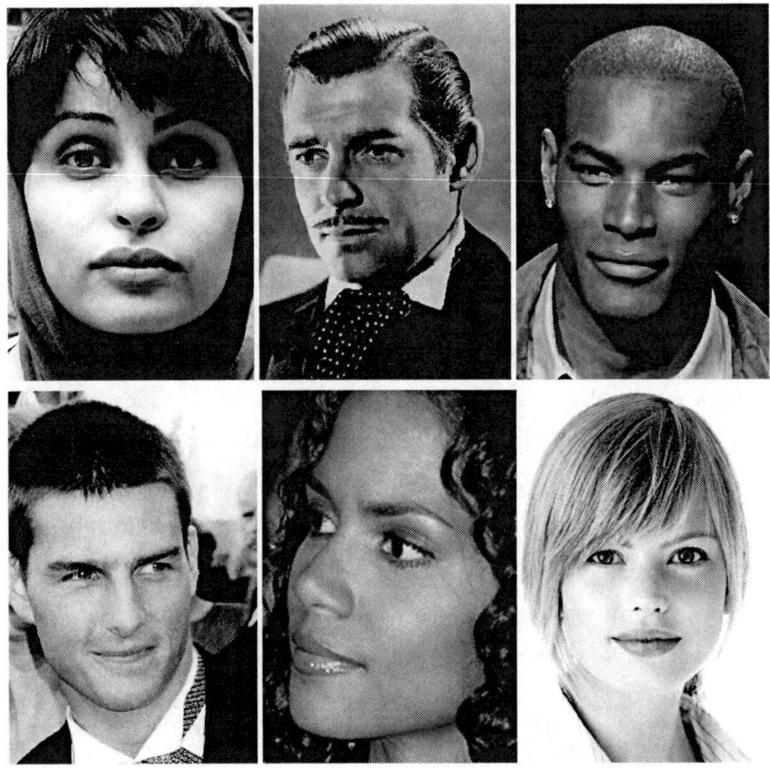

Figure 2. Variations on a Theme. Highly attractive people not only share characteristic features including broad faces, high cheekbones, wide jaws, full lips, and angular brows, they also grew in accordance with a code that has fascinated scholars since ancient times.

cal development has no social consequences. Less attractive people rate themselves as less popular,[39] less happy,[40] and less healthy.[41] They are more depressed more often,[42] spend more time in jail,[43] and are less well paid as adults[44] than their more attractive peers.

All preconceptions aside, the evidence suggests that the same conditions that allow our DNA to create health also allow our DNA to grow beautiful people. I call this phenomenon *the package deal effect* because beauty and health are just that—a package deal. The more you have of one, the more you probably have of the other.

You may, on some level, have already suspected this. In high school you may have noticed, as Rod Stewart sang in the '80s, *Some guys have all the luck.* Case in point: your homecoming king. No doubt he was popular, but was he also athletic? And did he get pretty good grades? What about your prom queen? Was she attractive? Smart? The epitome of good health? And was your valedictorian also attractive? I'm going to guess that, just as with my high school, the answers are all *yes.* But why should this be so? What is it about beauty that makes something not only look better, but function better? And why do we want it so badly?

Like the laws of engineering, chemistry, and physics, the laws of physical attraction emerge from the fabric of the universe and can best be understood using the language of mathematics.

The Man Who Discovered the Perfect Face

The desire for beauty is so great that some of us take matters into our own hands—or rather, into the hands of a professional—to get a larger helping of its sweet rewards. In 2005 more than 11 million cosmetic procedures were performed by more than 5000 plastic surgeons in the US alone. Most procedures involve moving fat, skin, and muscle around the face and body, but an extreme makeover can require breaking and resetting bone. As these doctors permanently rearrange our looks, what standards, do you suppose, guide their decisions? The answer is *none*—that is, none aside from their own personal aesthetics and experience. Thankfully, their skills usually leave the patient looking better rather than worse. But their training does not provide them with instructions for rebuilding faces according to any universal standard of ideal facial architecture.

Why not? Simply put, it's complicated. Each person's face has a distinct 3-D geometry that our brains can interpret. We don't know how exactly, and most of us don't need to worry about it. But if plastic surgeons want to build better faces reliably, and if they want to know whether or not they will be repositioning a jaw, a tooth, or an eyebrow in a functional, attractive location, they must find a way to describe functional, attractive facial geometry. Such was the thinking of a bright, young maxillofacial surgeon at UCLA named Dr. Stephen Marquardt.

One evening in the late 1970s, Dr. Marquardt couldn't sleep. In two days time he would commence an operation on a woman who'd been in a terrible car accident. It was his job to reconstruct her badly damaged lower face. But one question nagged him all night: *How can I be sure she'll be happy with the results?* In those days there were relatively few plastic surgeons, even in LA, and patients would receive their particular surgeon's trademark work—say Audrey Hepburn's nose—with results so consistent that other surgeons could tell who the patient had seen. Dr. Marquardt realized Hepburn's petite nose, as undeniably cute as it is, might not be the right nose for just anyone. How could a doctor know which nose, or chin, or jaw line is best proportioned for the face of the person on the operating table? Marquardt wondered why there weren't some rules or standards to follow. Would he always have to guess, fingers crossed, or might there be a more dependable approach?

In a search for answers, Dr. Marquardt went to a museum and spent the day examining great works of art. At the end of the day he had a stack of sketches, but no definitive set of rules. He wanted to know what, if any, principle guided the creation of all great works of art. Over the next several months he studied rules of beauty in architecture, art, music, and more. Still, no consistent theme had yet emerged.

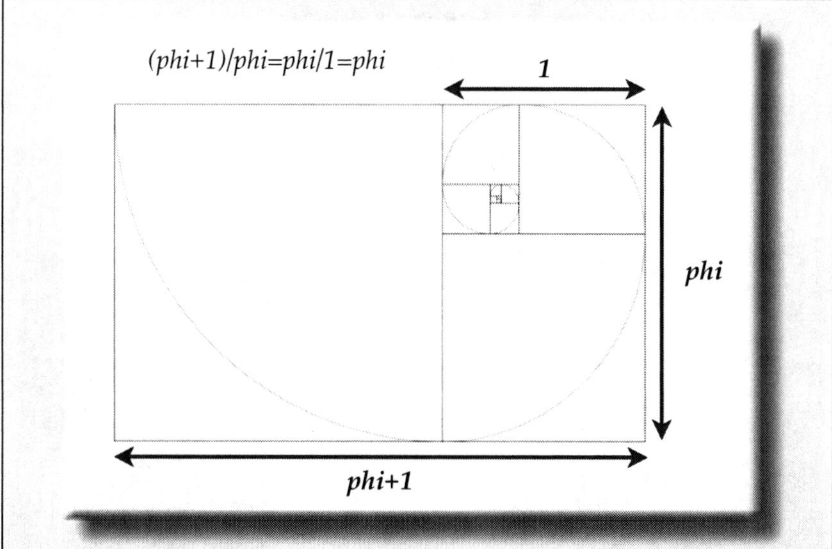

Figure 3. Golden Rectangle. The golden rectangle is divided in such a way as to create a square and a smaller rectangle that retains the same proportions as the original. Because of the amazing symmetry of *phi*, this process can be repeated over and over ad infinitum. Drawing a radius equal to the length of the side of the square across each square generates a golden spiral.

Finally, he recognized that he kept running across formulas, like the triangle on the color wheel, and the Rule of Threes in photography. He'd been studying individual subjects to find a common link, and that link was mathematics. At the core of the mathematical principles of beauty lay a set of numbers named after the Italian who first discovered it in the 11th century—the *Fibonacci sequence*.

Beauty's Secret Code

You may remember the Fibonacci sequence from *The DaVinci Code* in which the cryptologist heroine discovers a series of numbers her grandfather wrote on the floor with invisible ink at the site of his murder: 1, 1, 2, 3, 5, 8, 13, 21. The sequence builds by summing the last two numbers on the end, growing forever. Had the dead man lived to write the next number, he would have written 34—the sum of 13 and 21. If one were looking for a uni-

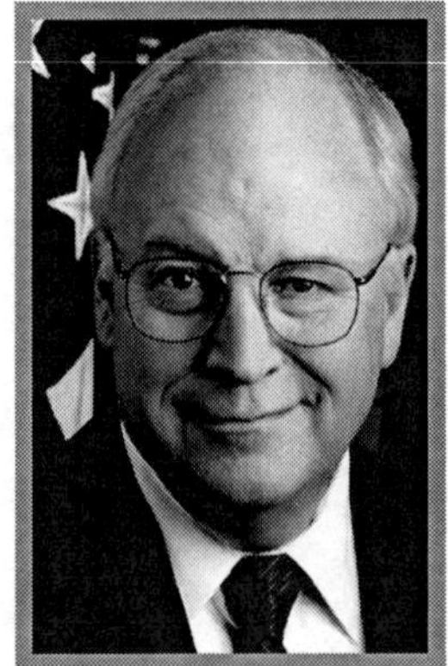

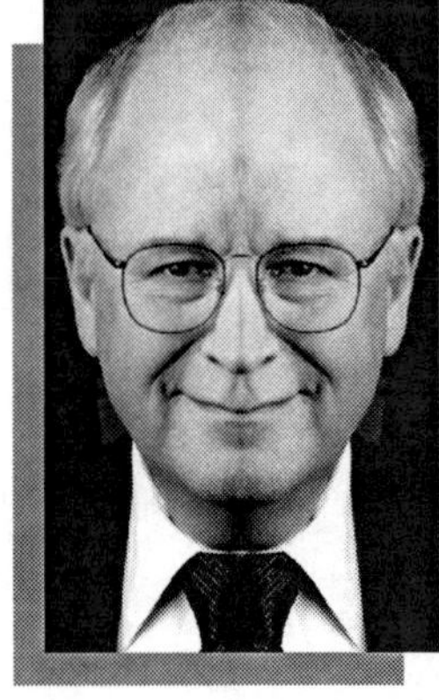

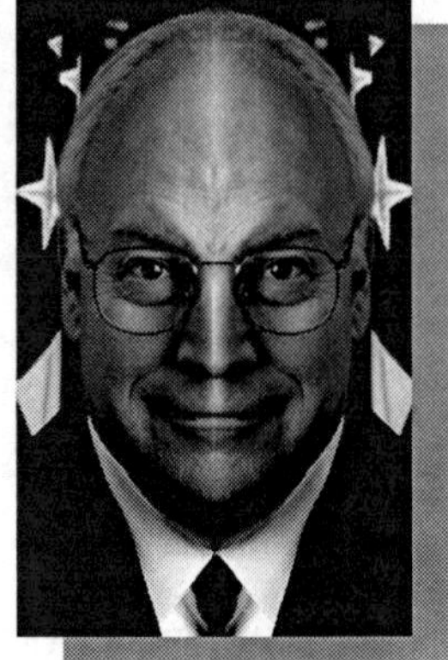

Figure 4. Biradial Symmetry Is Not What Makes Us Beautiful. Vice President Cheney (above) has been rendered biradially symmetric (lower) by reproducing each half of his face, flipping it, and pasting next to the original. If plastic surgeons could do this, it wouldn't necessarily make a person more attractive than they were initially. If, on the other hand, plastic surgeons could give our faces dynamic symmetry based on Marquardt's mask, Mr. Cheney would get a square jaw-line, larger zygomatic arches (cheekbones) and orbital ridges, his frontal bones (forehead) would be broader and, because dynamic facial symmetry creates bilateral symmetry, both sides of his face would appear equally presidential.

versal code of proportionate growth, this sequence of numbers would be the Holy Grail.

As you extend the sequence out to infinity, the ratio of the last two terms converges on an irrational number, approximately 1.618033988.... This is the *golden ratio*, used by the Greeks and Egyptians to design perfectly balanced works of structural art that mystify architects even today. The golden ratio is symbolized by the Greek letter *phi*: Φ. (Pronounced *fie*, rhymes with *pie*.)

In his pursuit of the perfect face, Dr. Marquart discovered that the golden ratio is uniquely capable of generating a special kind of symmetry, called *dynamic symmetry*. According to the theory of perception, there are two ways to create harmonic balance within an object or space. One is to divide it into equal parts, creating the symmetry of balance. The other is a division based on the golden section, creating the perfect from of *a*symmetry—perfect because the ratio of the lesser part to the greater part is the same as the ratio of the greater part to the whole. (See Figure 3.) This is *dynamic* symmetry. Interestingly, dynamic symmetry characterizes the growth of living matter, while static symmetry characterizes the growth of crystals.

The literature on human beauty is full of references to biradial symmetry, suggesting that, if one side perfectly mirrors the other, you've got a beautiful face. But that's a misconception, and here's why: Although dynamic symmetry often leads to biradial symmetry, biradial symmetry does not guarantee, or even imply, dynamic symmetry. Put another way, biradial symmetry is a necessary, though not sufficient, characteristic of an attractive human face. Living, growing beings are dynamic, and that's exactly the kind of symmetry that makes them beautiful.

The Egyptians and Greeks worshipped *phi* as a fountainhead of eternal beauty, calling it the *divine ratio*. The Parthenon and other great works of ancient architecture that still stand today do so in part because they were designed around this mathematic principle of ideal proportion, and architects to this day still study them with wonder. The philosopher Socrates saw geometry, in which *phi* plays a central role in relating various forms, not only as a guiding constant of the natural world but also as a potential source of life itself. DaVinci was obsessed with geometric relationships and the structure of the human form; his famous Vitruvian Man sketch of a man superimposed on a circle and a square illustrates his own quest for a code of nature that generates living forms. Like generations of scientists before him, Dr. Marquardt focused on *phi* as the essential clue. The divine ratio had to be buried somewhere in the proportions of the perfect human face.

If Hollywood were to set the action to film, they would show a montage of Dr. Marquardt at his desk holding his compass and protractor to a series of cover girl's faces, then a heap of dulled pencils in the foreground as he

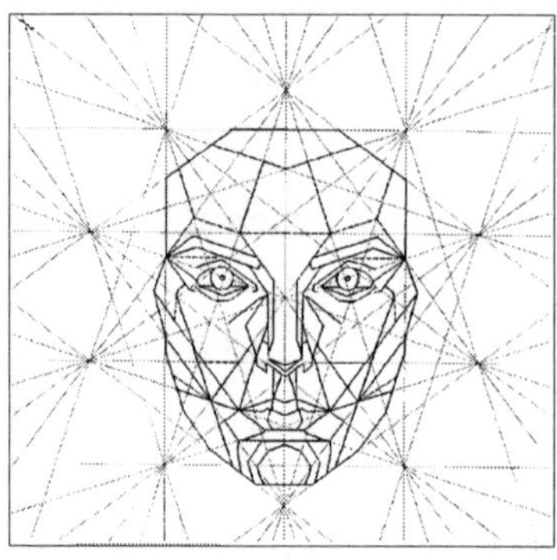

Figure 5. Beauty Emerges from Math. Every line of Marquardt's mask is geometrically plotted according to the dynamic symmetry of *phi*. When epigenetic conditions provide for optimal growth, facial features "crystalize" in a pattern that conforms to the mask. This is the female mask. According to Marquardt, the male mask is a variation on the female.

scratches out another formula involving square roots and algebraic variables. Until finally the moment of epiphany. Cut to Marquardt raising his cipher to the camera: a clear sheet of acetate on which his "Primary Golden Decagon Matrix" is printed in bold, black lines, the angulated mask of a perfect human face.

Marquardt's Mask is a matrix of points, lines, and angles delineating the geometric framework and borders of what Marquardt calls the Archetypal face, a plotted graph of the visual ideal our collective unconscious yearns for. Nested within the matrix are forty-two secondary Golden Decagon Matrices, each the same shape as the larger matrix, but smaller by various multiples of *phi*. These lock on to the primary matrix by at least two vertices.[45] The mask defines the ideal three-dimensional arrangement of every facial feature, from the size of the eyes and their distance from one another to the width of the nose, to the fullness of the upper and lower lip, and so on.

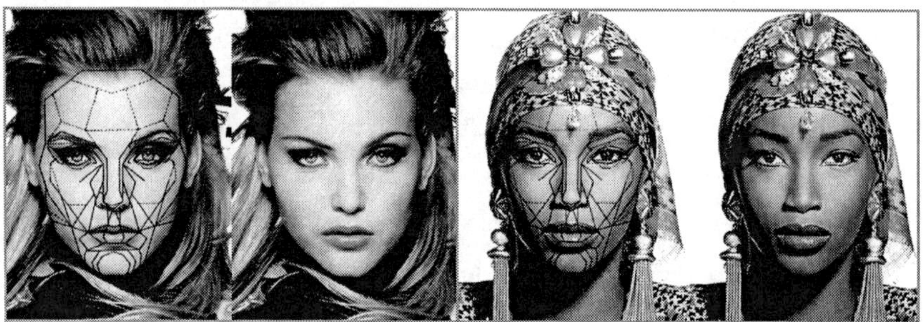

Figure 6. Blueprint for Beauty. Marquardt's mask fits neatly over beautiful facial architecture no matter what race.

In John Cleese's BBC series *The Human Face,* featuring Marquardt and based largely on his research, the mask transparency is placed atop separate photos of Mariyln Monroe, Halle Berry, and Elizabeth Taylor. Like a glass slipper sliding over Cinderella's foot, the mask fit each face perfectly, revealing the fact that, though each woman could be distinguished through skin tone and hair color, these icons of mega-stardom are all kin of consummate proportion who, by no coincidence, entered the world wearing the same archetypical mask. So much for beauty being in the eye of the beholder. Beautiful people exist not because of luck, but because all DNA is naturally driven to create dynamically symmetric geometry as it's generating tissue growth. Marquardt's work reveals the specific geometry that human DNA creates.

Like the Egyptian scientists thousands of years ago who found mathematical order extended throughout their landscape and out into the stars, I believe the same mathematic principles that give order to the universe also govern the growth of every part of every living thing. When that growth proceeds optimally, beautiful and functional biologic structures are the inevitable result. This is not a new idea; it echoes the writings of ancient philosophers from Plato to Pythagorus. What we can now understand that could not have been known in ancient times, however, is precisely how our brains recognize this math.

Why We Like Beautiful Things: Nature's Geometric Logic

Take a walk through a garden, in the woods, or on a beach, and you'll see all kinds of pretty things. If you look a bit closer, you'll notice patterns—curves, whorls, spirals, even repeating numbers. What's behind this? A new discipline, called *biomathematics,* is all about answering that question. Biomathematicians are confirming that *phi* and the Fibonacci sequence are encoded not just in the human face, but in living matter everywhere.

The shape of a pinecone, the segments of insect bodies, the spiral of the nautilus shell, the bones of your fingers, and the relative sizes of your teeth—everything that grows owes its form to the geometry of *phi.* When a plant shoot puts out a new leaf, it does so in such a way that lower leaves are

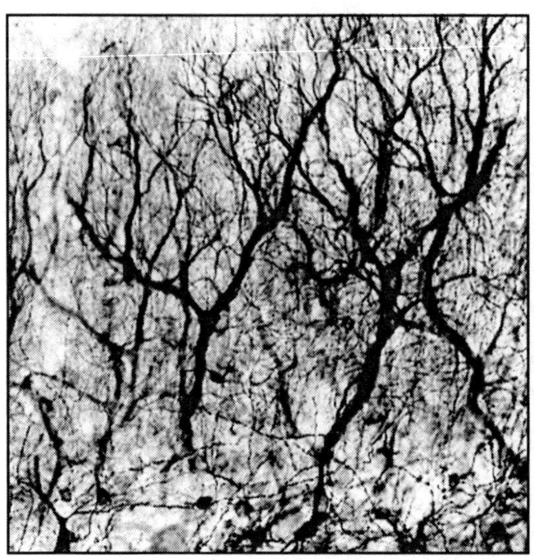

Figure 7. A Beautiful Mind. Usually used to describe the growth patterns of plants, phyllotactic growth patterns appear to drive the growth of neurons as well. This is a photomicrograph of a layer of the cerebellum. If dynamically symmetrical growth of these nerves allows them to resonate with one another in a more ordered fashion, then presumably *phi*-ordered geometry would be essential to optimal brain function.

least obscured, and can still receive sunlight. This is a benefit of a phenomenon called *phyllotaxis*, which describes the spiraling growth of stems, petals, roots, and other plant organs in 90 percent of plants throughout the world.[46] The angle of phyllotaxis is 137.5°, or $1/phi^2$ x 360 degrees. We can see the same pattern of branching, twisting, so-called dendritic growth when we look at nerve cells in the brain. All these instances of patterned growth are directed not by DNA but by the rules of math and physics, which act on living tissue automatically to create pattern. After the flow of genetic information has dropped off, like a lunar module floating through space, the organism's growth is now on autopilot.

As author, journalist, and TV producer Dr. Simon Singh explains:

> *Physics and mathematics are capable of producing intricate patterns in non-organic constructions (for example, snowflakes and sand dunes). They can offer a range of patterns which will emerge spontaneously, given the correct starting conditions. The theory which is currently gaining support says that life operates by using DNA to create the right starting conditions, and thereafter physics and maths do all the rest.*[47]

Biomathematics offers us a fundamentally new perspective of the universe and the living world. It is allowing us to recognize that recurring patterns seen throughout our living landscape are more than just coincidences. They seem to reflect the elemental structure and order of the universe itself.[48,49]

This organizing force, which helps sculpt a beautiful face, also functions during development of the organ with which you recognize beauty: your brain. Within the jelly-like matrix inside our skulls, neurons in the human brain form bifurcating tendrils, called dendrites (meaning branches). We call them dendrites because the earliest scientists who peered at neurons under a microscope were reminded of stately, graceful trees. For us to think and learn, these trees must be properly proportioned. This enchanted forest is the hidden landscape where beautiful minds are born.

Why would phyllotactic patterns of growth form inside the dark vaults of our skulls? The most obvious answer is, *Because every healthy part of every living thing follows the same basic formula for growth in order to function.* Just as the golden angle delineates phyllotactic growth and helps plants capture more sunlight, the same dynamic symmetry may allow our brains to pack in as many nerve connections per cubic inch as possible, making best use of the limited real estate between our ears. More complex than any computer and more efficient, the network in your brain works because each brain cell is connected to thousands of others. Those connections enable you to recognize faces, flowers, food and other familiar objects. How? With *pattern*.

Cognition is what mathematicians would call an *emergent property*. Emergence refers to the way complex systems and patterns arise out of a multiplicity of relatively simple interactions. Your thoughts and emotions are, likewise, not based on any individual brain cell's contents, but on the resonance frequencies that arise when millions of interconnected neurons are stimulated.[50,51] *Phi* may help our brains work better using its nimble mathematic flexibility to allow resonance to occur more often. When our nerves are structured so as to contain the maximum internal symmetry, not only can we sustain more complex perceptions, we can better comprehend the relation-

Figure 8(a) Why Attractive People Entrance Us

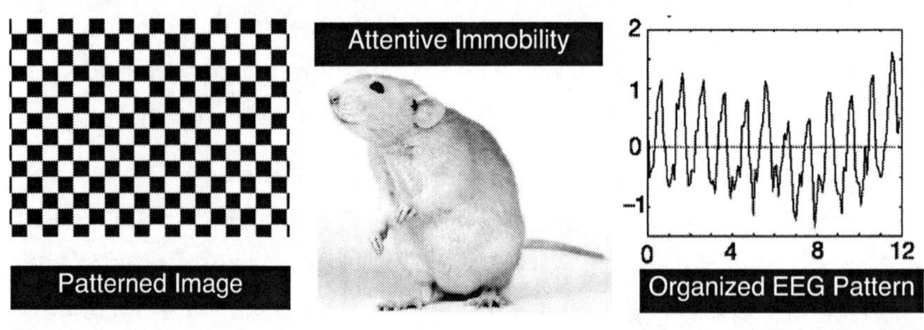

We presume we are entranced by beautiful faces because we are sexually attracted, but it may be that we are attracted to their patterns. When animal researchers show rats checkerboard patterns, the resulting brain waves demonstrate *rhythmic spikes* (upper right panel), which are said to reflect a state of "attentive immobility." While staring at the checkered image, blood flow to the pleasure center of the brain is increased, suggesting the rat enjoys looking at the pattern. Researchers believe this kind of brain activity allows for the "optimization of sensory integration within the corticothalamic neural pathways," which helps the rat "learn" the pattern.

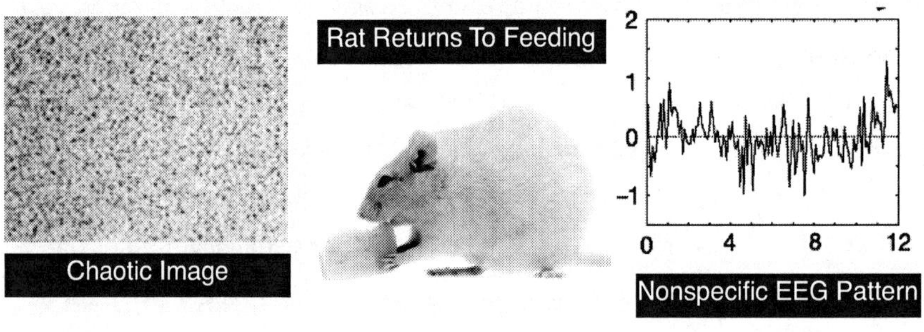

ships between perceptions, memories, thoughts, and other cognitive phenomena. In other words, every specialized sub-portion of our entire brain can function as an interconnected unit, and *poof!* consciousness emerges.

The pleasure we derive from looking at attractive people may offer us more insight into how the brain works. If beautiful faces share the same fundamental proportionality as the connections in our brains—*phi*—then they may trigger a more ordered series of recognizable resonances than faces with less symmetry, which may enable us to recognize the image as a distinctly human face that much faster. The biology of our brains may be such that our

Figure 8(b) Why Attractive People Entrance Us

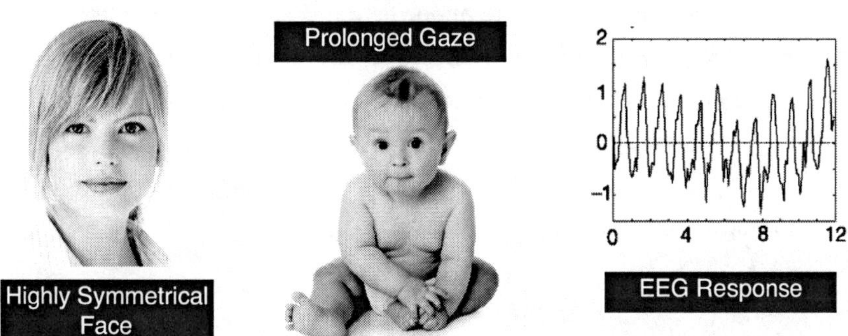

We are attracted to pattern at birth. Researchers studying infants find that babies gaze at more symmetrical faces longer and learn to recognize them faster, supporting the idea that pattern, both within the structure of our brains and within the objects our senses explore, enables us to make sense of the world. At puberty our brains begin to associate certain patterns with sexual promise, enabling us, instinctively, to select the most fit mates.

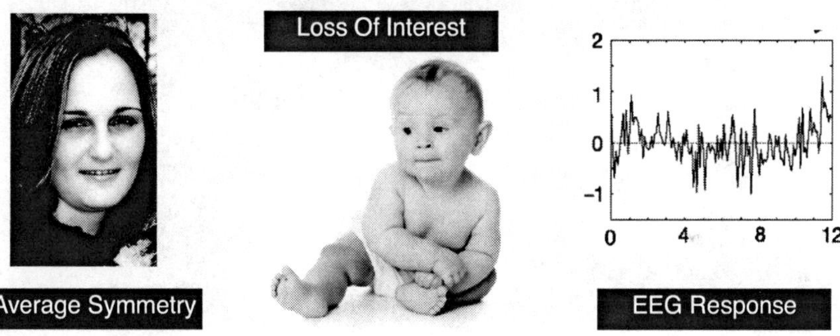

brains experience pleasure on having solved the puzzle of sorting out just what it is we're looking at. Every time the brain is presented with an image or sound it is, in essence, being posed a kind of mathematic riddle. The more pleasing the image or harmonious the sound, the fewer the barriers standing between the beholder and the pleasure of the epiphany of a solution. The Fibonacci sequence may facilitate this process, enabling us to solve these visual or acoustic riddles faster by serving as a template that helps order our minds and orchestrate our thoughts. Not only, then, does *phi* offer us beauty, it also seems to arrange our nerves in ways that facilitate intelligence.

Instinctive Attraction: The Myth of the Eye of the Beholder

The fact that the architecture of our neural tissue so closely mirrors that of dynamically symmetric, and therefore attractive, objects in the outer world helps to explain how our brains work. It also explains why our brains would prefer images of this same symmetry over others: Their familiar geometry resonates instantaneously with our own, making beautiful objects easier to perceive. Suggesting that beauty recognition seems hardwired into

Beauty: Tantalizing Math

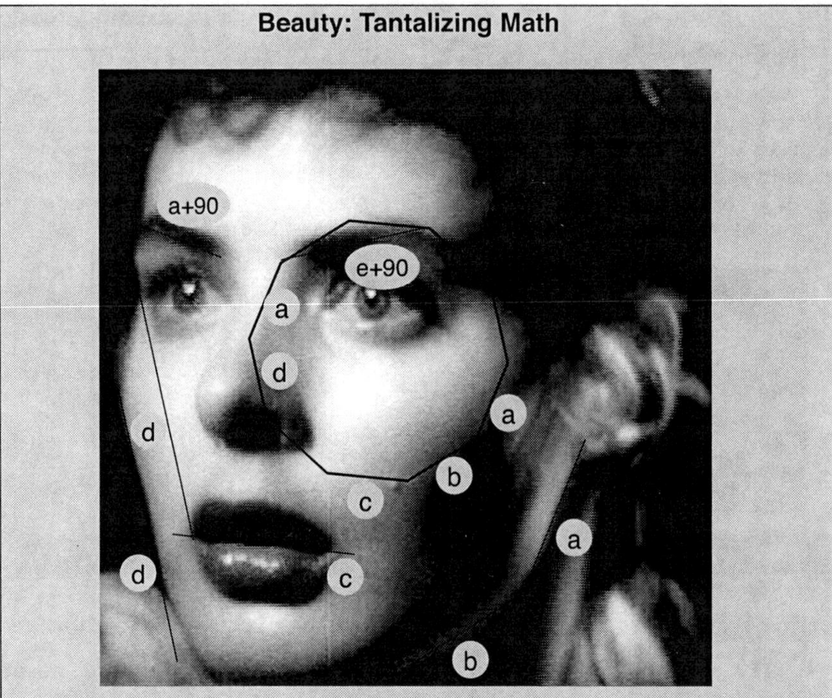

Figure 9. Repeating Patterns Draw the Eye into Ingrid Bergman's Perfect Face. Here we see how dynamic facial symmetry means that, from whatever angle we view a perfect face, its basic decahedral structure will generate repeating patterns, which may be what keeps us enthralled. If a decahedron is positioned, for example, to line up with the angles of Ingrid Bergman's eyebrow, as shown, the other major planes of her face line up in parallel with sides of the decahedron, as do imaginary lines between landmarks such as the edge of the right eye and the right edge of the lips. This is not the case with my face. Bergman's internally symmetrical facial geometry is an artifact of recursive growth in which patterns reflect themselves within themselves. Were she to turn her head or change expressions, a new set of symmetrical relationships would develop. (Letters a, b, c, represent parallel lines.)

our brains, Nancy Etcoff, author of *Survival of The Prettiest,* tells us that "when babies fix their stare at the same faces adults describe as highly attractive, their actions wordlessly argue against the belief that culture must teach us to recognize human beauty."

Consider the complications that would arise if a cheetah sizing up a herd had to be trained to recognize the absence of health, to meticulously weigh the implications of a halting gait or an uneven coat, signs of injury and disease. Without a killer instinct, or an instinctive guide to health, predators would go hungry, social animals would put themselves in contact with disease, and good genes would be diluted with compromised DNA.

This idea that we humans instinctively recognize the form-function relationship and use physical appearance, and specifically dynamic symmetry, to gauge health is supported by studies in which people were shown a series of male and female faces, each with varying levels of symmetry, and asked to make judgments about who was healthiest. What emerged was an undeniable positive correlation between the possession of dynamic symmetry and the perception of health.[52] So whether we're a cheetah, a baby, or a doctor, as far as our brains are concerned, dynamic symmetry—and attractiveness—*equals* health.

Of course, the ultimate purpose of this subconscious appreciation of the form-function relationship is the perpetuation of our DNA through the act of reproduction. And when it comes to the mating game, our responses to attractive members of the appropriate sex will typically percolate from their origins deep in our psyche to reach the surface, where they can become all-consuming.

The Perfect Mate: In Search of Sexual Dimorphism

When looking for that perfect man or woman, research shows that facial features deviating from Marquardt's geometric blueprint even slightly make a surprisingly large impression—or lack of impression.[53] A set of lips that fall just a millimeter or two short of luscious fullness, or eyes just a fraction of an inch too close together, downgrade a girl from pretty to plain. Take a strong

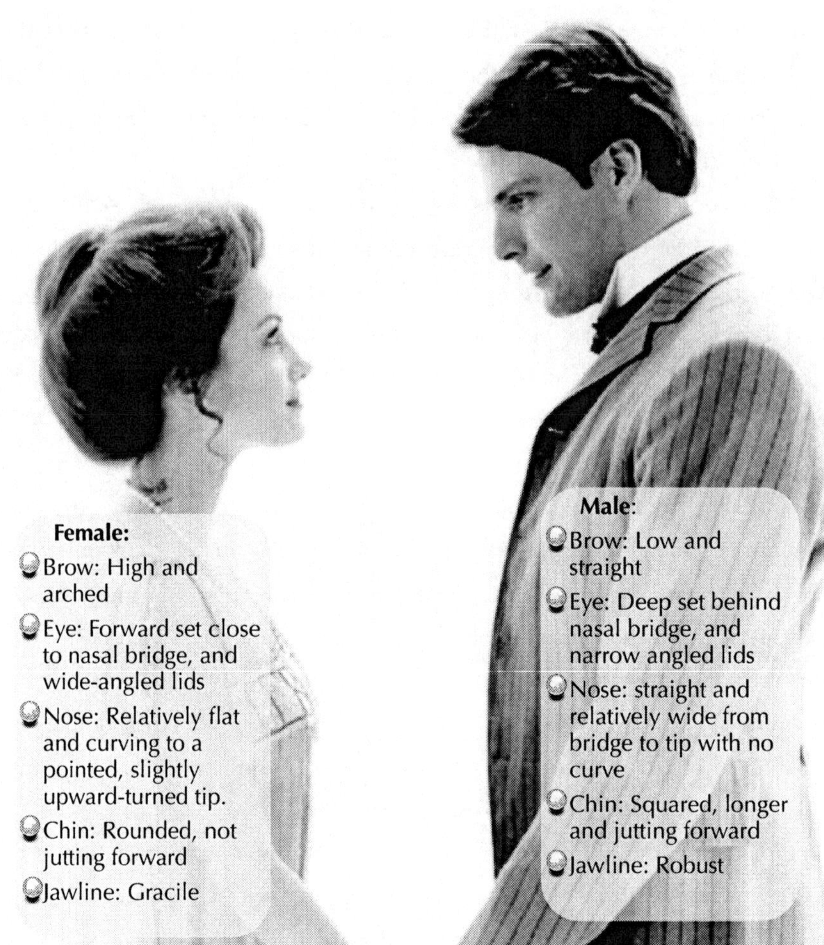

Figure 10. Sexual Dimorphism: Variations on a Theme. Like different species, male and females develop different features as we grow. But just as with different species, as long as we are healthy, both male and females demonstrate the same degree of dynamic symmetry.

brow and chin and pull them both back a tiny bit, and you change a handsome, dominating man—the kind you might envision as CEO of a company, or captain of the ship in an adventure movie—into a docile-looking office drone. Every curve of our features is sculpted under the influence of nature's tendency toward perfection. Our minds, too, are tuned by the ratio of *phi*, and so we desire dynamic symmetry, and pursue it with great tenacity. The extreme attraction we have toward sex objects exists because, during pu-

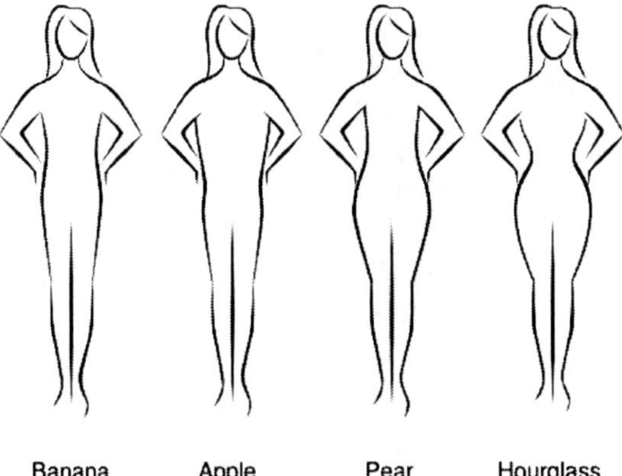

Figure 11. Female Body Types. The hourglass represents normal female sexual development, while the banana develops when sex-hormone receptivity is blunted. While the apple and pear can be found among women with normal body weights, the apple most commonly develops when women with banana-shaped bodies put on weight, and the pear when women with hourglass-shaped bodies put on weight.

berty, our grey matter is tuned to lust after a well-defined set of sex-specific variations on Marquardt's mask (Figure 10). These variations on the theme of human attractiveness are collectively called *sexual dimorphism*. While sex-differences in our facial and skeletal development exist in childhood, they become much more pronounced at sexual maturity. The package-deal effect predicts that those bodies which develop the full gamut of sex-specific features are the healthiest, and research correlating female body type with health bears this out.

Female Body Type and Health

Beauty researchers have divided female body types into four categories. In order of declining frequency they are: banana, apple, pear, and hourglass. Several studies performed in 2005 showed that apple-shaped women (with short waists and narrow hips) had almost double the chance of dying during the study compared to women with more generous curves.[54,55] Why would that be?

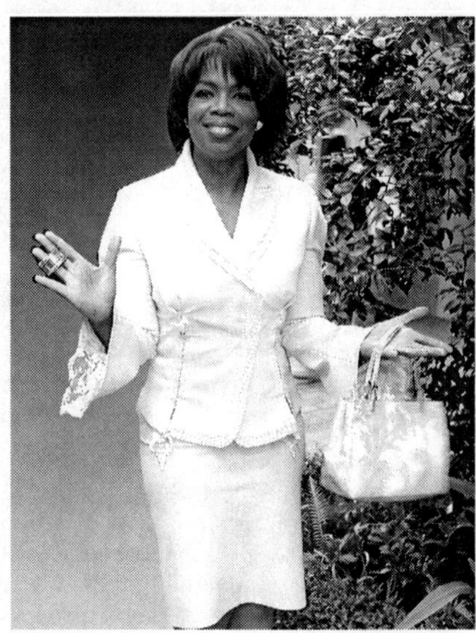

If Oprah reads Chapter 10, she'll learn how to take complete control of her weight. If she sticks with the current dietary dogma, she'll continue to face the same challenges of other yo-yo dieters. But Oprah has one key advantage: Her extra weight goes to the right places. So unlike more than 90 percent of us, she will retain her hourglass shape. Studies say this means she'll live longer. I say it means she's got healthy genes.

Figure 12. World's Wealthiest Hourglass

Voluptuousness is an indication of healthy female sexual dimorphism, while a lack of voluptuousness indicates a problem. Normally, the hips and bust develop during puberty as a result of a healthy surge in sex hormones. These developments involve expansion of the pelvic bones along with the deposition of fat and glandular tissue within the breasts. But women whose genetics are such that their spines are abnormally short or their hormonal surge less pronounced—or whose diet is such that it interferes with the body's *response* to hormones—end up with boxier figures. If they're thin, they'll end up as bananas. If they put on weight, it gets distributed in a more masculine pattern—in the belly, on the neck, and around the upper arms—and they'll become an apple. Today, after three generations of trans fat consumption (which interferes with hormone expression, see Chapter 8), and with daily infusions of sugar (which interferes with hormone receptivity, see Chapter 9), hourglass figures have become something of a rarity. According to a 2005 study commissioned by Alva products, a manufacturer of designer's mannequins, less than ten percent of women today develop the voluptuous curves they're supposed to.[56]

In a world of apples, pears, and bananas, Writer Nancy Etcoff has suggested that the most beautiful among us are "genetic freaks." It's not an insult: She is merely referencing the statistical improbability of someone growing up to look like, to use her example, Cindy Crawford. But the suggestion seems to capture Etcoff's general thesis accurately: When a stunningly beautiful person is born, it's largely the result of (genetic) chance. These select few, the thinking goes, played the genetic lottery and won big. But I couldn't disagree more. Why would biology program us to be hot for "genetic freaks"? It seems to me far more probable that we are attracted to beautiful bodies because they advertise health. In keeping with this idea, researchers studying the effect of these four female body types on life span find that women with the most attractive of the four body types, the hourglass, live the longest. Women with the least attractive figure, the blocky, often overweight apples, have the shortest life spans, frequently dying from complications of diabetes.[57]

Why Aren't All Bodies Perfect?

So far I've shown you a good deal of evidence that beauty is not incidental, not an accident of fate. It is the default position, the inevitable product of natural, *unimpeded* growth whose progress conforms to rules of mathematic proportion. Just as the laws of physics dictate that six-sided crystals inevitably result when clouds of water vapor form in freezing air, generations of optimal nutrition prime human chromosomal material for optimal growth. If optimal nutrition continues throughout childhood development, the laws of biology dictate the final result: a beautiful, healthy person. But if beauty emerges naturally from well-ordered growth, then why aren't all of us beautiful?

In October 2006, at a meeting in his Huntington Beach home, I asked Dr. Marquardt his opinion. His answer was, "We are." When I said I was surprised to hear this from a person who makes his living correcting facial anomalies, he elaborated: "If you put the mask over the population, you'll see that many people are not that far off from a perfect fit, though we wouldn't regard them as highly attractive." The variability we do have, he believes, stems from the fact that "we've evolved past the point of efficiency." In other words, societal safety nets allow people who aren't perfectly healthy or functional to reproduce whereas, in the past, they would simply have died off.

Marquardt's pragmatic explanation sheds some light on the origins of our current, historically unprecedented level of attractiveness variability. If we examine human history and focus only on access to nutrients, we would find that with civilization and sedentism (not migrating) came food shortages and disease. But sedentism was also less physically demanding than the wandering, hunter- or herder-gatherer lifestyle, and so it acted as a kind of safety net. Living in settled, relatively crowded cities began to chip away at our genetic programming, leading to the rise of disease while simultaneously enabling people with damaged genes, who might otherwise have died, to survive and give birth to less healthy children with less dynamic symmetry. Bit by bit, the genetic wealth created by thousands of years of successful survival in the wild was squandered as poverty or plague denied genes the nutrients they needed. During each period of nutritional deprivation valuable epigenetic programming was lost.

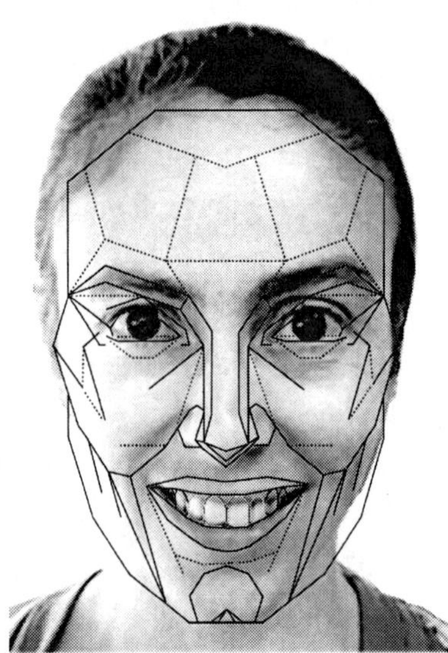

Figure 10. An Average Face. Marquardt tweaked the formula to get the mask to fit my face. If facial growth is disrupted, horizontal (X) and vertical (Y) planes grow disproportionately and perfect dynamic symmetry is lost. According to Marquardt, narrow faces are common, suggesting that when nutritional conditions are suboptimal, the coordination of growth planes) is uncoupled, and the X plane shrinks. But if conditions are bad enough, the growth coordination *within* a plane begins to fall apart. That's why, even with the mask adjustment, my jaw is still too narrow to fit.

As time has passed, we have required more and more safety nets and invented correctives like glasses, braces, and thousands of medications. Some would argue this physiologic fall from grace has not yet proved to be maladaptive for people living in modern industrialized societies, as we are still successfully reproducing. But that might be changing. Like many doctors in this country, I'm seeing more young couples frustrated by infertility. How widespread this problem will become remains to be seen.

I'm certainly not suggesting that only supermodels should have babies. And since I have argued that the genes of all people of every race and every walk of life carry the potential of extraordinary beauty and health, the implications of this chapter run about as far from the specter of eugenics as you can get. What I am saying is that—in the same way that I tell women trying to get pregnant to stop smoking and drinking, take their folic acid, and avoid medications known to cause birth defects—there are nutritional choices you can make to help ensure that your baby be born healthy and beautiful if that is what you desire. Of course, parents can choose to smoke and drink and ignore their doctor's advice. But I think every one of us deserves the best, latest, most complete information with which to make choices.

So if eating right can practically guarantee perfect, beautiful, growth, then *what are the nutritional prerequisites for healthy growth?* Believe it or not, this question had already been asked and answered in the early part of the 20th century by a man who didn't know about *phi* or epigenetics, but nevertheless found all the information he needed by studying people's teeth.

Four

The Greatest Gift

The Creation and Preservation of Genetic Wealth

Egyptologist Mark Lehner walks across what appears to be the smooth surface of a backyard patio until we see that it's actually a giant precision-cut stone in the middle of an abandoned desert quarry. At 137 feet long, it would have been the largest obelisk ever made had it not cracked before being raised from its stone cradle. The obelisk had lain ignored for nearly four thousand years, until archeologists considered just how difficult making it—and then moving it—would be. Over the past few decades, similarly impressive artifacts around the world have evinced ancient civilizations in possession of technologic abilities far exceeding our own. Piecing such history back together again will be challenging because, as an article in *Ancient American* theorizing on whether the Incas had found a way to sculpt solid rock using concentrated sunlight explains, their best technology was highly prized. "These stonemasons weren't giving away any secrets, or writing them down. Judging by the Freemasons, architects and builders who, some say, trace their lineage back to mystery schools of ancient Egypt, they were a secretive lot."[58]

There is, however, another kind of ancient technology that has had far greater impact on all our lives. Very much like the jealously guarded trade secrets of ancient stonemasons and civil engineers, the most powerful nutritional secrets, too, were kept close to the chest. Nutrition as a tool for optimizing human form and function, and for protecting the integrity of family lineage, was every bit as evolved, refined, and perfected as the tools of mathematics and engineering. The remnants of these great achievements are not waiting to be unearthed. They are walking among us, visible on TV and movie screens, and printed on the covers of *Vogue, Cosmo,* and *People* magazine. If there were as many scientists researching the rituals performed in ancient kitchens as there are researching examples of ancient civil engineering, it would be common knowledge how to use nutrition to create our own "great works," sculpted in bone and flesh. And if women wrote more of our history books, schoolchildren might learn something with more practical application than lists of battles won by various kings. They might learn something along the lines of what a dentist named Weston Price discovered when he traveled the world nearly a century ago, in search of the lost secrets to health.

Body by Ecosystem

In the early 20th century, Westerners were tantalized by the possibility that superhuman races lived just beyond the boundaries of the map. One of the most talked about groups of people were the Hunza, a sometimes-nomadic band of goat and yak herders living in the mountains of what are now Afghanistan and Pakistan. British explorers to these parts claimed to have encountered a rarified land where cancer did not exist, where nobody needed glasses, and where it was commonplace to live beyond 100. If these accounts were true, then such people would present Western medicine with a mystery. What was their secret? Pure air? Mineral-rich glacial water? Caloric restriction? True or not, enterprising businessmen soon discovered the word "Himalayan" was bona-fide magic—at least when it was printed on the tonic water bottles they were selling. Amid this circus of conjecture, capitalism, and hucksterism, one extraordinary dentist from Cleveland, Ohio was determined to inject some much-needed science. This man of introspection and quiet charm invested his own money in an amazing series of journeys, attempting to either verify or impeach these rumors. If people possessing extraordinary fitness were found, he planned to systematically analyze what made them so different than people in Ohio.

Price was not exactly the kind of man you'd expect to see rounding mountain trails on a mule. But there he was, a bespectacled, slightly pudgy man of average build pushing sixty. A reserved, meticulous man, his data collection was equally detailed and methodical. His passion for truth was driven by adversity, having lost a son to a dental infection, and growing, in his words, distressed by "certain tragic expressions of our modern degeneration, including tooth decay, general physical degeneration, and facial and dental-arch deformities."[59] Price couldn't countenance the idea that human beings should be the only species so riddled with obvious physical defects—like teeth growing every which way inside a person's mouth. After years of studying the source of orthodontic problems in active clinical practice as well as in his lab (animal research was a common aspect of early 20th century medical practitioners), he recognized that nutritional factors lead to the same kinds of facial deformities in animals that he was seeing in his patients. Crooked teeth didn't come from "mixing of races," being "of low breeding," bad luck, or the devil. There was a better explanation.

Price's preliminary work in the lab had helped to convince him that human disease arose far more readily from the "absence of some essential factors from our modern program[.]"[60] And now, halfway around the world, he was in search of those missing factors. Why the need to travel? Using the now-dated language of his time, he reasoned that the clearest path to understanding would be "to locate immune groups which were found readily as isolated remnants of primitive racial stocks in different parts of the world" and analyze what they were eating.[61] His plan was simple: count cavities. Count them in mouths of people living all over the globe. Whichever group has the fewest cavities, and the straightest teeth, wins. No fillings or orthodontics allowed. Price was betting that healthy dentition could be used as a proxy for a person's overall health—an assumption that proved correct—and so the number of cavities could be used as an objective, inverse measure of health across people of any racial and cultural background. It was an elegant and efficient plan.

The expeditions involved lugging several 8 X 10 cameras, glass plates, and a full complement of surgical dental equipment. Fortunately, Price had help from a seasoned explorer often featured in *National Geographic*, his nephew Willard DeMille Price, who no doubt greatly enhanced the elder man's ability to return with equipment intact. The resulting tome, *Nutrition and Physical Degeneration*, lays out the products of Price's exhaustive research along with his conclusions. Price was right. Not only were there entire groups of people who enjoyed perfect, cavity-free teeth and spectacular overall health, their finely tuned physiology owed itself to the fact that their traditions enabled them to produce foods with spectacular growth-promoting capacity. Of course, from their perspective, there was nothing extraordinary about their fantastic health. To them, it was only natural.

Price didn't know about *phi*, and he wasn't especially interested in finding beautiful people, per se. As a dentist, he was looking for beautiful sets of teeth. But after staring into his subjects' mouths, Price stepped back to notice that something undeniable was staring back at him: beauty. The beautifully aligned teeth he'd been looking for belonged—with rare, if any, exception—to beautiful people. Beautiful faces with beautiful cheekbones, eyes, noses, lips, and *everything* else—the total package, the physical representation of physiologic harmony.

In each of the eleven countries Price visited, people who had stayed in their villages and continued their native dietary traditions were consistently free of cavities and dental arch deformities. Price couldn't help but notice they also were just plain healthy. So healthy that on his first outing, to Lotchental, a Swiss mountain village isolated by a palisade of towering mountains, he seems as awestruck by the townspeople as by the scenery. "As one stands in profound admiration before the stalwart physical development and high moral character of these sturdy mountaineers, he is impressed by the superior types of manhood, womanhood, and childhood that Nature has been able to produce from a suitable diet and a suitable environment."[62] He

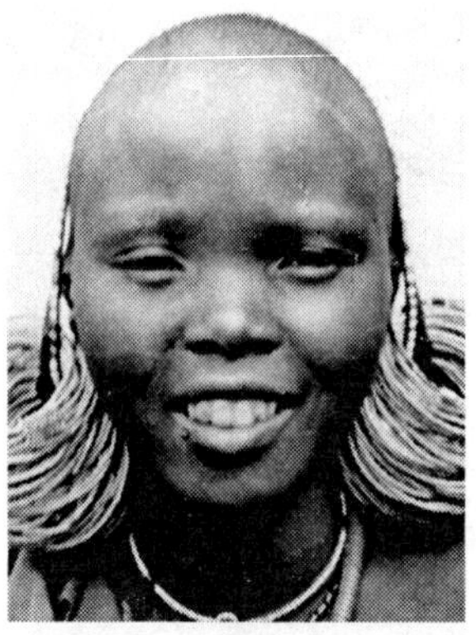
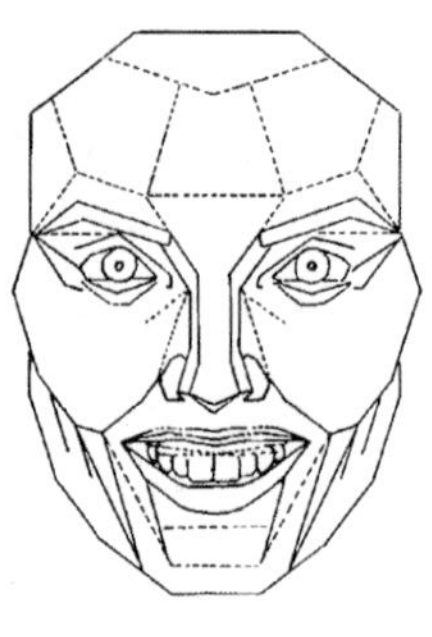
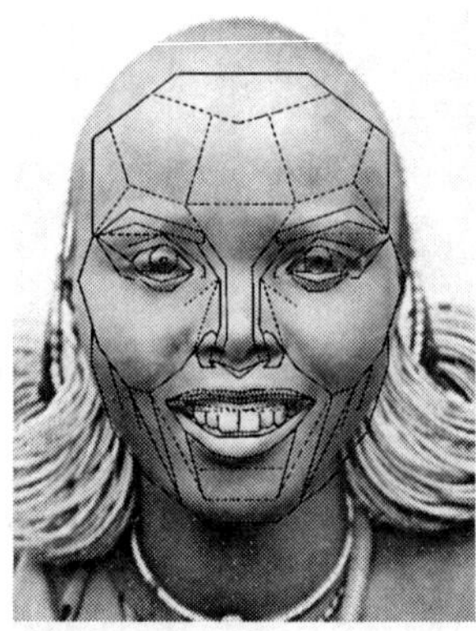

Figure 1. Price Meets Marquardt. A very high percentage of Maasai and other people Price photographed displayed similar bone structure to this attractive young lady. (Looking into the sun, she is squinting a little bit.)

Photo © Price Pottenger Nutrition Foundation, www.PPNF.org

Marqardt Mask © Stephen Marquardt, www.beautyanalysis.com

repeats this theme again and again, as he travels the world. It seems as if the beauty and vitality of a given landscape can be conducted into the bodies of those who populate that landscape through the foods they draw from it.

Form and Function: Another Package Deal

From the beginning of humanity's historic record, one can find numerous references to the idea that physical beauty and health are related. And although social taboo currently proscribes explicitly discussing that relationship—so much so that it delayed the publication of this book—to many it remains patently obvious. True, you may remember your high school football star as less than handsome, riddled with acne, wearing thick glasses and braces, and dependent on pills and an inhaler. But usually our high-school heroes receive recognition, admiration, and jealousy as a result of good looks and superior athletic skill. In the last chapter, I described the package deal in terms of physical appearance. But because form implies function, another hallmark of good genes is exceptional stamina and coordination. The genius of Price's book is that it dares to scientifically examine all these realities, to study the beauty-health connection with the same systematic approach we bring to bear when studying any other biological phenomenon.

The preference for beauty (in our own and other's faces) emerges as a result of the instinctive pattern recognition process described in Chapter 3. And it serves a survival function as well because, as unfair as it seems, less attractive people have more health problems. Price recognized that underdeveloped mandibles don't just look unattractive, they don't hold teeth very well, and that makes it hard to chew and increases the risk of cavities. What's more, people who aren't considered good looking tend not to see as well (on average) as their more attractive counterparts. To our animal minds, these traits represent potential liabilities, a weakness in the tribe bordering on contagion. This reaction is deeply ingrained, and it may be why even health professionals are reluctant to investigate the root causes of these physical problems. But Price felt differently. He rejected the age-old notion that the blessings of health and beauty are reserved for those few with the purest souls—the biological equivalent of "Divine Right." His thinking was truly "outside the box" and even today his research findings are ahead of their time.

If you'd like to get a taste of the kind of vitality Price discovered, what people looked like and how they lived, do a quick Internet search for indigenous tribes. Start with the San, Maasai, Himba, Kombai, Wodaabe, or Mongolian Nomad. Or watch any TV show about tribal life. When you look at the people's faces, notice how particularly well-formed their features are, and how their geometry resembles what Marquardt found. That is because their diets still connect them to a healthy living environment whose beauty, in a very real sense, expresses itself through their bodies.

One of the first documentary films ever made is called *Grass: A Nation's Battle For Life* filmed by Meriam C. Cooper (who later made *King Kong*). Cooper documents the lifestyle of the Baktiari tribe in the Zardeh Kuh Mountains of what is now Iran. It tracks one leg of the 200-plus-mile journey the tribe made twice a year in the seasonal search of fresh pasture for their goats and pigs. Up and down the rocky mountainsides, old men, pregnant

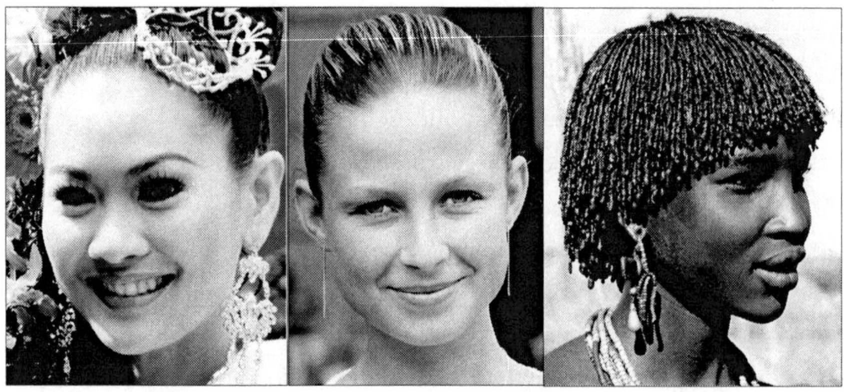

Figure 2. Profiles in Genetic Wealth. Native Thai (left), Danish barmaid (middle), Ethiopian woman (right). Notice their well-formed features, indicative of ideal geometric facial construction. Whether a people draw nutrition from the family farm, the sea, or the savannah, real food acts as a kind of conduit through which the beauty of the environment can be communicated into our bodies and expressed as human form.

women, and little children herd their stubborn, hungry animals, some breaking through waist deep snows in bare feet. Five thousand people travel with all their belongings across the 200 miles in a little over a month. In distance alone, they cover the equivalent of twenty marathons a year. How did they do it? Genetic wealth. Our 20th century Western perspective calls on us to label this lifestyle as subsistence since they lacked the accoutrements associated with prosperity. But they didn't carry their gold in leather satchels. Their treasure was safely hidden inside the vaults of their genetic material, and it had endowed every member of the tribe with chiseled features, strong joints, healthy immune systems, and the stamina to achieve athletic feats that few of us would dare even attempt. And remember, they did this every year.

How They Were Built: Exceeding the RDA by a Factor of Ten

Contrary to what Westerners tend to assume, indigenous people of the past were not merely scraping by, skinny and starving, desperate to eat whatever scraps they could find. Their lives did revolve primarily around finding food, but they were experts at it, far more capable than we are of making nutrient-rich foods part of daily life. By fortifying the soil, they grew more nutrient-rich plants. By feeding their animals the products of healthy soil, they cultivated healthier, more nutrient-rich animals. And since different nutrients are stored in different parts of the animal, by consuming every edible part, they enjoyed the full complex. They used their own version of biotechnology to create the most nutrient-dense foods possible, foods that functioned to design every sinew and fiber of their bodies, and upon which we have now come to depend.

At eleven locations around the world, Price secured samples of indigenous communities' staple foods for lab analysis. His nutritional survey rivals that of our best nationally sponsored programs in having tested for all four fat-soluble vitamins A, D, E, and K, and six minerals, calcium, iron, magnesium, phosphorus, copper, and iodine. Here's what he found:

> *It is of interest that the diets of the primitive groups [...] have all provided a nutrition containing at least four times these minimum [mineral] requirements; whereas the displacing nutrition of commerce, consisting largely of white-flour products, sugar, polished rice, jams [nutritionally equivalent to fruit juice], canned goods, and vegetable fats have invariably failed to provide even the minimum requirements. In other words, the foods of the native Eskimos contained 5.4 times as much calcium as the displacing foods of the white man, five times as much phosphorus, 1.5 times as much iron, 7.9 times as much magnesium, 1.5 times as much copper, 8.8 times as much iodine, and at least a tenfold increase in fat-soluble activators [Price's term for vitamins].* [63]

He continues, listing the findings for each of the other groups he studied. There was a clear pattern: The native diets had ten or more times the fat-soluble vitamins and one-and-a-half to 50 times more minerals than the diets of people in the US. It is obvious that diets of people living in what doctors at the time would have called "backward" conditions were richer than those living in the technologically "advanced" US by an order of magnitude.

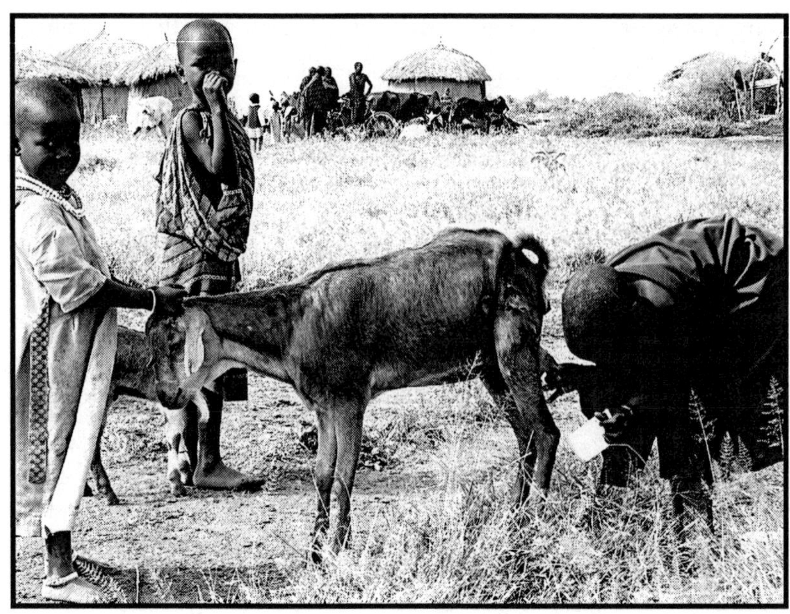

Figure 3. Old-fashioned Breakfast. Fresh, Local, and Unprocessed. This milk is rich in nutrients bioconcentrated by the goat, which is free to graze on the choicest shoots growing over vast plains of mineral-rich soil. Many small farmers in the US still raise their animals on pasture, offering the customer a healthy alternative to milk produced by grain-fed animals.

Though his laboratory was dismantled over 50 years ago, I consider Price's data a more accurate indication of how much nutrition we need than the RDA, or Recommended Daily Allowance.

What makes his 60-plus-year-old data superior to the state-of-the-art nutrition science today? Chiefly, the fact that today's state-of-the-art nutrition science leaves much to be desired. While Price's data may be old, he identified the healthiest people he could and then systematically analyzed the nutrient content of their staple foods. But if you ever look into how today's RDAs are set, you'll find a hodge-podge of differing opinions, unstandardized techniques, and poorly thought-out studies. For instance, the RDA of vitamin B_6 for infants younger than one year old was set at 0.1 mg per day based on the average B_6 content in the breast milk of only 19 women. Six of these women did not even themselves consume the RDA of vitamin B_6 for their age group, and their breast milk contained only one tenth of the B_6 of the women with healthier diets.[64] So you might wonder, then, if a third of the women were by our own definition undernourished, shouldn't they have been excluded from the study? The fact that they were not suggests to me that the researchers in charge of this study were not interested in what a baby might need to be healthy, but merely in calculating the averages and getting their job done quickly. This is just one example of the poor quality research that defines state-of-the-art, modern nutrition science. (It also determines what gets put into infant formula—and what gets left out.)

If you believe Price's data, which I do, then clearly our bodies seem accustomed to a far richer stream of nutrients than we manage to sip, chew, swallow or scarf down on the way to work today. Our need for nutrients is, apparently, quite extraordinary. But what is more extraordinary is the totality to which indigenous cultures, and presumably also our ancestors, involved themselves in the production of these foods. In contrast to our general attitude of nourishment as a necessary evil demanding expediency, traditional life seemed to revolve around collecting and concentrating nutrition. To this end, no methodology—and no recipe—was too bizarre.

I will give a few examples from Price's book to demonstrate how fully people immersed themselves in the production of food, and a few of the wonderful ingenuities that streamlined this undertaking. In the Scottish Isles, people built their houses using, chiefly, the grass that grew abundantly on the moors. The roofs were loosely woven and chimneyless so that the smoke from their cooking fires would pass directly through the thatch. When the roof was removed and rebuilt in spring after having been infused with mineral-rich ash all winter, the smoke thatch made fantastic fertilizer for their plant crops, chiefly oats. Their oats, in turn, were super sources of minerals and were incorporated into many dishes. One of the most important was a fish dish made from baked cod's head (rich in essential fatty acids) that had been stuffed with oatmeal (rich in minerals) and chopped cod's livers (rich in vitamins). On the other side of the world, in Melanesia, the original arrivals to the islands had brought with them a member of the pig family bred for its self-sufficiency at finding forage in the muddy and mountainous landscape. They'd released their hogs into the wild so they could colonize the forests. Soon, the hogs' numbers had grown to the point that one could be hunted down just about anywhere. Every part of the quarry—from snout to tail—would be cooked, or smoked, or otherwise prepared and eaten. Another Melanesian favorite was the coconut crab, so called because of its ability to sever coconuts from the trees with monster claws. To catch the well-armed crabs as they came down from the trees, natives would quickly girdle the tree with grass about 15 feet from the ground. Upon reaching the grass girdle, the crab—convinced it had reached terra firma—would release its grip, and fall. Stunned, the crab could be easily gathered. It would be tempting to eat them then and there. Nevertheless, the crabs were first confined in pens for several days and allowed to gorge on all the coconut they wanted—generally enough to burst their shells. According to Price, "They are then very delicious eating."[65] Around the world again to Northern Africa, he found Maasai life revolved around producing healthy cattle, used primarily for their milk and their blood and only occasionally for their flesh. Maasai men spent nearly a decade learning to tend their animals. This education included everything from identifying the best grazing grounds based on rainfall patterns, to selective breeding, to regularly drawing blood from the jugular vein using a bow and arrow with surgical precision. As the Maasai ate neither fruit nor grain, this milk, either fresh or curdled (and bacterially-enriched), was their dietary staple. Recent studies have shown that Maasai milk contains five times the brain-building phospholipids of American milk.[66] In the dry season, when milk yields are low, they fortify the milk with blood to make another staple drink.

As focused as people once were on the production of healthy food, the chief crop—and the ultimate prize—was the next generation of healthy children. Traditional cultures made a science of it. As we'll see in the next chapter, step one was planning ahead. Around the world, traditions reflected extensive use of special foods to boost a woman's nutrition before conception, during gestation, for nursing, and for rebuilding before the next pregnancy.

Some cultures thought it prudent to fortify the groom's diet in preparation for his wedding ceremony.[67] The shreds of surviving information suggest such knowledge was quite sophisticated. Blackfoot Nation women utilized the still-unknown nutrient systems found in the lining of the large intestine of buffalo (and later, cow) to "make the baby have a nice round head."[68] To ensure easy delivery, many cultures reinforced pre-conception and pregnancy diets with fish eggs and organ meats—loaded with fat-soluble vitamins, B_{12}, and omega-3—as well as special grains carefully cultivated to be high in important minerals.[69] The Maasai allowed couples to marry only after spending several months consuming milk from the wet season when the grass was especially lush and the milk much denser in nutrients.[70] In Fiji, islanders would hike miles down to the sea to acquire a certain species of lobster crab which "tribal custom demonstrated [to be] particularly efficient for producing a highly perfect infant."[71] Elsewhere, fortifying foods didn't just facilitate pregnancy; they made the difference between the baby making it to term or not. The soil of certain areas around the Nile delta is notoriously low in iodine, the lack of which can lead to maternal goiter and infant malformation. Tribes of the Belgian Congo knew that burning water hyacinth (rich in iodine) produced ashes capable of preventing these complications.[72]

These ingrained traditions existed throughout the world and, until recently, dictated the ebb and flow of daily life. This kind of dedication, study, and wise use of natural resources is what was required to amass and protect the genetic wealth that enabled people to survive in a very different, and harsher, wild, wild world. Of course, these days, most of us spend our time fighting traffic, not wild boar. But the same nutritional input that toughened and fortified the physiologies of these indigenous peoples can still be accessed today for the attainment of extraordinary health. Were the medical community to bring the same enthusiasm to the engineering and maintenance of healthy bodies as archaeologists bring to their study of ancient architectural wonders, they would soon call for a radical revision of what we understand to be a healthy human diet. The construction of a beautiful, sound building is not a matter of chance, but of planning, good materials,

Are We Really Living Longer?

People often say we're living longer than ever. But is that really true? According to an article called *Length of Life in the Ancient World*, published in the *Journal of the Royal Society of Medicine* in January 1994, from circa 100 BC until 1990, we have managed to tack an additional six years onto the life span. This modest increase is easily attributable not to better nutrition or even better health, but to emergency room care, artificial life support, life-sustaining pharmaceuticals, vaccines, and other technology, not to mention the many leaps in accident prevention. Presuming that it's sensible to gauge health by longevity of life span as opposed to longevity of function, the numbers still tell a surprising story. Even though the *average* life span has increased slightly, according to the US census, in the past 200 years the *percentage* of people living a really long time may actually have gone down:

Percentage of Americans aged 100 in 1830: 0.020

Percentage of Americans aged 100 in 1990: 0.015

Percentage of people living today expected to live to 100: 0.001

(From Wise Traditions Vol. 8 No.1, 2007 p13)

and reference to the collected body of relevant science. Winning the genetic lottery depends upon those very same prerequisites.

Today, at every stage in the process of producing food, we do things differently than our sturdy, self-sufficient ancestors did, wasting opportunities to provide ourselves with essential nutrients at every turn. We fail to fortify and protect the substrate on which the life and health of everything depends—the soil. We raise animals in unspeakably inhumane and unhealthy conditions, fill their tissues with toxins, and color the meat to make it appear more appetizing. Being raised on open pasture is no guarantee that an animal's body, and ultimate sacrifice, will be put to full use; typically, only the muscle is consumed. Much of the nutrients, bioconcentrated over the animal's life, are thrown to waste. Grains—even those grown on relatively healthy soil—are too often processed in ways specifically damaging to the most essential, and delicate, nutrients. Once in the kitchen, the consumer takes one last swing at whatever nutrition has survived, through overcooking and the use of cheap, toxic oils. Finally, since we've not been told that certain vitamins and minerals are more bioavailable when combined with acids or fats (see Chapter 7), many of them pass right through us.

Given that we drop the ball at every stage in the process of bringing food to the table, it's not surprising that recent studies show, far from exceeding the RDA as we should be, few—if any—people even meet it. For vitamin A, only 46.7% of healthy females meet the RDA,[73] and levels are low in 87% of children with asthma.[74] For vitamin D, 55% of obese children, 76% of minority children, and 36% of otherwise healthy, young adults are deficient.[75] For vitamin E, 58% of toddlers between one and two years old,[76] 91% of preschoolers,[77] and 72.3% of healthy females do not consume enough. Zero percent of breastfed infants were found to have achieved the minimum recommended intake of vitamin K.[78] For the B vitamins, only 54.7% consumed adequate B_2 (riboflavin);[79] for folate, only 2.2% of women between the ages of 18-35 and 5.2% of women aged 36-50 achieved the recommended intake; and for calcium, fewer than 22% of African-American adolescent girls consumed the RDA.[80] There are more studies, but you get the idea. Not one study shows 100% adequacy of any single nutrient, not to mention adequacy of all measurable nutrients. Presumably the vast majority of Americans are deficient in more than one, if not all, known vitamins, minerals, and other nutrients.

Many of my patients suffer from symptoms that could be attributable to poor nutrition, problems as common as dry skin, easy bruising, runny noses, yeast infections, and crampy digestive systems. Unfortunately, testing for vitamin adequacy is not easy. We haven't even defined what "normal" levels are for many nutrients, including essential fatty acids and vitamin K. For those that have been so defined, the normal range may extend all the way down to zero. That's right: You may have none of an essential nutrient in your bloodstream, yet still be considered to have consumed an adequate amount. So why bother testing? And since many vitamins are stored in the liver and other tissues, even if blood levels are adequate, overall body stores may be low. As far as I can tell, the best way to assure nutrient adequacy is not with testing, but with adequate nutrient consumption—itself no simple matter.

Aside from building a time machine and transporting back to the halcyon years of nutritional bounty, in the face of so many barriers to good nutrition, what is an ordinary American to do? Is it remotely possible, in this day and age, to get the nutrients you need without breaking your bank?

Absolutely. You can grow a garden, shop for fruits and vegetables by smell (as opposed to appearance), and buy animal products from farms that raise them humanely—on pasture and outside in the sun. In the coming chapters, I'll go into more detail about special ways to make your food as nutritious as possible. But I can tell you right now, you'll get the most bang for your buck, and the fastest return on investment, if you learn to enjoy something that many kids in many countries aside from this one will fight each other for—the organ meats.

These were the original vitamin supplements, and they comprise key components of almost all truly traditional heritage dishes. They are the missing ingredients whose disappearance from our dinner tables explains many of our health problems, and whose replenishment would go a long way towards improving those dismal nutrition statistics. But like most middle class Americans, for most of my life I assumed such odd tidbits and wiggly things were best fed to my cats and dogs. I might have thought differently had I been raised some place where traditions of self-sufficiency are still alive and kicking. Some place where children can learn cherished recipes from their parents. Some place where there's plenty of land and open water per capita, where the weather invites people to spend time outdoors with their extended families. Someplace like Hawaii.

Crossing the Culinary Divide

The south side of Kauai is known all over the archipelago as Filipino territory; in our neighborhood about one in three households speaks Illokano. Luke, a devout meat-eater whose favorite meal is a blood-rare steak, considered himself a serious carnivore until he met these guys. People who catch wild boar with hunting dogs and kill the tusked beasts with knives (not guns, mind you) experience a fuller meaning of the word. Here, the majority of households, young and old, can make short work of a large carcass or a sturdy goat leg. Being an unworldly American, the culture struck me as slightly terrifying.

Then the inevitable happened: We were invited to a neighborhood buffet for a crash course in local, "any kine" Filipino cuisine. I'd heard about these parties and I knew what kind of stuff awaited us on the rough-hewn picnic table out on the patio behind the sliding glass doors. At the potluck, kids gathered inside to watch and to laugh at the *molikini Ha' Oles* (newly immigrated white folk) trying to cope. Thankfully a sweet eight-year-old girl took pity on us. Graciously highlighting key ingredients, Kiani guided us through the mystery casseroles, greasy open plates, and bowls of soupy chunks.

First up, *morcon,* a meat, egg and cheese wrap sliced into neat cross-sections, beautifully setting bright-yellow yolk against deep maroon liver. Next, one of those suspiciously chunky soups: tan-colored *paksiw na pata,* pork knuckles and pork meat braised in a mixture of soy sauce, sugar and vinegar, and flavored with dried lily buds. I couldn't get past the knuckles. More soupy chunks, this time in green and tan, of *balon-balonan,* chicken gizzards softened in vinegar and mixed with water spinach. Beside that, a duo of honeycomb-tripe and vegetable stews—*goto and callos*. I felt as if I'd wandered into a Klingon delicatessen. But then I noticed, at the far corner of the table, a single lonely looking bowl of sweet potato soup. This I could manage.

Luke was a more enthusiastic guest. The weirder the dish's ingredients, in fact, the more he slopped onto his compartmented Styrofoam plate. This was enormously entertaining to our younger hosts, every scoop generating louder giggling until the adults' attention was drawn to Luke's selections. By the time the table tour was over, he had piled on an unbelievable ten dishes that were, sadly, melding into one. Onlookers volunteered approval with a round of claps and cheers.

While Luke transformed the contents of his overflowing plate into a small pile of bones, I began to develop the suspicion that I had been living in a cloistered world. The feeling followed me home, and resurfaced each time I hiked past the goatherds that dot the rolling green hills of Lawai.

I'd worked in Thailand and trekked in Nepal. I'd eaten at hundreds of ethnic restaurants, and in the homes of friends from all over the world. But the potluck had really been outside my normal experience of eating. There were things on that table I didn't know you could eat, let alone would want to. At the age of 33, I had learned there's more to meat than meat. While I'd been in my kitchen sprinkling chicken extract powder over re-hydrated ramen noodles, just down the road, my Filipino neighbors were stuffing hoofed feet into a boiling cauldron. I wasn't so much horrified as I was envious.

Shortly after this initiation buffet, I would fall sick from the infection in my knee and learn that I'd developed the problem due in large part to nutrient deficiencies. Had I been raised, like my same-aged cohorts here, on such wild gastronomic safaris rather than the standard middle-class fare of white meat, margarine, and frozen vegetables, my life would most certainly have been different. I would be healthier. In addition to avoiding the chronic connective tissue problems during my athletic career (we'll learn more about connective tissue health in Chapter 11), I would also very likely look different. The slim waist, luscious lips, doe eyes—and other traits my grandmothers both possessed—could have been mine.

In the chapter preceding this, we learned that these are the characteristic features all of us want because they are ingrained in the collective memory of our DNA, indicative of normal growth, and vital to health—so vital that just looking at them stimulates the pleasure centers of the brain to release the happy juice. In this chapter, we learned how much more nutrient-dense our ancestors' diets were compared to ours, and why these traditional diets enabled them to grow healthier, stronger bodies that were highly resistant to disease. Not surprisingly, having been fabricated without all the normal ingredients, people today are developing "old age" diseases in early or mid life, and other health problems previous generations never even heard of. (*Harrison's Principles of Internal Medicine* from 1990 doesn't even list attention deficit disorder or fibromyalgia in the index, and I didn't hear much about either in medical school. Now, both are common.) If the genetic intelligence needs more nutrients than it's currently getting, and if Price was right, and perfect faces grow where good nutrition flows, you'd expect to see facial form progressively diverging from Dr. Marquardt's definition of the ideal. I think that's exactly what's happening. In the next chapter, you'll read evidence that, not only does facial degeneration predictably develop from poor nutrition, the effects are so immediate that you can see it happening within the space of a single generation.

PREPARATION.—We will tell here how to cook a whole salmon, from about 8 to 10 lbs. and it will be exactly the same with any other fish or part of fish to be cooked "au court bouillon." 1st. Clean and wash your fish, remove the gills and the fins, but preserve the tail, place the fish in a fish kettle (with a grate in the bottom so as not to break it, when you take it from the kettle) with 2 carrots, 1 onion sliced, some thyme and laurel. 6 grains of whole pepper and enough water to cover the fish well. 2d. Let heat and *as soon as it boils* place the fish pan on a corner of the stove and let simmer for about 1 hour without letting boil. 3d. Serve in a long dish on a folded napkin and dispose around the fish or serve apart 2 nice potatoes for each guest, boiled in slightly salted water and carefully carved. Serve the sauce apart. For the sauces see Nos. 151-152-159.

67. SAUMON OR TRUITE AU COURT BOUILLON.

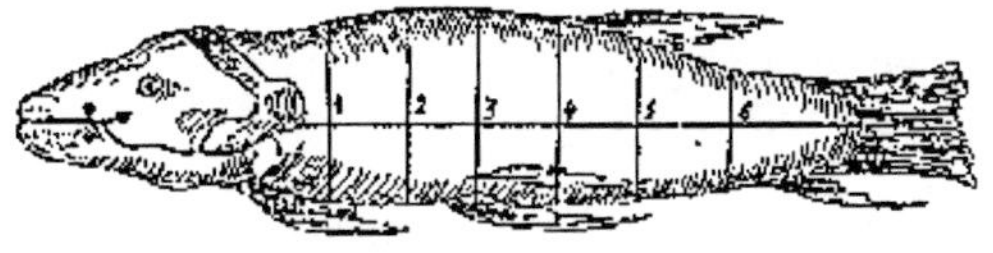

BOILED SALMON OR TROUT.

Figure 4. Recipe from *French Cooking for Every Home*, by Francois Tanty, Chef de Cuisine for Emperor Napoleon III. Usually when we buy fish these days it's already filleted and sani-wrapped. But how much closer to the source of your food would you be, and how much more like a top chef would you feel, if you knew how to clean and prepare a beautiful, whole fresh salmon all by yourself?

Five

A Mother's Wisdom

Letting Your Body Create a Perfect Baby

Almost nothing gives a woman more pride and confidence than the birth of her first child. After one successful pregnancy, there is an understandable expectation that a second pregnancy will go even more smoothly. And perhaps it will, at least for mom; more distensible pelvic tissues do facilitate a second labor. But unless the mother gives herself ample time and nutrients for her body to fully replenish itself, child number two will not be as healthy as their older sibling. And so, while big brother goes off to football practice, or big sister gets a modeling job, these children will be spending time in the offices of the local optometrists and orthodontists. It's not that they got the "unlucky" genes. The problem is that, compared to their older sibling, they grew in a relatively undernourished environment in-utero.

Timing is Everything

Why does being born second sometimes mean a child's body is second rate? For one thing, most American women have no idea how badly they're eating. One study shows that "[o]verall, 74% of women are falling short on nutrients from their diet."[81] However, I think that's being optimistic (see last chapter's statistics and below). If most mothers-to-be aren't even taking in enough nutrients for themselves, how can we expect them to properly provide for a growing baby, not to mention one right after the other? But the biggest reason there's often such a difference between number one and number two in cases of rapid-fire conception has to do with how the placenta works.

Even minor nutritional deficiencies can hamper baby's growth. So to better protect baby, nature has provided a built-in safety mechanism, allocating as many resources to the placenta as it can get away with, even if it means putting mom's health at some risk. The baby-protection mechanism is so powerful that even on an all-McDonald's diet, a woman can expect to produce a baby with ten fingers and ten toes. Dr. John Durnin of Glassgow University describes the mechanism vividly: "The fetus is well protected against maternal malnutrition—that indeed it behaves like a parasite oblivious to the health of its host."[82] If mom's diet is deficient in calcium, it will be robbed from her bones. If deficient in brain-building fats—as horrible as this sounds—the fats that make up the mother's own brain will be sought out and extracted.[83] Pregnancy drains a woman's body of a wide variety of vitamins, minerals, and other raw materials, and breastfeeding demands more still. As you might expect, the demands of producing a baby draw down maternal stores of a spectrum of nutrients, including iron, folate, calcium, potassium, vitamin D, vitamin A and carotenoids, magnesium, iodine, omega-3, phosphorus, zinc, DHA and other essential fatty acids, B_{12}, and selenium.[84] To the placenta, mom's central nervous system, for instance, is simply a warehouse full of the kinds of fat needed to build baby's central nervous system. Studies show maternal brains can actually shrink, primarily in the hippocampal and temporal lobe areas, which control short-term memory and emotion. These brain regions are not responsible for basic functioning, like breathing or blood pressure regulation, and so are relatively expendable. This marvelous nutrient scavenging ability of a human placenta means that even in conditions of insufficient maternal nutrition the *first* child may come out relatively intact. Meanwhile, mom's body may be depleted to the point that before and after pictures reveal her spine to have curved, her lips thinned, and she may have trouble remembering and learning new things, or feel anxious and depressed—as in postpartum depression.

It may sound harsh, but it's just the "selfish gene" at work. Successful genes behave like greedy pirates, commandeering maternal nutrient stores

Number One Son—Why So Lucky?

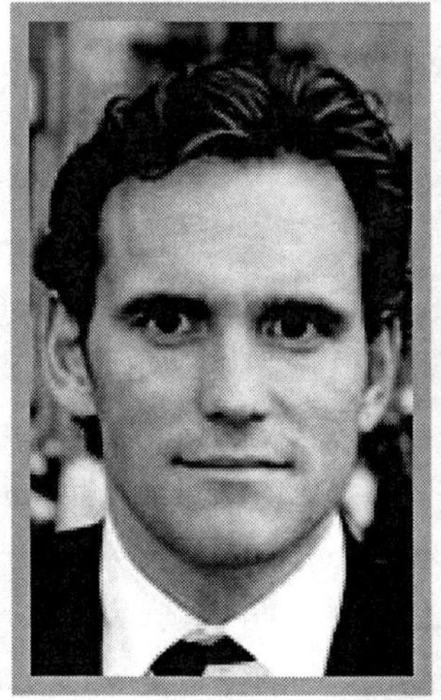
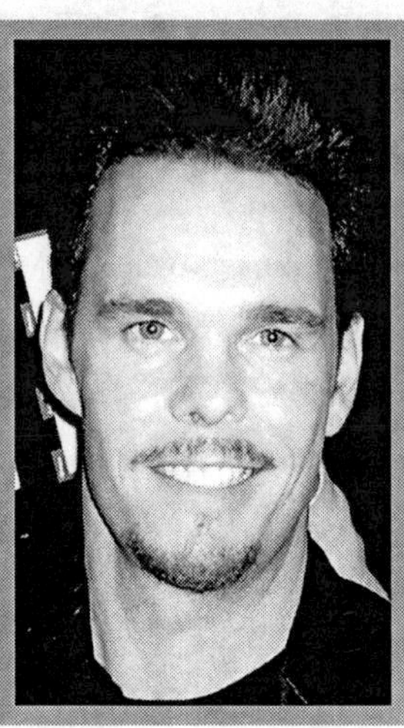

Figure 1. Two Famous Brothers. On the left is Matt, who has been starring in movies since his teens. On the right, the incredibly talented Kevin, eighteen months his junior. Both men were 43 when photographed. Why does Kevin look older, and why has he rarely been cast as a romantic lead? The answer: Second Sibling Syndrome.

for the benefit of their own optimal replication. However, any child conceived in too short a time for those storehouses to be refilled will be at significant disadvantage. In such depleted conditions, were baby to extract from mother all the nutrients its genes would like it to have, this would put mom's life at significant risk. Following the utilitarian calculus of genetic survival, biology pragmatically chooses not to kill the mother while a baby is gestating and opts, instead, for a compromise. This second baby will be constructed as well as possible in the depleted conditions in order that mom may pull through. Tragically, this exposes the child to a variety of health problems, which can become increasingly noticeable, and even debilitating, as they grow older.

Here's something else to consider. Sugar and vegetable oils act like chemical static that blocks the signals our bodies need to run our metabolisms smoothly. Most women's diets today are high in sugar and vegetable oils, adding to the growth disturbances already caused by missing nutrients. Not only does sugar and vegetable oil consumption disrupt maternal metabolism and lead to gestational diabetes, pre-eclampsia, and other complications of pregnancy, the sugar and vegetable oils streaming through a developing baby's blood block signals in the womb, disrupting the sequence of highly sensitive, interdependent developmental events that contribute to the miracle of a healthy birth.

The consequences of not getting enough nutrients and the introduction of toxins are primarily brought to bear through changes in the infant's epigenome. As we saw in Chapter 2, the epigenome consists of the set of molecules that attach themselves to DNA and other nuclear materials that control when a given gene is turned on or off. These genetic switches inform every aspect of our physiologic function. Diseases previously assumed to be due to permanent mutation—from cancer, to diabetes, to asthma, and even obesity—actually result from mistimed genetic expression. And since the proper timing of gene expression requires specific nutrients in specific concentrations, if a second sibling gestates in a worse nutritional environment than the first, their epigenetic expression will be suboptimal, and growth and development will be impaired. We know, for example, that low birth weight, often due to mom's smoking or high blood pressure (both associated with poor nutrition), puts children at risk for low bone mass and relative obesity for the rest of their lives.[85] Abnormal epigenetic responses due to nutrient deficiency may explain why children of subsequent births are at higher risk for disease, from cancer[86] to diabetes[87] to low IQ and birth defects.[88]

Our skeletal development depends on normal genetic expression too. Because normal facial growth demands large quantities of vitamins and minerals,[89,90] and short inter-pregnancy intervals make it unlikely that mom's body would have been given adequate time to replenish all the vitamins and minerals the first baby used up, children born in close succession might reasonably be expected to look different. But I could find no study addressing the potentially life-changing influences of birth order on facial development. So I designed one myself.

How Birth Order Affects Our Looks

I began by looking to the stars—TV and movie stars, that is. A glitterati's face is loaded with instances of a special kind of symmetry, called dynamic symmetry, which we recognize by instinct. The actor with "screen appeal," the actress with "that certain something," the up-and-coming journalist groomed for the anchor seat because of her "fresh" face, the photogenic author with the winsome smile—what we're really talking about, here, is geometry. As we saw in Chapter 3, our brains are exquisitely sensitive pattern detectors, capable of assessing the architecture of a human face with NASA-like precision. And as NASA was reminded with Hubble, a hair's breadth can make all the difference. Deviations of just a millimeter from the ideal create features that fail to align perfectly with Marquardt's mask, and we can take all this information in instantaneously. We prefer to fix our gaze on faces with broad foreheads balanced by strong jaws, prominent brows above deep-set eyes framed with nice, high cheekbones—those are the characteristics which tend to bend the angles of the human face toward a more perfect proportionality. As you might have guessed, models and movie stars from Greta Garbo to Angelina Jolie have a habit of hoarding more than their share of dynamic symmetry. And often they are the first born of their family.

In contrast, their younger siblings' faces are often noticeably less symmetrical. Most are characterized by a narrowing of the mid-portion of the face, rounded, indistinct features including noses, cheekbones and brows, and a weakening of the chin and jaw. Are A-list movie stars always the oldest child in the family? Certainly not. As you'll see later, in the setting of maternal malnutrition, sometimes the uterus doesn't work quite perfectly the first time around. But with few exceptions (notably, Tom Cruise), those who had older siblings had three or more years spaced between them.

Of course, superstar looks are rare (in the modernized world), and the chance for any family to produce even one stellar beauty is vanishingly small. The statistical improbability of one stunner following on the heels of another would predict, with rare exception, any consecutive child to be less attractive than the first. This would explain a fair, though miserly, rationing

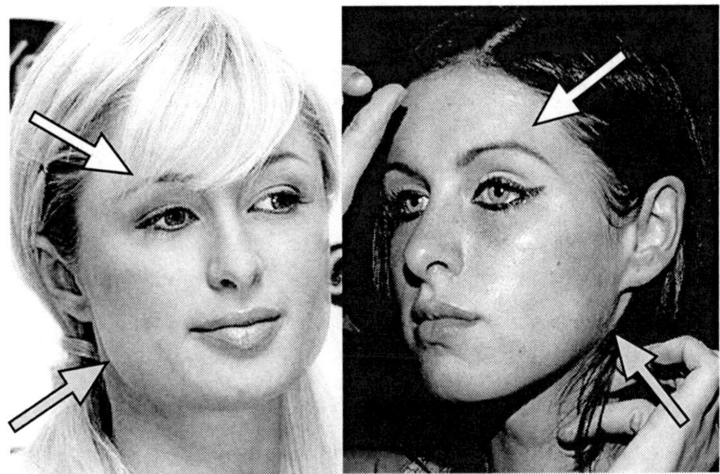

Figure 2. Different Geometry. Left Paris Hilton (b 1981) Right Nicky Hilton (b 1983). Both girls are lovely, however one's fame far outshines the other's. Arrows shown indicate two of the features that differentiate these attractive women. Grey arrows indicate the corner of the mandible (lower jawbone) called the gonion. Paris has a nearly 90 degree angle within the bone structure of her mandible, while Nicky's is more oblique and her gonion is located much closer to her ear, indicating a smaller, relatively underdeveloped jawbone. White arrows indicate the inflection point of the eyebrow. Paris' eyebrow is angulated, while Nicky's eyebrow is simply curved, indicating less angular orbital bones. Subtle nutritional deficiencies create subtle growth imperfections of the underlying bone.

of young stars and starlets throughout the general population, but it would fail to account for the fact that the most attractive, most successful siblings are typically the oldest or, in families of three or more, one of the first two. It seemed to me that better nutrition was the simplest, most likely explanation for first-born children with favorable looks. But before exploring that further, I first wanted to see if the second sibling phenomenon could be found not just among the supermodels of society, but also among the rest of us in the general population.

So I expanded my research. With the generous help of office mates, patients who supplied stacks of high-school yearbooks from 1969 to 2006, and graduate students from the University of Hawaii, I compiled several hundred groups of siblings, cutting and pasting their senior photos (to control for age) and organized them in family groups. Some were large and some were small. But all the families included in the study had at least two siblings born within two years of each other. Just as with the celebrity siblings, among those pictured in the yearbooks, family beauty generally faded according to the same pattern: From oldest to youngest, the jaw grew narrower and receded, the cheekbones flattened out, and the eyes were less deeply set. The closer in age the siblings, the more striking the changes. But spacing alone does not prevent this effect. With anything short of an optimal dietary context, if mom's body is asked to produce large numbers of children, then each subsequent baby uses up more of her reserves so that, even with three to four years between births, her body continues to lose nutritional ground. This can magnify the effects of second sibling syndrome down the line. The implications for the younger children are obvious.

There is, however, one additional twist on the second sibling syndrome worth mentioning—as I alluded to earlier. It seems to result not from nutri-

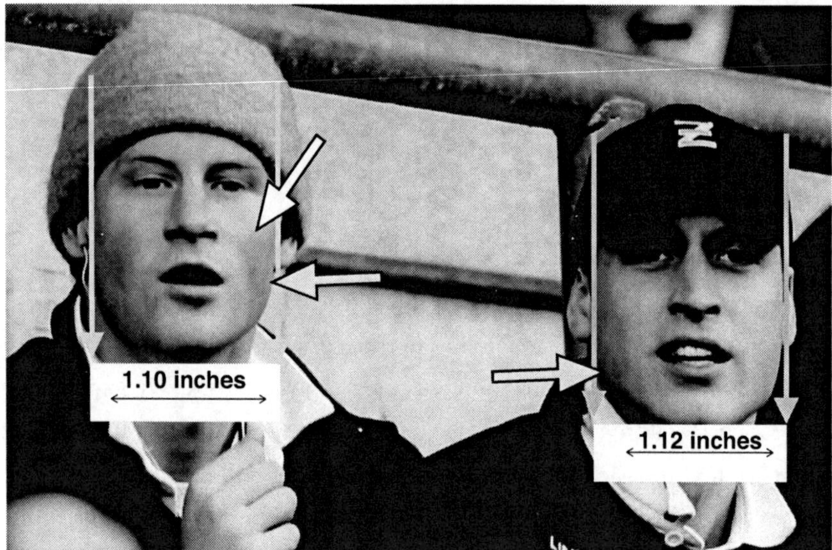

Figure 3. Royal Jaw Development. Prince Harry (left, b 1984). Prince William (right, b 1982). The younger Prince's lower jawbone and mouth are subtly narrower than his older brother's. The .02 inch difference in the distance between the base of their ears in the photo translates to approximately 1/8th of an inch difference in real life. As with Paris and Nicky, Prince Harry's gonion is higher than his older brother's (grey arrows). The shadow on Prince Harry's cheek indicates the presence of a subtle hollow under his cheekbone (white arrow), absent from Price William's face. The small gap between Prince Harry's teeth formed after he wore braces and likely needed a few molars pulled, one of the consequences of a narrow jaw.

ent deficiency per se, but from chemical interference (from sugar and vegetable oil) delaying signal transmission between mom's body and her own uterus. Some second-born females have fuller lips and more sexually appropriate chins and eyebrows than their older siblings—a woman's chin being a little more pointed, less squared, than a man's, and a woman's eyebrows being more arched while men's are lower and straighter. The pointier female chin and gracefully curved eyebrows are examples of *sexual dimorphism*, the differential development between males and females. Human males, in addition to strong, squared chins, tend to have broad shoulders while women, with their more petite and rounded chins, also have slender shoulders, wider hips, and fatty breast tissue. So what would explain these second-born girls with the more attractive, sex-specific features?

A woman's body undergoes a miraculous change soon after conception. Under the influence of a new physiologic directive, the functioning of every organ is altered by waves of hormones, all generated by the tiny collection of rapidly dividing cells. Many of these changes are permanent. Of course, no organ is affected more obviously than the uterus. But a modern diet interferes with hormonal signaling, as we'll see later, so the uterus especially can't perform quite so well, at least not at first. Blunted uterine (and placental) estrogen signals could explain why estrogen's effects on a *first* baby girl appear diminished. Subdued estrogen effects lead to relatively masculine features: slightly too prominent brow and chin, aggressive-looking eyebrows, and lips not quite filled out. She may be handsome, but she won't turn heads. With uterine systems already existing the *second* time around, estrogen's effects are optimized. The first baby girl's younger sister (Christy Turlington is a perfect example, see Figure 4), gifted with the similar bone structure but feminized and with the felicitous addition of full, rounded lips, will present a face whose image will leave men hopelessly enthralled, haunted by her image as if evolution had specifically wired them to be susceptible to its charms. Incidentally, if the second sibling were a boy, the burst of estrogen receptivity may still create a feminizing effect, sharpening the center of the chin, arching the eyebrows, rounding the forehead, and plumping the lips.

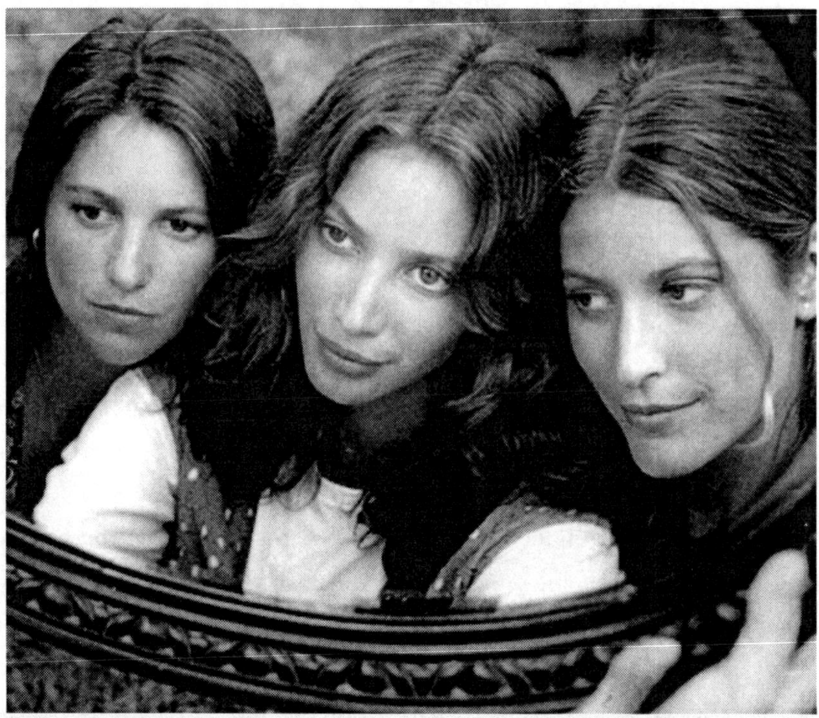

Figure 4. Benefits of an Experienced Uterus. Christy Turlington with sisters Kelly and Erin. Erin (right) is older, and Kelly (left) is younger than supermodel Christy (middle). Notice Erin has slightly masculine features, while Kelly's are slightly childlike. Christy's siblings are both very attractive women, but they lack the "certain something" that talent agents seek. Christy's full lips and feminized bone structure result from improved uterine blood flow in comparison to older Erin. Younger Kelly, whose features are less sharply defined than her sisters', will never develop the dramatic angles and tantalizing symmetry of a supermodel.

So what does this mean? Well for one thing, though the development of a beautiful, healthy baby is—as we are so fond of saying—miraculous, it's not a mystery. This spectacular orchestration of events is as dependent upon a strict adherence to a program of good nutrition as it is vulnerable to its breach. Studying siblings enables us to see *why* we aren't all perfect. It enables us to see that nutrient deficits change a child's growth in ways that are both predictable and easy to measure. I call it second sibling syndrome not because it only affects second born children, but simply because the effects of maternal malnutrition on a child's growth are most readily visible in the faces of children born in a short time period after an older sibling who, presumably, shares similar genes and thus serves as a kind of control. But as I just described, no child, not even the firstborn, is immune from second sibling syndrome because the underlying problem is not birth order; it's malnutrition. In the younger children, maternal nutrient deficiencies result in relatively less material to build bone, nerve, and so on, impairing hormonal receptivity and thinning and flattening their features to create a worn-down look. In the older children, static interference from sugar and vegetable oils often blunts placental hormone production, reducing sexual dimorphism.

If you read Chapter 4, then you already know that the vast majority of Americans—and I mean just about everyone—isn't merely malnourished, but severely malnourished. Which should make you wonder: *Doesn't that mean we're* all *suffering from second sibling syndrome?* Most of us are, which is why there seems to be so few lottery winners walking around. And what explains them? How did they, raised by parents who, presumably, followed the same advice my parents did, and ate the same steady diet of frozen, canned and vitamin-poor fruits and vegetables, mystery meat from poisoned animals, grains grown on mineral depleted soils, margarine, and everything else that makes our modern diet unhealthy, curry Mother Nature's favor? *They* didn't. Their great-great grandparents did, by eating such nutrient-rich diets that they imparted the family epigenome with *genetic momentum*, the ability of genes to perform well with suboptimal nutrient inputs for a finite amount of time. And their placentas did, by sending an especially urgent message to mother's bones, brain, skin, muscles, glands and organs, to release every available raw material for the benefit of the baby. In these one-in-a-million cases, the fetal genome operating in mom's belly can do what it's been doing for a hundred thousand years: create the miracle of a perfectly symmetrical *Homo sapiens* body.

What Mothers-To-Be Need To Know

I'd like to believe that most mothers want what's best for their child and I am convinced that, once made aware of the profound impact of nutrition on their child's future, the vast majority will use the knowledge to make bet-

The Fabulous Fiennes

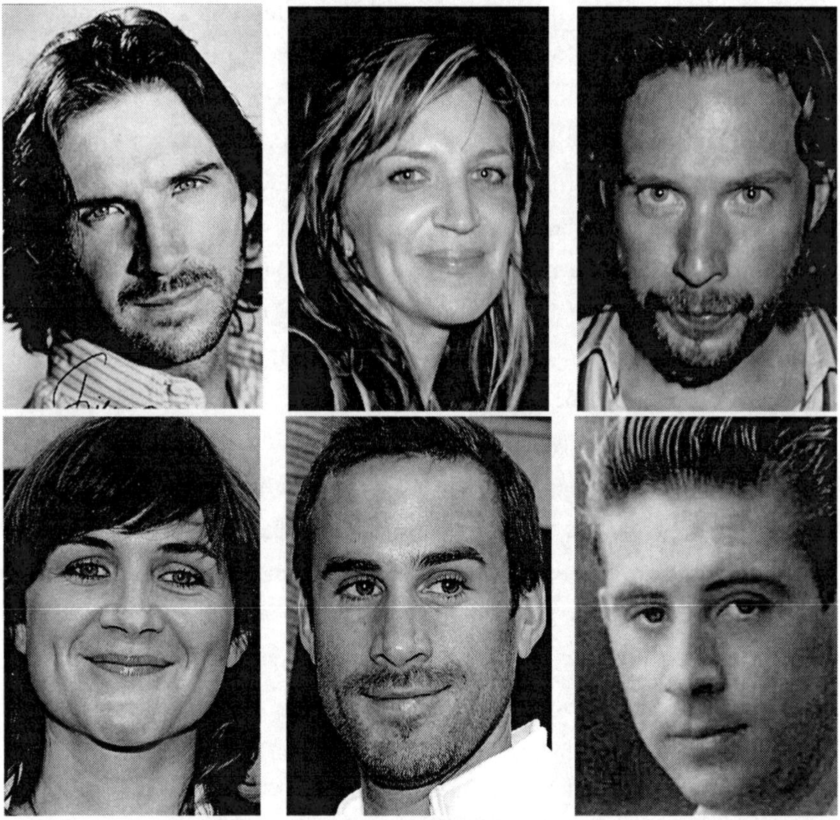

Figure 5. Left to right from top: Ralph (b 1962) Martha (b 1964) Magnus (b 1965) Sophie (b 1967) Twins Joseph and Jacob (b 1970). Notice how features morph from eldest to youngest: Eyes gradually move closer together, the brow softens and becomes less distinctive, the nose shortens and narrows as does the lower jaw, and the cheekbones drop, move inward or disappear altogether. Joseph may have benefitted from the fact that placental blood flow to twins is often unequally distributed, giving one child relative growth advantages.

ter decisions about what to eat. But I miscalculated the barriers to disseminating this kind of information by way of the medical establishment.

Doctors get their information from researchers. Researchers can only do research when they can get grant funding. These days, grants come from industry or special interest groups, and tend to support either the use of expensive medications and technology, or a demand for more medical coverage for one of many special interest groups. I didn't know research had to fall into one of these two categories to be funded until Luke and I took a plane trip to California to meet with researchers at UCLA and UCSF. There, I met with over a dozen doctors and PhDs to bring up the possibility that there might be an obvious, though currently overlooked, relationship between modern food and disease.

The trip was a real eye-opener. These researchers held fast to the idea that their primary directive was improving human health. But it soon became clear that their more immediate goal, by virtue of the realities of economics, was the acquisition of grant funds, necessitating never-ending compromises between the exigencies of financing and the integrity of the science. I learned from an epidemiologist that various agricultural interests funded most of his research in nutrition, and out of financial necessity, he was directed toward the promotion of the largest crops: fruits.[91] As an epidemiologist, he was unaware that excess fruit consumption leads to health problems due to the high sugar-to-nutrient ratio in fruit. And he was surprised when a colleague pointed out that she'd found, after advising her patients to eat the recommended three to six servings of fruit a day, that doing so raised their triglycerides to unhealthy levels.[92] Hoping to drive home the point that our bodies demand more nutrition than we can get from fruits, vegetables, grains, and low-fat meat, and hoping to stir up interest in doing more research on nutrition and optimal fetal and facial development, I described the results of a pertinent study. It showed that one in three pregnant women consuming what mainstream research suggests would be a healthy diet nevertheless gave birth to babies with dangerously low levels of vitamin A in their blood.[93] Vitamin A deficiency is associated with eye, skeleton, and organ defects. The epidemiologist was fascinated but admitted that his reliance on funding from fruit growers bound him to continue producing more and more research just like he'd already produced—showing that fruits are "good for us." I learned that neither he nor anyone else at UCLA would likely be able to pursue this new nutritional issue or anything similar because there was no giant industry to support it.

Ironically, another researcher at UCLA was examining so-called "Hispanic paradox," a term referring to the mysterious finding that recent immigrants from Latin American countries (with a more intimate connection to the products of a traditional diet) have healthier babies than their Caucasian counterparts. Might the mystery be explained by the fact that our Mexican, South American, and other Latin-nation friends are still benefiting from their healthier, homeland diet? The physician I spoke to said that while my argument was plausible, he had not considered the possibility. However, he considered it unlikely that superior Hispanic nutrition was the reason for superior Hispanic maternal-child health. His idea was that Hispanics enjoy a greater network of social supports (in spite of the fact that many have immigrated to this country from thousands of miles away, which fractures families). And he felt that somehow social supports translated into fewer premature births and birth defects. In his publications, he points out that networks of social support are reinforced by community medical clinics. Where did his money come from? State-funded grants for medical clinics serving Hispanic immigrants. I left UCLA impressed by the spirit of optimism but demoralized by the misdirection of its pursuits and the sheer volume of intellectual and financial capital expended on generating the logical contortions necessary to earn funding from various state and industrial entities.

Hoping to find greener pastures elsewhere, Luke and I traveled north to speak to a perinatology expert at UCSF. There, I was thrilled to meet with an MD/PhD with a special interest in prenatal health. We discussed the pattern of facial changes I saw in younger siblings and their implications for improving maternal nutrition. Once again, I was taken aback. The well-respected researcher agreed that there was a relationship between nutrient depletion and skeletal development, but he was unconvinced that the *pattern* of skeletal changes could be due to anything other than chance. In her view, which reflected the general attitude I found at UCSF, it was unlikely that children born in the US, let alone in the relatively affluent Bay Area, could be exposed to any significant levels of deficiency. Why not? "Because," she explained, "pretty much every pregnant woman is given a prenatal vitamin."

And that's true. Obstetricians and primary care doctors like me routinely write prescriptions for prenatal vitamins to help reduce a woman's risk of pre-eclampsia (an immune system disease causing mother's body to partially reject the baby and give birth prematurely) and to decrease the child's risk of low birth weight and neural tube defects like spina bifida. However, a large study completed in the US showed that pregnant women using their prenatal pills still develop "combination deficits" of niacin; thiamin; and vitamins A, B_6, and B_{12} that persist throughout each of the three trimesters.[94] Other studies show that prenatal vitamin pills don't solve many nutritional problems. The following are just a few examples:

- Vitamin D deficiency. Studies in which over 90 percent of participants took their prenatal vitamins, 56 percent of white babies and 46 percent of black babies were vitamin D insufficient. Insufficiency in early life increases the risk of schizophrenia, diabetes, and skeletal disease. [95]
- Long chain essential fatty acids. As of the date of this writing, there is no recommendation about how much of these to consume, and most people who don't supplement get almost none. But supplementing with cod liver oil during pregnancy has protective and lasting effects on the baby's intelligence.[96]
- Choline. Gestational deficiency of choline is associated with life-long learning deficits.[97] One survey showed 86 percent of college-age women were lacking adequate dietary choline.[98] Choline is not part of any prenatal vitamin supplement commonly marketed in the US.

While the prenatal pill partially addresses the issue of nutrient deficiency, it does nothing to address the over-consumption of sugar and vegetable oil, both of which interfere with signal transmission required for normal growth and development.

The sad truth is many, if not most, of the best minds in the research business are satisfied with the status quo. There appears to be very little sense of urgency in the prevention of unnecessary suffering from physiologic default or disease, and little humility brought to the reality that, in the battle against common childhood and adult diseases, medical research has by any objective account failed miserably. We are told to accept the idea that facial deformities—even relatively minor changes like those I study—occur randomly, all products of the whimsical nature of the "genetic lottery." There was a time when the facial deformities now known to be associated with fetal alcohol syndrome (FAS) were written off as unpreventable. Doctors went on telling their pregnant patients to drink to settle their nerves. And there was a time when the spinal cord and brain malformations, which we now prescribe prenatal pills to prevent, were believed to occur by chance. That is, until 1991, when *The Lancet* published an article entitled "Prevention of Neural Tube Defects."[99] Provided with unambiguous evidence that folic acid deficiency played a role and that better nutrition could prevent problems like spina bifida physicians ultimately adopted measures of prevention. We are all served by science's affinity for explanations to natural phenomena. Without it, we are guided only by magical thinking and superstition. The witches of Salem weren't possessed; they were poisoned. Hurricanes aren't retribution for sinful behavior; they are explicable meteorological phenomena. Likewise, physiologic deficiencies occur for a reason and most can be easily prevented.

I'm sorry to say that such professional complacency is increasingly common in medicine. Although we tell pregnant patients to quit smoking and drinking and to take their prenatal pill, and we screen for certain diseases, the list of childhood epidemics keeps stacking up. That's a tragedy. But for the most part, we physicians simply go about our business assuming someone else will someday do something about it.

This apathy toward prenatal care has affected the way the general public thinks, as well. I brought up the prenatal pill earlier, so let's look at that as one example. A woman recently came to see me already seven weeks pregnant with her third baby in less than three years. Most women have no idea that the prenatal vitamin pill works best when taken *before* conception because it helps to boost a woman's vitamin levels to prepare for the first ten

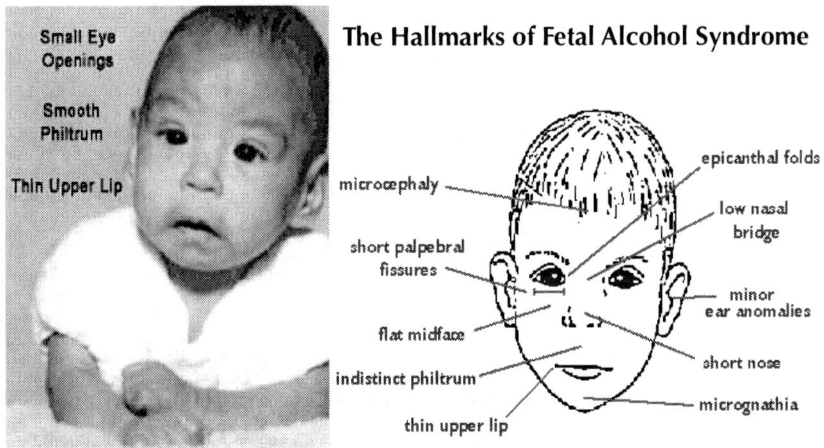

Figure 7. Fetal Alcohol Syndrome: How much is really malnutrition? Both pictures show characteristics of FAS. As with Second Sibling Syndrome, we find tall, narrow skulls, minor ear anomalies, small jaw, thinned lips, and flattened cheekbones (here described as flat midface). Alcohol's toxic effects occur largely due to cellular membrane damage.* Sugar and toxic fats also damage cell membranes (see Chapters 8 and 9). Either mechanism would be expected to block signal transmission and thus impair growth.

*Effects of low concentrations of ethanol on the fluidity of spin-labeled erythrocyte and brain membranes. Mol. Pharmacol. 13:435 – 441, 1977.

weeks of pregnancy, the time when the most fundamental decisions about how to shape the baby's body are made. After that window of opportunity has shut, though it can still improve birth weight, the vitamin pill can do little to prevent most major birth defects.[100] This mother's third child will be at high risk not just for disfiguring facial changes but also for skeletal and organ defects which will likely turn him or her into another chronic disease statistic before graduating high-school. Still, this is likely the first time you've heard this bit of information about prenatal vitamins, which tells us something about the dissemination of critical child development information in our country. (It might help if we called it a "pre-conception" pill.)

The young mother-to-be certainly had heard nothing of it, but it's not her fault. Her attitude emerges from living in a society that treats the decision to grow another baby as casually as picking out a video for the week-end. Not only are we missing the opportunity to do the very minimum—getting women on prenatal pills prior to conception—we're also missing the opportunity to truly prepare her body with solid nutrition, giving her baby's genes the materials they need to compose their physiologic masterpiece. Of course, that would involve more than taking a pill. It would require improving the nutrient content of her food.

Synthetic vitamin pills are, of course, a step up from no nutrition at all, but they are a sorry replacement for real food for the following list of reasons: 1) They're not the same as what nature makes. Many vitamins exist in nature as entire families of related molecules, only a few of which can be recreated in a factory. For example, there may be over 100 isomers of vitamin E, but only about 16 are put into tablets.[101] 2) The processing of synthetic vitamins necessarily involves the creation of incidental molecular byproducts, the effects of which are largely unknown. About half of the content of vitamin E tablets are isomers that don't exist in nature, which might explain why some studies show taking vitamin E pills increases mortality. 3) Without the proper carrier nutrients in the right balance, many vitamins are not absorbed. 4) Many vitamins work synergistically with other nutrients in ways we don't fully understand. 5) Who knows what else is in that pill? The entire supplement industry is essentially unregulated, and supplements have been found to be contaminated with toxic compounds including lead, or dangerously high levels of copper.[102] But, again, there is some benefit to taking certain supplements, especially in pregnancy, because the food supply is so bereft of nutrients when compared with foods from only seventy years ago.

A real danger of the prenatal pill is its psychological effect, how it implies to mothers that the nutrition issue has been addressed and been safely removed from their "to do" list. This prenatal vitamin pill, part of "advanced" prenatal care, is widely believed—by health professionals and patients alike—to make up for the fact that today's modern diet is so wantonly lacking. The general idea is that, whatever our mom-on-the-go can't provide to her baby through whatever she's eating, the prenatal vitamin pill can, thus implicitly giving her permission to continue with the standard diet and expose her body to foods which could not be better engineered to deprive a growing child. In my practice, I give all pregnant women who see me a prescription for a prenatal multivitamin, but I make sure they know that it's no magic bullet. If they want to have a healthy, beautiful baby, they have to learn how to eat. (See Chapter 7.)

Studies like those cited here, showing how poorly nourished we actually are, have presumably been conducted so that perinatologists and other specialists can familiarize themselves with, and begin to address, childhood disease and physiologic deficiencies that result from malnutrition. However, taking action based on what a given study recommends would require personal initiative on the part of individual healthcare providers. But as corporate culture goes, so goes medical culture. We live in the age of consensus and groupthink, where otherwise curious and capable professionals avoid being singled out by huddling in the center of the herd. The herd, in turn, waits for an authority figure to lead the way. So if there is no authority figure acknowledging the importance of a given article's findings, nothing happens. It's as though it were never written.

Long before any of today's ivory towers had been built, and long before a diploma was proof of wisdom, people were making their own observations and drawing conclusions, acting on those conclusions, and passing that wisdom down to their children. Much of that accumulated knowledge pertained either directly or indirectly to the production of healthy babies, yet only a few scattered snippets still remain. These whispers from the past help explain how people used to avoid the problems of second sibling syndrome. And they can still help anyone hoping to become a parent, providing a plan of action to better ensure good fertility, a smooth pregnancy, and a healthy, beautiful child.

Native Intelligence

A group of social workers studying access to healthcare in Africa in the 1970s were surprised to discover resistance to the building of more hospitals and clinics from—of all people—local village grandmothers. It's not that these women didn't care about health or feared new technology. They felt the influx of Western ideas had already caused harm to their children and grandchildren. The new order smacked of an insidious form of imperialism. So when these independently minded African women were politely asked to relinquish their roles as protectors of the community genome, they bridled at the idea.

> *Today we don't make any decisions about spacing the births of our children[...].Our ancestors had stronger children because they were not born too close together. Today parents no longer worry about their children getting sick. They think that they can always buy medicine and then the child will get well. This is why couples no longer separate their beds after the birth of a child, as they used to do in the time of our ancestors.*[103]

When social workers examined how these traditions eroded away, they uncovered an explanation not entirely irrelevant to us: Westerners, including mine owners, officials, missionaries, and doctors working with these groups, judged the traditional practice of spacing childbirth to be at odds with their long-term goals of expansion and did not support its continuation.[104] "Intimate Colonialism: The Imperial Production of Reproduction In Uganda 1907-1925" suggests rather provocatively that when companies need workers they care more about sheer numbers than the quality of workers' lives or their longevity.[105] Such concerns become irrelevant given a large enough pool of potential workers to draw from. And so the systematic spacing of children that was once an "important feature of the control of excellence of child life"[106] is tossed aside as an anachronism, a fractured artifact of female empowerment. But it is not just a women's issue, and it extends beyond the political. We all gain from children's good health, which requires giving mom's body at least three, preferably four, years to refortify her tissues with a generous supply of nutrients.

Nearly a century ago, Mahatma Ghandi preached self-sufficiency as a prerequisite of self-government, reminding his countrymen that "to forget how to dig the earth and to tend the soil is to forget ourselves." FDR later echoed this principle, saying, "a nation that destroys its soil destroys itself."

Two of the most important resources we have are the land that provides us with food and the farmers who work it on our behalf. If the idea of refortifying a mother's body between births and doing the same with soil between crop cycles strikes you as related concepts, you're right. Just as we are all custodians of the genome, traditional farmers (described as "subsistence farmers" when they work in places like China and India) are the frontline custodians of the land, going to great lengths to replenish the ground between crops and to replace all the minerals required for healthy growth of the plants—even to the point of layering recycled outhouse waste over the ground to recapture nutrients that would otherwise grow depleted. The modern technique is to replace only a few of the many nutrients crops draw from the ground each year. As a result, our food supply is of much lower quality now than it was before industrial farming, which in turn makes fortifying mom's body a tougher task.

While the fact that we still produce bumper crops year after year makes for good press, in reality the nutrient content of American-grown plants and animals is far worse than it was during the dustbowls of the 1930s. One report showed that packs of sliced green beans have only 11% of the vitamin C claimed on the package. Another report comparing mineral levels of 27 fruits and vegetables from 1930 and 1980 found modern produce to be depleted by an average of 20 percent, with calcium dropping 46%, magnesium 23%, iron 27%, and zinc 59%. Meat and dairy, which ultimately depend on healthy soil, have declined commensurately in quality between 1930 and 2002, with iron content in meat falling an average of 47%, milk 60%, and lesser declines in calcium, copper, and magnesium.[107] When plants and animals are reared on mineral-deficient soil, not only are they missing nutrients, they're not as healthy. And their cells are, in turn, less able to manufacture the vitamins and other nutrients that would benefit us. If we could somehow view these grocery staples as they now exist nutritionally, they would look like ghostly afterimages of their former selves, semi-transparent shapes of apples, cucumbers, the various cuts of beef. Of course, in real life it all looks relatively fresh and appetizing. It had better: Most are grown and engineered with eye appeal in mind. But these pretty displays hide the fact that it is more difficult to purchase nutritionally rich foods today than any time in recent history.

Without healthy soil to nourish them, plants are unable to use the energy from the sun to manufacture optimal levels of vitamins. Without vitamin- and mineral-rich plants for animals to eat, they can't add the next layer of chemical/nutritional complexity *we have evolved to depend on*. We are here today because our ancestors taught their children how to garden, hunt, and prepare their food so that they could one day raise healthy children of their own. Their hard work and due diligence in building and maintaining a healthy environment to support a healthy human genome can, however, only take us so far. We are coasting along on the nutritional momentum left over from millennia of enacted nutritional and environmental wisdom. If our food is composed of far fewer nutrients than it was four generations ago, it's a fair bet that our physiologies—our connective and nervous tissues, our immune systems, etc.—have taken a hit. What about our genes? Might they be affected as well? What might be the expected effect of generations of nutritional neglect on our own children?

That depends, in large part, on the choices each of us makes. But there is little doubt that physicians, like me, are going to be very, very busy.

The Omega Generation

Here in Hawaii, four generations sometimes come in to my clinic for an office visit all at once, giving me a front-row view of the impact of modern food. Quite often, this is what I see: Great-grandma, born on her family's farm and well into her 80s, still has clear vision and her own set of teeth. Her weathered skin sits atop features that look as though they were chiseled from granite. More often than not, she is the healthiest of the bunch and has a thin medical chart to prove it. The youngest child, on the other hand, often presents symptoms of the whole set of modern diseases: attention deficit, asthma, skin disorders, and recurrent ear infections. Like many of today's generation, one or more of his organs wasn't put together quite right. Maybe there's a hole in his heart, or maybe he needed surgery to reposition the muscles around an eye. While the exact effects may be hard to predict, what is predictable, given the dwindling dietary nutrients and proliferation of toxic materials, is some kind of physiologic decline.

Within a given family, the earlier the abandonment of traditional foods for a diet of convenience, the more easily perceptible the decline. I'm thinking of one little boy in particular, the great-grandchild of one of Hawaii's many wealthy missionary families who developed an ear infection during his visit to Kauai from another island. This little boy bears none of his great grandmother's striking facial geometry. His jaw is narrow, his nose is blunted and thin, his eyes set too close, and his cheekbones are withdrawn behind plateaus of body fat. The lack of supporting bone under his eyes makes his skin sag into bags, giving him a weary look. His ears are twisted, tilted, and protruding out, and his ear canals are abnormally curved, predisposing him to recurring external ear infections.

Narrow face, thin bones, flattened features—sound familiar? This is second sibling syndrome. But the young child sitting on my exam table wasn't a second sibling, though he exhibits the familiar characteristics. He's the fourth-generation product of a century of nutritional neglect and the consequential epigenetic damage. According to a landmark 2003 CDC report, this child, like all others born in 2000, has a one-in-three chance of developing diabetes, a condition which reduces life expectancy by between ten and twenty years.[108] What is going unreported is the fact that it isn't just diabetes on the warpath. Every year, growing battalions of familiar diseases are cutting a wider and wider swath of destruction though the normal experiences of childhood.[109]

Whereas in previous centuries part of a parent's responsibility was to work hard to prevent their children from getting sick, today so many of us are sick ourselves that we've grown to accept disease as one of life's inevitables—even for our children. Today's kids aren't healthy. But rather than make such a sweeping and terrifying declaration, we avert our eyes from the growing mound of evidence, fill the next set of prescriptions, and expand our definition of normal childhood health to encompass all manner of medical intervention. This latest generation of children has accumulated the epigenetic damage of at least the three previous generations due to lack of adequate nutrition along with the over-consumption of sugar and new, artificial, fats found in vegetable oils. From the point of view of the family genome, it's been getting battered relentlessly for almost a century—even during key, delicate periods of replication. The physiologic result of these accumulated genetic insults? Distorted cartilage, bone, brain, and other organ growth. Many physicians have noted an apparent increase in young couples complaining of problems with fertility which, given the implications of epigenetic science, should come as no surprise. Children born today, I'm afraid, may be so genomically compromised that, for many, reproduction will not be possible even with the benefit of high-tech medical prodding. This is why I call these children the Omega Generation.

Born by cesarean section (often necessitated by maternal pelvic bone abnormalities), briefly breast-fed (if at all), weaned on foods with extended shelf-lives—the human equivalent of pet foods—these Omega Generation children see the doctor often, and even the first-born suffer from obvious signs of second sibling syndrome. In the same way we talk about bracing for the aging baby boomers' medical needs, we had better reinforce the levies of our medical system for the next rising tide: medicine-dependent youth. These children will age faster, suffer emotional problems, and develop never-before-seen diseases. In my experience as a doctor, parents have an intuitive sense that their children are already dealing with more health problems than they ever did, and they worry about their future, for good reason. But no parent is helpless. If you have children, or are planning to, I can think of at least one child who can do something to avoid all this illness and start getting healthy—yours.

Restoring Your Family's Genetic Wealth

If having an Omega Generation baby sounds terrifying, you can do something about it. You can get off the sugar and vegetable oils that would block your child's genetic potential. That means cutting out processed food, fast food, junk food and soda. And you should give yourself at least three, preferably four, years between pregnancies and make every effort to fortify your body with vitamin-rich foods (or if you can't, at least use prenatal vitamins) *before* conception. Those who want to do everything possible to have a healthy baby will find additional instruction throughout this book. But this discussion opens up a new question: *If I do everything right, how beautiful and healthy can I expect my child to be?*

My first answer to that question is that, of course, *all* children are beautiful. But if you're asking if your child will have *extraordinary* health, excel scholastically and in sports, and be so physically striking as to elicit the envy of peers, then the answer is *it depends*. It depends on how much *genetic wealth* you gave him. Which, in turn, depends on what you inherited from your parents.

Genetics is all about information. Your genetic wealth is a function of how much of the information in your genes has been damaged or remains intact, and how well the supportive epigenetic machinery is able to express the surviving data contained in your genetic code. To gauge the present condition of your genetic data, you can begin by asking your parents and grandparents what they ate when they were little. Find out if you were breast-fed. Were they? Learn whatever you can about who was born when (including birth spacing). Dig up as many family pictures as you can find to look for the telltale signs of second sibling syndrome. The more you know about your family history, and the more objectively you measure your health and appearance along with that of your partner, the more clues you will have to assess your genetic, and epigenetic, health.

Let's give it a try. Let's attempt to gauge a person's genetic momentum using Claudia Shiffer as our case-subject. Though both her parents were tall and reasonably attractive, you wouldn't guess they could produce the superstar beauty they did. Their genetic equation was complicated by the fact that her father and mother were born during the depression and raised under the conditions of post-war food shortages. Claudia's secret weapon of genetic wealth may be that her great-great grandmother grew up in the most wholesome and remote of farming communities in Austria, a town near Elbigenalp, which had changed very little for thousands of years.[110] This close relation to someone living in a successful, stable, indigenous society is truly a rare gift. Adding to this, Claudia's father's family was affluent, meaning that (during their formative years) he and his parents presumably had access to the best foods of the early 20th century. Put the two together, and keep the good food coming, and *voilà,* a genome operating under moderate duress for a spell is effectively rehabilitated. Along these lines, if Kevin Dillon (Matt Dillon's younger brother) was to marry say, Carole Ann Schiffer (Claudia's younger sister), and these two were fully dedicated to their perfect diets and provided the same for their children, chances are good they would right the genetic ship and produce a child of nearly ideal physiologic proportion and outstanding health.

Let's look at a broader example of genetic rehabilitation, this time dealing with height. Height is one of the most desirable proportions for a man. Aside from the obvious social and mating advantages, the professional advantages gained with every additional inch of height are well documented. Studies show that tall men take home higher salaries, obtain leadership positions more often, and get more sex.[111] Hawaiian archeological evidence shows that, for hundreds of years, a man's stature helped to secure him a better official position in the class hierarchy. Our language—big shoes to fill, big man on campus, someone you can look up to—reflects society's universal preference for the tall. The positive perception of the taller among us often extends to women, as well. I am not suggesting that taller people are better, only that height affords certain physical and social advantages. With that in mind, can relatively diminutive parents who want those advantages for their children have a baby who might someday walk tall and rise above the fray to stand head and shoulders above the rest?

Absolutely! This potential is encoded in our genetic memory. We've all heard that we used to be a lot shorter, how few of us could fit into one of those little suits of armor worn by medieval knights. But around the world, evidence is accumulating that, thousands of years prior, our Paleolithic

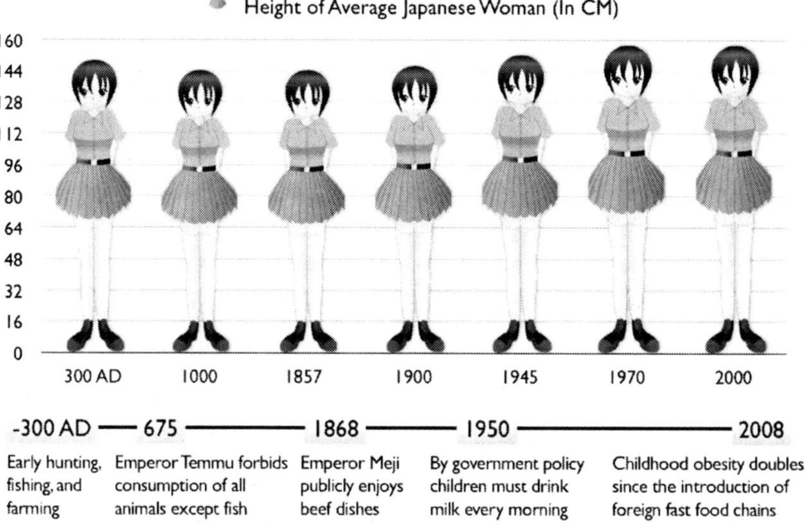

Figure 8. Skeletal Response to Diet Change. Short-stature may be a kind of biologic "choice," an epigenetic adaptation to inadequate bone-building material in a previous generation's diet. Rather than build weak, breakable bones, the genome makes bone of the same strength, only less of it. When the nutrient supply increases, the genes respond again, taking advantage of the extra material to build a bigger frame.

predecessors were at least as tall, if not taller, than most of us are today. Even in the early Middle Ages, 1,000 years ago, European men were nearly as tall as they are now. What caused the temporary skeletal shrinkage? As the population grew, crowding reduced access to nutrients until stature reached an all time low in the early 1700s.[112] Improvements in agricultural technology, most notably the series of inventions attributed to lawyer-turned-farmer Jethro Tull, revolutionized the process of tilling soil, vastly increasing productivity.[113] By the late 1700s, having recovered some of its former nutritional inputs, the European genome rebounded—and with it the average European's height. But it would probably have dipped again, so that a tall man today might measure just over five feet, were it not for the early 20th century invention of refrigeration. The ability to freeze food meant that fisherman could travel as far as they needed and fill their hulls to brimming. Refrigeration also meant that even during winter, wealthy countries could reach down to the tropics for summer fruits and vegetables, making it profitable for millions of acres of rain forests around the globe to be converted over to crop production. For the past 100 years, industrialized nations have had consistent access to enough nutrition to achieve our Paleolithically preprogrammed height. Of course, height doesn't equal health. But generally speaking, when a genome has access to a *surplus* of complex nutrition, it is far better positioned—and may be said to have a built-in preference—for the production of offspring with more robust, larger frames.

The two basic steps to accomplishing genomic rehabilitation are 1) stop eating toxins, and 2) start eating according to the Four Pillars of World Cuisine. Later, we'll learn more about how sugar and vegetable oils, the two most common toxins in the modern diet, prevent you from being as healthy and beautiful as you otherwise would, and how avoiding them can improve your own and your children's health both immediately and in the long run.

Avoiding toxins seems like a pretty sound idea. But how, exactly, to do that? It gets confusing because a product can call itself healthy when there's not enough nourishment in it to keep a rat alive. I'm not kidding. According to industry insider Paul Stitt, author of *Fighting The Food Giants*, a popular cereal company did a study in the 1940s that showed its puffed rice product killed rats faster than a starvation diet of water and minerals.[114] Similar puffed and processed whole-grain products are still sitting on store shelves today, sold under every major brand label. In fact, even store-bought granola, loaded with unhealthy oils and sugar, is an unhealthy way to start your day. Much better, alternatives can be found in the fresh food departments (as we'll learn in Chapter 7). To understand the depth to which our food supply is saturated with products that keep us barely alive, I'll take us back in time to understand where and when things started to go wrong with the way we think about food.

Six

The Great Nutrition Migration

From the Culinary Garden of Eden to Outer Space

But if thought corrupts language, language can also corrupt thought.
—George Orwell

In 1987, my friend Eduardo was called to Laetoli in northern Tanzania to restore fossilized footprints left by a wandering family of hominids some 3.5 million years ago. Befriended by local tribesmen, Eduardo soon found himself immersed in a world both unimaginably vibrant and deeply spiritual. By day, Eduardo used hypodermic needles to inject poison into tiny plant shoots that threatened to break apart the footprints left by our *Australopithecus afarensis* ancestors. By night, he shared food—on one memorable occasion, the still-beating heart of a goat—with Tanzanian herder-gatherers, known as *Maasai,* whose culinary rituals had remained largely unchanged for thousands of years.

Hearing Eduardo describe his time with the Maasai, I was reminded of the kind of awe with which Price described the cultures he visited and the people he studied. Eduardo was most impressed by the tribal chief who, while rumored to have been over 70 years old, was still an absolute physical specimen, standing over six-foot-five, completely free of wrinkles, and still able to keep the peace among his several wives. It seems that few people who journey to visit the Maasai have returned home without feeling profoundly changed. Jen Bagget, a travel writer, describes her visit to Tanzania as if she'd discovered Shangri-La. "With distinctively tall and willowy frames and striking facial features, the Maasai are easily the most beautiful people we've seen in the world. We were instantly captured by their friendly dispositions, open manner and natural elegance."[115]

The Maasai represent one of the rare surviving intact and functional indigenous cultures. These societies are, in essence, windows into our past. Reading accounts of travelers who've spent time among people like the Maasai, one could get the impression that—as far as human health is concerned—*once upon a time* really existed. In the good old days, people enjoyed an almost idyllic physiologic prosperity. This prosperity was earned, in large part, by the maintenance of an intimate relationship between themselves and the land, their animals, and the edible plants that rounded out their diets. As a result of this intimacy, they talked about food differently than we do. To us food is primarily a fuel, a source of energy, and sometimes a source of guilty pleasure. To people who remain connected to their culinary origins, food is so much more. It is part of their religion and identity. And its value is reinforced with story.

> *In the beginning, Ngai [the Maasai word for God, which also means sky] was one with the earth. But one day the earth and sky separated, so that Ngai was no longer among men. His cattle, though, needed the material sustenance of grass from the earth, so to prevent them dying Ngai sent down the cattle to the Maasai .... No Maasai was willing to break the ground, even to bury the dead within it, for soil was sacred on account of its producing grass which fed the cattle which belonged to God.*[116]

In a few sentences, this story articulates the cattle's central position in Maasai life and the necessary injunction against harming the land. As startled as Eduardo was when invited to take his share of a still-beating goat heart, he might have been more unnerved had they started talking about the total number of calories in their meal, the percentage of their daily intake of protein, carbs, and fat, and the benefits of eating fiber. Such reductionist terminology would have been out of step with the way the Maasai see the world. If they did start talking that way, as a physician, I'd be concerned. Because, no matter where you live, talking about—and then envisioning—food in such arbitrary categories is bad for your health.

Of course, here in the US, we talk about food that way all the time. These days, very few of us participate in any deeply rooted culinary traditions, let alone share mythical stories connecting the food we eat to the environment it came from. Like everything else, foodspeak has to meet the requirements of a sound bite culture and is limited to grunting imperatives such as "eat your veggies," "watch your carbs," and "avoid saturated fat." Having lost the old ways of talking about food, we've also lost the physiologic prosperity that once endowed us with the gift of perfectly proportionate growth. Orwell warned that the acceptance of newspeak is no small matter; it can ultimately convince us to trade liberty for totalitarianism. So what have we lost by accepting the reductionists' foodspeak?

Driven from the Garden—A Record in the Bones

Along the western coast of South America, the powerful Humboldt current sweeps north from near the South Pole until its frigid water is blocked by a coastline of sandy plains descending from the high peaks of Peru's Cordillera mountains. The resulting upwelling current helps to produce several months a year of rain-rich clouds and, in terms of sustaining sea life, is one of the richest currents in the sea. This food-producing confluence of geographic and oceanographic elements helped give rise to the great civilizations of Peru, whose ancient cities are thought to have supported up to a million people.

In the mid 1930s, Weston Price, interested in the effects of nutrition on jaw structure, was drawn to the area by mummies—some fifteen million of which had been buried in mounds and preserved by the succession of seasonal rains on the dry sand. Grave robbers had previously unearthed many of them, so on his arrival it appeared as though the objects of his intended study had come to greet him. "As far as the eye could see the white bleaching bones, particularly the skulls, dotted the landscape."[117] He was interested in those skulls because, at that time in America, from 25 to 75 percent of the population had some deformity of the dental bones or arches, and he suspected that rate of malformation was an historic anomaly.[118] His visit proved to be illuminating. In a study of 1,276 ancient bones, he "did not find a single skull with a significant deformity of the dental arches."[119] What's most striking about Price's visit to Peru is that when he left the desert mummies to study modern city dwellers, he found the people's structural symmetry and balanced growth patterns had melted away, replaced by what he described as "a sad wreckage in physique and often character."[120] The Peruvians had changed. Using anthropologic methodology (studying skull structure), Price showed that when a farming population adapts a city lifestyle, this shift can affect bone structure. But how? What was the root of the problem?

Price's discovery was not entirely new. Physical anthropologists have long recognized the diversity of human cranial development, and the anthropologic literature is full of discoveries that link skeletal modifications to dietary changes. For example, when Native Americans migrated down the coast from Alaska to California and the consumption of animal products dropped, the average women's bone size shrank by nine percent and the men's thirteen within just a few generations. Meanwhile, brain size dropped five and ten percent respectively.[121] Elsewhere, in South Africa, two distinct episodes of skeletal shrinkage occurred, one 4,000 years ago, the other 2,000. The first coincided with population pressures and the second with the use of pottery, indicating an increased dependence on farming. In the intervening years, absent of farming artifacts, the skeletal size (including the skull and brain-space) appears to have recovered.[122] And in the southernmost Andes Mountains, precisely where plants were first domesticated in South America, the fossil record again reveals "farmers hav[ing] a smaller craniofacial size than hunter-gatherers."[123]

Not only is it a consistent finding in the anthropologic record that modifications in diet coincide with modifications in human growth, but there seems to be a general downward trend in size. That is, as groups of modern humans have moved from hunter-gatherer to agricultural-based lifestyles, their bodies shrink. Why would that be? Bioanthropologists, who consider nutrition in their studies, suggest that "our hunter-gatherer forbearers may have enjoyed such variety of viands that they fared better nutritionally than any of their descendants who settled down to invent agriculture."[124]

The development of farming has long been thought to represent one of humanity's greatest achievements, the cardinal technologic leap that would set us on course to living easier and healthier lives with every passing century. But this assumption has been challenged lately by both skeletal and living anthropologic evidence. It appears that the hunter-gatherer and herder-gatherer (like the Maasai), who lived in greatest harmony with natural cycles, may have enjoyed an easier lifestyle than all but a few of the wealthiest families today. In fact, Marshal Sahlins, an anthropologist at the University of Chicago, calls hunter-gatherer-style communities (of old) the "original affluent society."[125] In his treatise on hunter-gatherer life, he paints an Arcadian image:

> *A woman gathers in one day enough food to feed her family for three days, and spends the rest of her time resting in camp, doing embroidery, visiting other camps, or entertaining visitors from other camps. For each day at home, kitchen routines, such as cooking, nut cracking, collecting firewood, and fetching water, occupy one to three hours of her time. This rhythm of steady work and steady leisure is maintained throughout the year.*[126]

Embroidery? Entertaining visitors? Visiting your neighbors and trading gossip over tea? Though it might sound like something out of *Martha Stewart's Living,* this is a fieldworker's description of an average day in the early 20th century life of the Hadza, a nomadic band of hunter-gatherers who have lived in the central rift valley of East Africa for perhaps a hundred thousand years. Many other accounts corroborate the fact that the ecology in certain locations once provided more than enough bounty for the hunter-gatherer to simply sit back and enjoy, at least on the average day.

Hunting and gathering requires a lot of moving around, wandering from place to place chasing seasonal abundance. Farming, on the other hand, enabled us to stay put. Along the banks of the world's mightiest rivers, on some of the world's most fertile soils, societies grew larger and more stratified, developed more tools and technology, and embarked upon ambitious engineering projects like the pyramids. But there was a tradeoff. All the while, agriculturalists struggled to provide the level of nutrition to which their hunter-gatherer genes had grown accustomed. Over generations, this drop-off in nutrition would impair growth so that stature would diminish relative to that of their hunter-gatherer counterparts. You could say that, for the sake of developing agrarian civilizations, these societies chose to swap some of their vitality, toughness, and robusticity for aqueducts, large buildings, and other public works. Of course, if any group of people were to break away from city life and return to nomadic hunting or herding and gathering, they would reclaim the physique they'd given up; Their bodies would grow larger, and their skulls tougher and more robust.

This ability to adjust stature to better match a given nutritional context lends more support to the idea of an intelligent, responsive genome (as the operating mechanism) than to the suggestion that physiologic change depends solely on random mutation. If evolutionary change were dependent on random mutation, then it would be exceedingly unlikely that responses to nutritional change would be so consistent and quick to appear. If however an intelligent genome had recorded in its epigenomic library which physiologic adjustments were most appropriate in any given nutritional context, then the epigenomic librarian (see Chapter 2) could simply read the instructions on what to do next. And this is why we see that "[t]hroughout the course of human evolution, features of robusticity like supraorbital and occipital tori [boney ridges], have been acquired, lost, or changed in different groups."[127]

If you want to be poetic about it, you could say that the shifting and morphing skeletal and facial features represent the genomic artist at work. Each set of subtle skull feature modifications that have distinguished all the equally beautiful nationalities of human beings is a painted portrait, each one created using different nutritional pigments in varying proportion and displayed on the canvass of world geography. In this way, the intelligence in our genes has generated numerous variations on the theme of human attractiveness. The striking cheekbone, the slender waist and graceful legs, the delicate female chin, and the powerful brow of a dominant male face—all these universally desired features are tweaked a tiny bit to generate the continuum of anatomical variation that is *Homo sapiens*.

But if you look at these anatomical variations the way Dr. Marquardt does and focus on the basic blueprint of our skeletal plan rather than the embellishments, you'll see that in reality very little has changed over time. Though our statures and the prominence of individual facial features may vary, thanks to the genetically programmed growth preference for *phi*-proportionality, everything fits neatly together. Every part has maintained its functional relationship to every other part. Everything works. This is true of people living everywhere around the world. Or rather it *was* true. Very recently, something changed.

Which brings us back to Price, and those perfect skulls he found scattered on the Peruvian sand. On Price's visit, he recognized that a precipitous drop in proportionality of Peruvian skulls had taken place in contemporary history. There was a key difference in the dentition of ancient and modern Peruvians (and up to 75 percent of the American population) that indicated a process entirely distinct from the nuanced skeletal variations present throughout evolutionary time. That difference: a loss of proportion. Why is that so significant? As we've seen in the preceding chapters, health and beauty are all about proportion. *Dis*proportionality disables the body's ability to function.

In Chapter 3 we defined a perfect face—and the bones beneath it—as a face that has grown in accordance with a mathematic formula called *phi*, which defines healthy growth in numerous species of plant and animal life. Dr. Marquardt, the plastic surgeon who discovered how *phi*-based growth occurs in the human species and created a mask to illustrate it, has shown us that balanced growth occurs in three dimensions, the X, Y, and Z facial planes. When that balanced *phi*-proportionality is lost, the resulting growth distortions lead to problems. In my own face, the loss of *phi*-proportionality in the horizontal (or X) dimension narrowed my skull so that my wisdom teeth didn't fit into my head and had to be pulled, and my disproportionately sized eye sockets distorted the shape of my eyeball, forcing my lens to focus light to a point in front of (rather than on) my retinas, blurring my vision. A mid-face that is more severely narrowed than mine may pinch the airway, causing sinus problems. When skull narrowing affects the Z-plane (visible in profile), it may foreshorten the palate, increasing the likelihood of *sleep apnea,* a condition in which a person's own soft tissues collapse inward and periodically suffocate them, causing fatigue, memory problems and heart disease.

Phi seems to be the universal template nature uses to ensure that optimal proportionality drives development, even under conditions of varying nutritional inputs. Over the past century or two, however, the typical human diet has diverged so far from anything before that our growth patterns can no longer adhere to the template. The switch from hunting and gathering to farming was accompanied by nutritional sacrifice, yes. But it did not block the ability of the *phi*-template to continue generating perfect proportionality. Why not? As I've suggested, modern historians have vastly underappreciated the value of traditional nutritional knowledge. I believe it was this wisdom that enabled people who'd made the shift from hunter-gatherer life to settled life to continue to make (mostly) sound decisions about what kinds of foods they needed to feed their children and expectant parents in order to ensure optimal health. Though history's most celebrated inventions—like trigonometry, plumbing, and the plow—helped give rise to the visible artifacts of civilization, none of this could have been possible had we been severely undernourished. The extraction of adequate nutrition from grains, for instance, required advanced *biologic* technology. These vastly undervalued strategies enabled growing populations to maintain nutrition adequate for healthy growth even after leaving the relative bounty of the hunter-gatherer pasts behind. And they did this by using the Four Pillars of World Cuisine.

The skeletal record evidences the success of traditional dietary regimes around the world—which universally include all four of the Pillars. If we were to create a visual timeline of the entire human story from nearly 500,000 years ago until today by lining up human skulls on one long table, we would find that, as *Homo sapiens* progressed, migrating across continents and oceans—some finding tiny, isolated islands to call home—all the while changing size and varying features, some skulls, like Paleolithic *Homo sapiens*, would be heavy and robust and others, like recently discovered *Homo floresiensis*, diminutive. But with every skull in our lineup, we'd see teeth well aligned and free of carries[128], square jaws, and *phi*-proportionate construction in the X, Y, and Z facial planes.[129] This math is what gives rise to deep and wide eye sockets, powerful male brow ridges and delicate female chins, broadly arched zygoma (cheekbones), and all the other features anthropologists use to define a skull as belonging to a former *Homo sapiens*. These features would be clearly visible in every skull on our table. Until, that is, we walk to the end of the table where the lineup is still being built. In the skulls from the past 100 years or so, we'd see an abrupt change.[130]

Of course, human skulls have recorded within their features every switch from farming to hunter-gatherer lifestyle and every migration from place to place. But our healthy and proportionate bodies had been maintained and protected as if under the aegis of a kind of nutritional Garden of Eden. So what happened to those skulls at the rightmost end of the table, the ones with the disfigured dentition and disrupted proportion? An examining anthropologist might conclude that we'd left the Garden for good, completely abandoning the diets that had protected us throughout history, and made a pilgrimage to the nutritional equivalent of a barren and inhospitable country. But what no anthropologist could discover by sorting through the bones is *why?* What nutritional sin had we committed?

The answer to that riddle can be found in the pages of a cookbook written over 100 years ago. You see, in order for a burgeoning food industry to convince people to make this journey—this exodus from nature—and to give up traditions with thousands of years of success without a battle, it needed to change the way people talk about food.

You Say Potato...

Have you ever heard someone say, "I've been trying to cut out carbs"? Or a TV chef say, "Now, all this dish needs is a protein"? Carbs? A protein? When did we start talking about our foods like chemists? The answer is, not coincidentally, right around the time of the industrial revolution.

The *Fanny Farmer 1896 Cook Book* introduced this new food terminology to a large audience: "Food is classified as follows: Organic or Inorganic," with organic being composed of the following, "1. Proteid (nitrogenous or albuminous). 2. Carbohydrates (sugar and starch). 3. Fats and oils." This new, simplified breakdown of food immediately began influencing our approach to food and diet, and not in a good way. What was once understood holistically—rabbit, potatoes, or hand-pressed oil of *known* origin—would now be seen as so much protein, starch, and "one or more of the following" vegetable oils. Don't get me wrong. Francis Farmer's cookbook is considered a classic, and deservedly so. But the classification of complex organic systems based only on their more readily isolatable chemical components makes about as much sense as describing the Taj Mahal as so many tons of marble and stone. In terms of isolatable components, a bottle of Romanee-Conti isn't all that different from box wine, but the winemakers of Burgundy would likely argue that there's more to wine than its basic components.

Though you can boil, extract, and refine living tissue to isolate the protein, carb, or fat, you do so only at the cost of everything else that held the cells and organs together. Yanking certain components from living systems—as we do to make flour, sugar, protein slurries, and 90 percent of what's now for sale in the store—and expecting them to approximate their original nutritional value is like removing someone's brain from their body and expecting it to respond to questions. That is not science; it is science fiction. So is the idea that heavily processed food can be healthy.

So where does this terminology, this way of talking about food, get us? It gets us away from talking about the most important aspect of any food, its source. And that, by the way, is exactly how the mass producers of cheaply manufactured processed food products would have it. Now, we can say things like "Sweet potatoes are really nutritious!" without stopping to consider that some sweet potatoes—those grown in sterile, toxic soil—are nutritionally bereft. We can toss another package of farmed salmon into our shopping cart thinking that it's essentially the same, nutritionally, as wild. And we can buy beef from cows raised on petrochemcial-soaked corn, in deplorably crowded conditions, and tell ourselves that, as long as it's tender, it's every bit as good for us as the flesh from happy, roaming, grass-fed animals. Once they've got us believing such absurdities or, worse yet, buying our food reflexively as a thoughtless habit, they can get us to buy just about anything. Why, with a little marketing and the right package, they might even get us to eat dog food.

The Dog Food Aisle

Take a look at the back of a bag of dog or cat food, and here are the ingredients you'll see: corn meal, soy meal, (occasionally) wheat, partially hydrogenated soy or corn or other vegetable oil, meat and protein meal, and a few synthetic vitamins. But guess what? The animal pushing the shopping cart is buying foods with the same list of ingredients for himself. The main differences between donuts, breads and Cheerios are the quantities of hydrogenated oil and sugar. Cheerios, in turn, are nearly identical to Ramen noodles. Throw on a little salt, and you've got snack chips. Add tomato flakes and bump up the protein powder and—bam!—it's Hamburger Helper with Noodles! Add a pinch of meat byproducts, take away some tomato powder, and we're in the pet food aisle again, holding a 20-pound bag of grade A Puppy Chow.

We already know why manufacturers make food this way: It's cheap and convenient to reformulate the basic ingredients of protein, starch, and fat (there are those words again!) into a variety of shapes and textures, coat them in sugars and artificial flavor enhancers, and ship them just about anywhere. That's why they make it. But why would we eat it? Same reason: It's cheap and convenient. These days, a busy parent can buy a frozen lasagna dinner heavy enough to feed a family of five for about what it would cost to make from scratch. It comes in its own disposable aluminum pan so—no fuss, no muss—the dinner riddle is solved. Like other foods in the supermarket, it keeps forever (or at least a really long time) in the freezer, so if we don't eat it tonight, it'll be ready when we want it. And thanks to the fact that these convenience foods contain protein, fat, and carbohydrate plus some synthetic vitamins, we can survive on them for a certain amount of time. But that doesn't mean these foods aren't changing us. They are.

As I discussed earlier, whenever our ancestors moved from one place to another, their diets changed and, in turn, so did their physiologies. And, as you'll recall, each time they relocated from one natural locale to another, though that relocation influenced their stature and relative prominence of certain facial features, their skeletons generally remained perfect examples of function and proportionality. They didn't think of food in terms of carbs and protein and fat. They thought more in terms of good soil, healthy animal, freshly picked. And for this reason, their traditional cultural practices, and the foods they took into their bodies, kept them firmly tethered to the natural world. In other words, they stayed *connected.*

For eons, human beings maintained that connection thanks to the guidance of their cultural wisdom. But they couldn't have known all the possible consequences of cutting those natural ties. How could they? Until recently, the people of this planet benefited from a relatively stable climate without knowing how easily it could be thrown into chaos; we never had to think about it until it all started breaking down. Indeed, we might have remained blind to the underlying cause had it not been for a handful of prescient climatologists and geologists who, at great professional cost, made certain their warnings were heard. As a result, most of us are fairly well versed in the concepts of climate regulation and instability.

We know, for example, that the industrial revolution and subsequent commercial growth created massive CO_2 pollution, which magnified the greenhouse effect and is now making global climate warmer. What we don't yet appreciate is the extent to which the industrial revolution polluted the food we eat, leading to so many changes in our health and physiologies that it has altered the way we look. Over the past 100 years, we have completed the single most comprehensive dietary shift in the history of our race. This shift, a major dietary migration over vast nutritional territory, has gone on largely unnoticed—even by the medical community—for the following reasons: 1) It didn't involve moving from one geographic point to another; only our food has changed. 2) Except for the very well-off and the recently urbanized, few of us in America have been exposed to the products of culinary tradition and therefore don't know what we're missing. 3) Since the migration from real to fake food has occurred over five generations, even our parents were likely born into an environment bereft of culinary tradition. 4) Cheap and convenient products catch on quick, and we tend not to ask where they were made or what they were made of, so the easier and cheaper our food gets the less we think about it. 5) The merging of business and science into one corporate body means that medical science can no longer countenance advice incompatible with the interest of commerce. 6) A constant stream of new technologic fixes continues to buttress our collapsing physiologic infrastructure, which has so far masked what would otherwise be obvious maladaptive consequences of that collapse.

This last point is the most significant. If needing glasses killed us, we would no doubt pay keen attention to factors that render a child nearsighted. If having oral cavities killed us, we would steer clear of the things known to rot teeth as if our lives depended on it. If there were deadly consequences from inattention to nutritional detail, our nutrition science would be so advanced that it would be, dare I say, effective at preventing disease and capable of promoting health. It would be at least as good as it was in the past, when the knowledge of building healthy bodies with nutrition was, in fact, a matter of life and death, so highly valued that Dr. Price found many indigenous people reluctant to "disclose secrets of their race." As Price discovered, "The need for this [reluctance] is comparable to the need for secrecy regard-

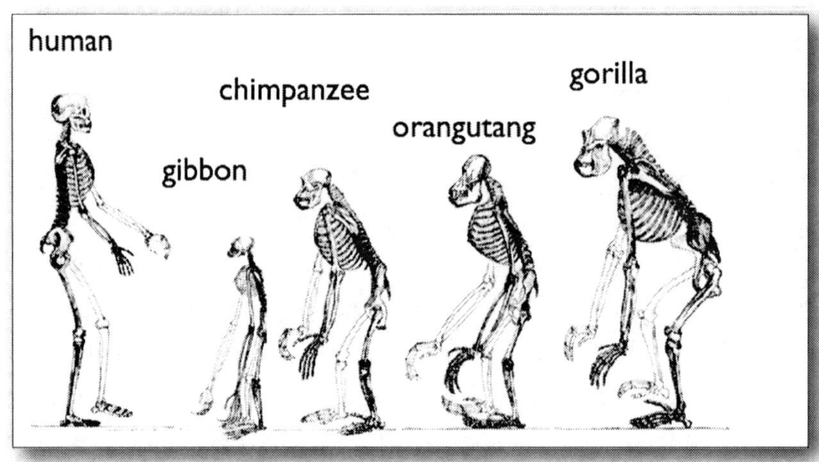

Figure 1. Changing Our Diet May Change Us. Big brains require brain-building fats like cholesterol, lecithin, choline, saturated fat, and long-chain polyunsaturated fats. These compounds are found in highest concentration in organ meats, cold-water fish, and fish eggs. Today these rich foods are primarily consumed by the wealthy, in high-end restaurants where foie gras, fresh oyster, lobster, crab and caviar are staple items. Our hominid ancestors consumed them in greater quantity than other primates.

ing modern war devices."[131] We don't think that way any more. And it's ironic that the kinds of technological advancements that allowed for the mass production of nutritionally wanting processed foods are now necessary to address the physiologic consequences of their consumption.

That's an irony I'd just as soon watch play out from a safe remove. And I'm not alone. *How do I put this delicately?* If you think the wealthy—members of the upper, upper social class—would even *touch* the foods we eat daily, the foods relentlessly touted as healthy, you'd be mistaken. No, the most privileged among us eat very much the way their great-great-great-grandparents ate. If we could fly past the iron gates guarding the White House lawn and peer through the dining room windows to see what the guests were eating at George Bush's inaugural lunch, we'd see this: *First course: lobster pie served in a rich, flaky crust. Main course: Roasted Missouri quail and chestnuts served with brined root vegetables. Or, an alternative choice: Petit filets of prime* [presumably pasture-raised] *beef tenderloin, presented over steamed green beans with Madiera demiglace. Third course: sour cream drop biscuits.*[132] Those dining on these sinfully rich foods represent the same government whose food pyramid forbids us regular folk from eating anything of the kind. And since we're all supposed to be watching our salt, we'd hardly risk touching our lips to something like brined root vegetables or demiglace. Have these culinary daredevils lost their minds, wandering so far outside the protective dietary shadow cast by the food pyramid? Or are their chefs the instigators, luring these susceptible victims over the cliff with the aroma of quail and hollandaise sauce? Whether through daring, by calculated intention, or by virtue of the same felicitous winds of fate that have caressed other aspects of their lives, one thing is sure: By maintaining their diet of real, traditional foods, the well-heeled have managed to ensconce their genomes inside the walls of a nutritional fortress and defend their physiologic dynasties against the hoi polloi—the swelling masses of the sick and enfeebled.

Given that the privileged can, and typically do, eat the way we all used to, and given that this shift in eating habits first occurred over a century ago and that the effects of continued nutrient deprivation are magnified with each generation, the widening gap between nutritional-physiologic classes should place the other issues of class differential well into the background. A hundred years ago, two nutritional roads diverged in an evolutionary wood. The less well off took the one never before traveled by, and—judging by the health statistics—that has made all the difference.

It is as if, at the beginning of the 20th century, ordinary working people were told to start packing their bags, leave their farms and fertile soil behind, and take their assigned seats in an enormous space cruiser headed for the moon. If ordered to make such a journey, most of us would hesitate, because we would know instinctively that the consequences for our health, and for the health of our children, might prove catastrophic. That is a good instinct because, even though our great-great-great-grandparents may not have known to follow it at the time, that instinct remains alive in every one of their descendants, and it will help get us back to Earth.

Life in Outer Space

If we did live confined in some kind of giant artificial life-support system on the moon, what would our diet be like? Would it really be so different from our own modern diets?

Most moon foods would need to have long shelf lives. Since the shuttle only comes a few times a year, the shipments must be able to last for months. You'll find that moon foods are high in shelf-stable ingredients such as sugar, flour, protein isolates and hydrolysates, and vegetable oil. ("Sports" and "nutrition" bars contain almost nothing else.) Though these products have been refined and stripped of living, reactive components, many contain toxic preservatives to make them last even longer, including BHT and BHA (the same chemical compounds, incidentally, used by plastic and tire manufacturers).[133] Since vegetable oil is particularly unappealing to micro-organisms (for reasons described in Chapter 8), you will find it incorporated into numerous products and nearly impossible to avoid while living on a moon food diet.

"Fresh" moon food's not too big on flavor, as the moon-dwelling children's distaste for it might remind adults. The space station environment can support the growth of a few assorted veggies, including iceberg lettuce and hydroponically grown tomatoes. The occasional shipments of carrots, bell peppers, broccoli, potatoes, apples and a few more fruits and vegetables give moon dwellers' meals the color that helps make people think they're getting real food, in spite of what their taste buds tell them. In reality, significant nutrient decay occurs during extended transport so that many "fresh" fruits and vegetables actually contain no more nutrition than their canned or frozen counterparts.[134,135] Many moon-ready fruits and vegetables are picked unripe, and so contain significantly lower levels of vitamins (less than half in some cases) than any physiologically mature product.[136] Research suggests such mass-produced products might taste bland because they contain little more than water and cellulose, some having just one tenth the vitamins or antioxidants of their organically raised cousins.[137]

Space is at a premium on the moon, so animals grown for human consumption there are denied access to pasture, sunlight, room to run, etc. There is no open ocean on the moon, and so fish—genetically engineered for prodigious growth—are farm raised on high-calorie pellets. Chickens, fish, cattle, and hogs are reared indoors in containers, fed a mash of corn or soy, and their more perishable fleshy parts (organs) and bones are saved for pet food or discarded.

The manufacturers on Earth know that the upper-end moon consumer is willing to pay a fraction more for products labeled "organic." Savvy producers have slightly altered their manufacturing process to reduce chemical inputs at the production end to comply with the labeling rules, enabling this demographic to feel that their shelf-stable, highly processed, low-flavor and low-nutrient foods are safer for their families. Moon shipments include a small portion of their volume as organic cereals, milk substitutes, meat and cheese substitutes, and desserts, to satisfy these consumers. Other health-conscious consumers—sensing the inadequacy of their diets—follow the astronauts' lead and take synthetic vitamins, lots of them, unaware that the vitamins manufactured in factories typically fail to approximate the real thing.

You get the idea. It is no great exaggeration to suggest that, as far as our bodies are concerned, most of us may as well be living on the moon—just as our parents, and their parents did before. Compared to the Maasai, who still root their genes deep within the same nourishing fruits of the Earth as their ancestors did 40,000 years ago, our genes are flailing in empty air. The milk the Maasai enjoy today is much the same as it was thousands of years ago when artists drew pictures of people with their cattle on the walls of caves in the Gilf Kabir in Northern Africa. More to the point, it carries the same information to their cells. The grey-white substance pumped from our sad cows? Not so much.

Fortunately, you don't need to join a nomadic tribe in the desert to start eating better. All you need to do is follow the recipes laid out in any truly traditional cookbook. Rather than give you a restrictive meal plan composed of a few acceptable recipes, you'll learn to distinguish traditional foods from their modern, Americanized substitutes so that you can pick the best recipes from the billions available in already published cookbooks and on the World Wide Web. We are going to rethink food. Rather than envisioning food in disconnected categories of often-flavorless chemical compounds, I want you to understand it as your ancestors did, and to appreciate that nourishment captures the power of nature and carries it into your being. Once you learn about the Four Pillars of World Cuisine, and how to reproduce them, you will be well on your way to making your genes perform the way you want them to and release your full genetic potential.

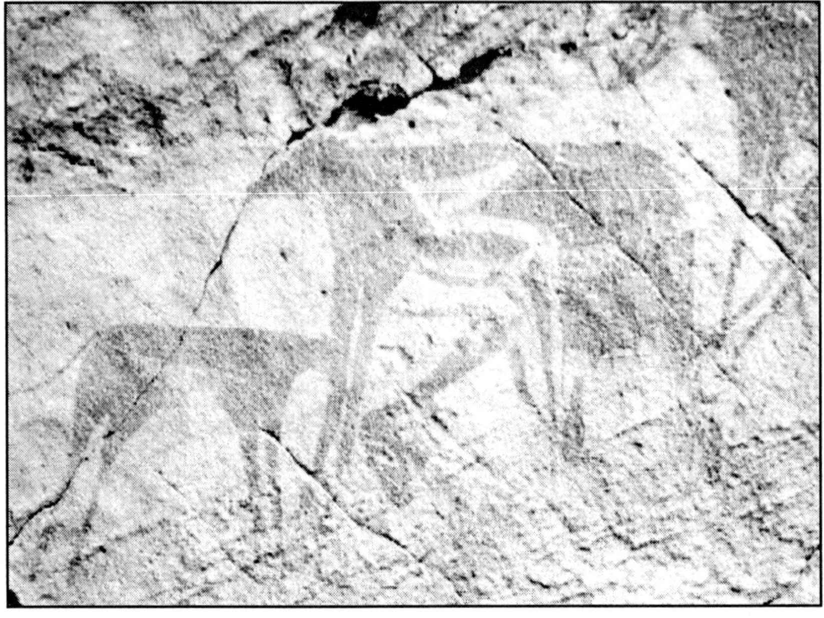

Figure 2. African Petroglyph. This depiction of a woman milking a cow can be found in the same "Cave of Swimmers" featured in the movie *The English Patient.* It is located in an area of Egypt known as the Gilf Kabir and believed to have been painted around 10,000 years ago, when the Sahara was a lush grassland. The woman on her knees appears to be collecting milk in a gourd with her left hand while holding off the calf with her right.

Seven

The Four Pillars of World Cuisine

Foods that Program Your Body for Beauty, Brains, and Health

If you've ever seen one of those museum exhibits of "ancient man," you might recall all sorts of arrowheads and spears. Or perhaps a diorama of hunters pointing weapons threateningly at a lumbering, large-tusked giant beast, while, somewhere in the background, women smoke meat around a fire. With this masculine view of history, one could easily get the impression that sheer aggression enabled early humans to hunt down more animals than their competitors, outliving and out-breeding them to be the ones to venture from Africa to every corner of the globe. But this tells only half the story. The other half is what happens after the animal is killed and hauled back home. This chapter rotates our historical stage 180 degrees, so that the cooks are placed in front as the true heroes of our shared historical journey.

The astounding invention, creativity, and study human beings have honed into the craft of culinary art deserves more scientific appreciation. Other animals can hunt, but only humans have learned to extract every last bit of nutritional content from the edible world around us. That knowledge—inherited, improved upon, and passed down—was born of trial and error and plenty of inspiration. Armed with these skills, the Julia Childs of the ancient world could fold a greater diversity of nutrients into the narrative of human evolution than what would otherwise have been possible. In this chapter, we will examine regional cooking traditions from all over the world, not to identify which is best, but to describe what they all have in common. If you've read everything leading up to this, you've no doubt gotten the impression that this physician finds the prerequisites of both health and sickness to be in no way mysterious. The rules of healthy living have been passed down freely. Anyone with curiosity and common sense can recognize their logic.

Along the same vein, we needn't scratch our heads wondering which fad diet we should follow and which—because experts now say so—we're all supposed to reject. We need only return to those foods that have shepherded us through the toughest trials by which Mother Nature mercilessly tests and fine-tunes her creations. It is not just a happy coincidence we instinctively prefer the taste of those foods proved successful over millennia—not just in preventing cancer, protecting our hearts, and keeping our immune systems strong enough to ward off disease—but those foods that have ensured the proper growth and health of our offspring, their children, and their children, and theirs. Every fad diet is ornamented with claims of success. But only the Four Pillars, these four classes of foods—the nutritional foundation of the species *Homo sapiens*—can be said to have made us who we are.

The Four Pillars: The Foundation of World Cuisine

One way you could reproduce a healthy diet would be to simply pick a single region's traditional cuisine and copy it precisely. The problem is, we don't do that. When you get books on, say, the Mediterranean or Okinawan diet and use those recipes, rarely are you creating the same dishes as the people actually living in those regions. Why not? Typically, the recipes are inaccurate. The authors reinterpret them, replacing difficult-to-obtain or unfamiliar ingredients with substitutes you can find at any Costco. Traditional fats, like lard, are replaced by government-recommended vegetable oils. (Why is that a problem? See Chapter 8.) Variety cuts, unfamiliar and often unavailable, are replaced with boneless, skinless, low-fat alternatives. Any meal that takes more than an hour to prepare is deleted from the list of possibilities. And if the recipe originally required homemade components—like bone stock, fresh pasta, or fermented vegetables—the instructions are rewritten in the name of convenience and you wind up with instructions for making foods stripped of the very things that made them tasty, authentic, and *healthy* in the first place. You get American food with exotic spices. I'm going to show you what all those cookbooks have been missing.

Those components of traditional cuisine removed from the typical diet or cookbook comprise the very components that every successful traditional diet has in common. I call these components the Four Pillars. These fundamental foods provide healthy people all around the world the consistent stream of nutrition that, no matter the regional culinary peculiarities, adequately provides the nutritional input our bodies have been programmed to require. Though each local interpretation appears unique, as far as your body's cells are concerned, healthy diets are all essentially the same, resting on the same Four Pillars: meat on the bone, fermented and sprouted foods, organs and other "nasty bits," and fresh, unadulterated plant and animal products.

To our palates, the spectrum of regional cuisines is as diverse as the ecology of our planet. In Hawaii before Captain Cook's arrival, the staple food was *poi,* a paste made of roasted and dried taro (a tuberous root vegetable) that could be stored for months, rehydrated on demand and then, as a final step, fermented. This staple was supplemented most often with fish, coconut, and banana. (Interestingly, the *alii,* or royal class, ate more fish and other high-nutrition foods than poi and were also taller. I suspect that, as with any society, the cause-and-effect relationship between height and access to the choicest foods went in both directions: Better foods made some people relatively tall; being taller offered access to better foods.) Until around 1940, the Netsilik Eskimo traditionally ate seal, fish, lichen, and not much else. In the Mongolian desert today, nomadic bands of camel breeders eat mainly dairy products, some grains, lots of tea, root vegetables, and meat. In the rain forest of Papua New Guinea, one of the last surviving hunter-gatherer groups, the Kombai, dine on fat grubs of giant flies, lizards, birds, pounded sago palm hearts, and—for special occasions—fattened pig. In West Africa, farmers known as the Mofu grow millet, beans, peanuts, forage for insects, and raise goats and chickens, just as they have for thousands of years. While each of these seemingly diverse diets contain foods that may strike you as bizarre, the nutritional content they represent is as familiar to your body, and to your epigenome, as salt or water. As far as your body's cells are concerned, vegetable oil and massive doses of sugar—now *that's* strange. If you've been eating a standard, food pyramid-compliant American diet, any authentic regional diet, no matter how exotic, along with the abandonment of vegetable oil and sugar, would bring your body, your cells, and your genes a welcome and long-awaited relief. But you don't have to move to get the benefits of these traditions. Simply include foods from each of the Four Pillars into your diet. Start with eating something fresh once every day. And work your way up to using foods from two or more categories daily.

French Cuisine

Although no region has cornered the market on health, French cooking is special. Against the backdrop of international food, French cuisine stands out for its variety, depth, and indulgent sensuality. The French literally wrote the book on culinary arts, as every chef trained in the Western tradition owes his or her skills to Escoffier and the culinary pioneers who preceded him. Some would argue that China deserves equal billing with France as a culinary epicenter, as it is the original source of so many foods we now take for granted. But unlike Chinese or Italian or Mexican food, French food served in the US and around the world is often prepared using age-old techniques, allowing it to retain unparalleled flavor profiles and healthful character. You could say that French cuisine stands firmly on all of the Four Pillars.

Of all the cuisines in all the restaurants in all the world, why would French food enter the 21st century looking very much the same as it did in Napoleon's court?

In a word, snobbery. This famously French attribute definitely has its good side because, without it, the universally celebrated gift of authentic epicurean expression would never have come to exist.

The early 19th century middle classes wanted to prove that they had been elevated beyond "the mere physical needs of nourishment."[138] The result was a new brand of cooking which the upwardly mobile, who could now afford to hire chefs, would come to call *grande cuisine*. *Grande cuisine* was, and is, a style of cooking offered by high-class restaurants. Chefs would seek out the best regional ingredients in season and perfect the techniques used to prepare them, not so much to maximize nutrition as to maximize flavor. "The *grande cuisine* attained its status because it emphasized the pleasure of eating rather than its purely nutritional status."[139] In spite of this new emphasis, *grande cuisine* originated at a time when real ingredients—as opposed to things like MSG and sugar—were the only edible materials available. So as these chefs concentrated real, quality ingredients to intensify flavor, they couldn't help but concentrate their nutrients at the same time.

The codification of *grande cuisine* in professional texts has encapsulated in amber centuries-old techniques for extracting flavor and nutrients from foods grown throughout Europe and Asia. By no coincidence, foods representing each of the Four Pillars appear again and again in classical French cooking. In Chapter 5, I told you about the "Latina Paradox," the fact that relatively less affluent, recently immigrated Hispanic women, eating traditional Hispanic foods, somehow still manage to have healthier children than the average American woman. As you know, the French have their own health "paradox"—relatively low rates of heart disease, despite a notoriously rich diet. Now that you understand why these traditional diets are actually far healthier than the typical American diet, you can see that there really never was any mystery at all. The answer is in healthy fats, very little sugar, and plenty of foods from each of the Four Pillars, starting with meat on the bone.

Pillar Number 1: Meat On The Bone

It's easy to enjoy well-prepared meat, but we're not born with the knowledge of how to make it taste good. That part, we have to learn.

Though the art of making meat taste great can be as simple as it is rewarding, if you've never seen a person do it, you'd never know the trick.

The secret? Leave it on the bone. Thanksgiving dinner is, for many, the most memorable meal of the year, which happens to be centered on a large bird, slow-cooked whole. When cooking meat, the more everything stays together—fat, bone, marrow, skin, and other connective tissue—the better. This section will introduce you to the simple techniques that primitive and haute cuisines use to make meat taste succulent, juicy, and complex. The better the material you start with, the better it tastes, and the better it is for you. For that reason, and more, animals raised humanely and pastured on mineral-rich soil are best. I'll show you the four rules you need to know to preserve and enhance the taste and nutrition of all our precious animal-derived items. And I'll show you the science that explains why mastering the art of cooking meat is the first step toward capturing the true power of food.

Cooking Meat, Rule Number One: Don't Overcook It

There are two kinds of people, those who like their steak rare and those who don't. If you're the medium-rare type, you'll know which side you fall on by answering this question: What would upset you more, if the steak you just ordered came to your table undercooked or overcooked?

When I started eating meat again after experimenting with vegetarianism in graduate school, Luke's opinion that well-done meat is wasted meat was unconvincing. But after studying the chemistry of well-done versus rare, I recognized that, once again, Luke's primal instinct was spot on. I can still recall the effort required to swallow my first bloody, glumpy, chewy bite when I crossed over to the other side of the culinary divide. Luke's delicious brown stock gravy helped my first time go much easier. Now, five years later and much the wiser, I find meat cooked as much as medium to be stringy, chewy, coarse and devoid of the savory flavor of juicy red blood. I'll never go back.

When it comes to steak, it's not the size that matters; it's the consistency and texture. Overcooked meat is tough because its fat, protein, and sugar molecules have gotten tangled and fused together during a wild, heat-crazed chemical orgy. The result is a kind of tissue polymer that requires more work to cut with a knife and more chewing, as well as more time to digest. The worst part is that so many of the nutrients we need are ruined.

Ruined nutrients don't just politely disappear. Once ingested, your body won't be able to simply flush them down some metabolic drainpipe. When heat kills nutrients, it does so by causing reactions *between* nutrients, forming new chemical compounds including known carcinogens (such as *aromatic hydrocarbons* and *cyclic amines*), as well as other molecular fusions that dam-

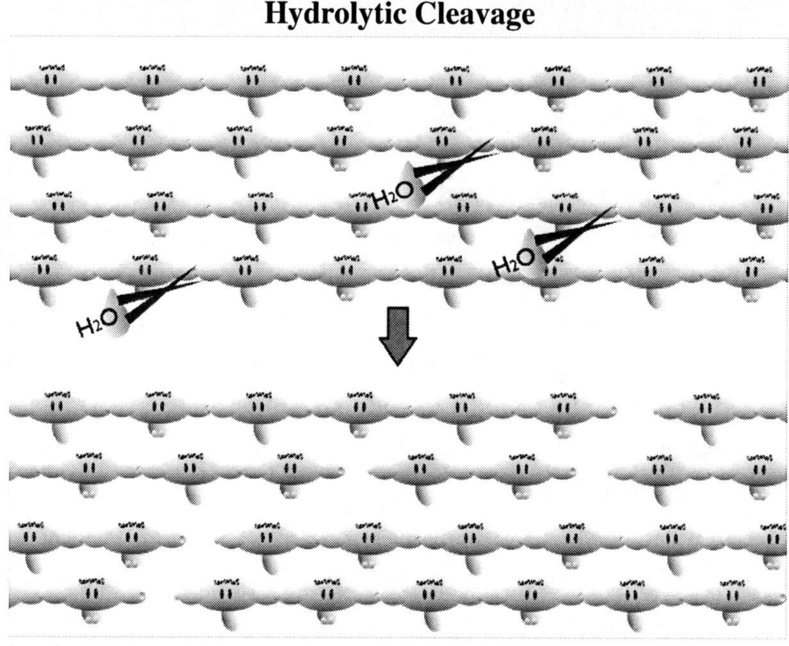

Figure 1. Perfectly Done. Gentle, moist heating clips just enough peptide bonds to break long protein chains into peptide segments, as shown. As long as the meat stays moist, the rows stay neatly aligned and separate. Trouble arises if the meat dries, or if the temperature rises above 170 degrees Fahrenheit. If the chef allows either to happen, hydrolysis stops, the chains themselves curl and bend around creating a tangle, and new, unbreakable bonds form between amino acids in distant chains, between amino acids and sugar, and between amino acids and fats. These undesired reactions create toxins, destroy nutrients, and make the meat tough to cut and chew.

age your kidneys and blood vessels.[140] When meat is cooked properly, fewer harmful reactions occur.[141] The nutrients and flavor compounds survive, and can now be gently released into the meat's juices where they are more bioavailable, and more readily tasted and absorbed.

So how much heat is too much heat? If, when you slice it, there's not even a trickle of juice, it's way overdone. Steak should be juicy and red. I recommend you work your way down to medium rare, and once you get used to that, go for rare. One last thought: If you're an Anthony Bourdain fan, you already know that restaurant patrons who order their steak well done get the oldest, least choice cuts. It's not that the chefs have it in for people who order their steaks brown. They have to save the freshest product for those palates that can taste the difference.

Cooking Meat, Rule Number Two: Use Moisture, Time, and Parts

Not long ago, at a party, I met a dark-eyed Peruvian woman with a sultry accent who had just discovered her slow cooker. She'd owned it for two years before a visiting friend released it from confinement in the back of the kitchen cabinet. That whole week they ate nothing but stews. After years of indifference toward it, my new friend had fallen in love with her slow cooker because "it giff so mush flavor!" When I told her that good, complex flavor means good nutrition, and that she should use it as often as she wants, she fell in love with me.

It is a little-known fact that when a chef talks about flavor, he's also talking about nutrients. When he says *some flavors take time to develop*, he's saying sometimes you have to wait for certain nutrients to be released. Cooking meat slow is the best way to turn an ordinary meal into something extraordinary—in terms of taste *and* nutrition. The potential flavor of meat, or any food, derives from its complexity. Depending on the cut, "meat" may include muscle, tendon, bone, fat, skin, blood, and glands—each a world of chemical diversity. When that diversity is released on your tongue you can taste it, and the rich, savory flavor means a world of nutrients are on their way.

You don't actually need a slow cooker to cook meat slowly and enjoy all the same benefits. All you need is moisture, time, and parts (as many different tissue types as possible: ligament, bone, fat, skin, etc.). Making soup, stewing, keeping a top on to trap the steam, basting often when cooking in the oven—all these techniques keep the moisture inside the meat, enabling water molecules to make magic happen. Here's how.

The transformation of, say, a cold and flavorless chicken leg into something delicious begins when heated moisture trapped in the meat creates the perfect conditions for *hydrolytic cleavage* (see figure 1). At gentle heating temperatures, water molecules act like miniature hacksaws, neatly chopping the long, tough strands of protein apart, gently tenderizing even the toughest tissue. And because water also prevents nearby strands from fusing together, keeping meat moist prevents the formation of the protein tangles that make overcooked meat so tough.

How does hydrolytic cleavage translate into taste? It's simple. Taste buds are small. The receptor site where chemicals bind to them is tiny. So things that impart taste (called flavor *ligands*) must be tiny, too. If you were to take a bite of a cold, raw leg of chicken, you wouldn't get much flavor from it. Cooking releases trapped flavor because, during the process of hydrolytic cleavage, some proteins are chopped into very small segments, creating short strings of amino acids called *peptides.* Peptides are tiny enough to fit into receptors in our taste buds. When they do, we get the sensation of savoryness food manufacturers call the "fifth flavor," or *umami.* (Sour, bitter, salt, and sweet are the other four major flavors.)

How does having additional parts (skin, ligaments, etc.) create additional nutrition? Water molecules tug apart the connective tissue in skin, ligaments, cartilage and even bone, releasing a special family of molecules called *glycosaminoglycans*. You will find the three most famous members of this family in nutritional supplements for joints: glucosamine, chondroitin sulfate, and hyaluronic acid. But these processed supplements don't hold a candle to gelatinous stews, rich with the entire extended family of joint-building molecules. What is more, cartilage and other connective tissues are nearly flavorless before slow-cooking because (just as with muscle protein) the huge glycosaminoglycan molecules are too big to fit into taste bud receptors. After slow-cooking, many amino acids and sugars are cleaved away from the parent molecule. Once released, we can taste them.

Slow-cooked meat and parts are more nutritious than their mistreated cousins for still another reason: minerals. Mineral salts are released from bone and cartilage during stewing, as well as from the meat itself. These tissues are mineral warehouses, rich in calcium, potassium, iron, sulfate, phosphate and, of course, sodium and chloride. It turns out our taste buds can detect more of these ions than previously suspected, including calcium, magnesium, potassium, and possibly iron and sulfate, in addition to the sodium and chloride ions that make up table salt.[142] Overcooking traps these flavorful materials in an indigestible matrix of polymerized flesh that forms when meat begins to dry out. You can only taste, and your body can only make use of, minerals that remain free and available.

A word about flavor complexity. Although we've been told that some taste buds taste only salty, others sour, others bitter, and others sweet, studies have revealed that, though taste buds may taste one kind of flavor predominately, one bud can in fact detect different flavor ligands simultaneously. It turns out, the more, different kinds of flavors there are, the more we taste each one. When peptides *and* salt ions bind at the same taste bud, the result is not a doubling of flavor, but a powerful thousand-fold magnification in the signal going to your brain.[143] In this way, our taste buds are engineered to help us identify and enjoy (nutritional) complexity. (This is why hot dogs, for instance—or better yet, actual sausage—taste better with *sauer*kraut and *bittersweet* mustard.)

Now, some of you might still pine for your Arby's or your Big Mac. But keep in mind, the MSG and free amino acids in fast foods are tricking your tongue. The artificial flavoring MSG (a free amino acid, called *glutamate*) binds taste receptors just as peptides in slow cooked meat would. MSG and other hydrolyzed proteins are manufactured by taking hydrolytic cleavage to its completion, fully breaking down plant or animal protein products into free amino acids while refining them away from other cellular components. Health food stores sell these taste-enhancers in the form of Bragg's Aminos, which is no better for you than hydrolyzed soy sauces. (*Brewed* soy-sauces derive flavor from peptides, which are safe.) The problem with these products comes from the fact that certain free amino acids have neurostimulatory effects that can lead to nerve damage (amino acids glutamate and aspartate are the most potent). When consumed in small amounts as part of a meal containing a diversity of nutrients, free amino acids are actually good for us. But when consumed in large quantity without their normal complement of nutrients (most notably, without calcium or magnesium),[144] these amino acids can cause temporary memory loss, migraines, dizziness, and more. This is why the concept of whole foods must be applied to animal products as well as plants. Simply refining the protein away from its source turns normal, healthy amino acids into potentially harmful compounds.

Cooking Meat, Rule Number Three: Use the Fat

We need to eat animal fat, just as we always have. Many people believe that the animals we eat today are unusually fat, but that's not true. While grain-fed animals do contain unhealthy fat (see Why Organic Meat Is Worth the Price), and lots of it where it's bad for the animal (like within the muscle), the animals humans historically ate were relatively chunky too because, whenever possible, people picked them at the peak of plumpness. Free-range deer, for instance, are as much as fifteen percent fat (by weight) in summer.[145] But by the time hunting season rolls around they've stuffed themselves for winter fasting and tip the scales at thirty to forty percent body fat.[146] According to early American explorers like Samuel Hearne and Cabeza de Vaca, North American Natives preferred the fattest animals, and valued their fattiest parts most of all. When hunting was especially good, they'd leave the lean muscle meat behind for the wolves.[147,148]

What are the nutritional benefits of our appetite for fat? For one thing, fat is a source of energy, like sugar. Unlike sugar, however, fat is a major building material for our cells, comprising 30 to 80 percent (dry weight) of our cell membranes. And unlike sugar, fat doesn't trigger the release of insulin, which promotes weight gain. Furthermore, a high-sugar meal damages our tissues, but a high (natural) fat meal doesn't (see Chapters 8 and 9). And this is something I was tested on in med school but forgot right after the test: We need fat to be able to absorb most fat-soluble nutrients, including vitamins A, D, E, and K. The fact that the presence of fat in meat also helps protect it during cooking—let's just call that a happy coincidence.

To be honest, though, it's not always just a coincidence. Since, to keep meat moist, fat must be located on the outside of a cut of meat, good butchers strive to produce cuts encased inside a neat layer of rich, tasty fat. In smaller, leaner animals like birds, most of the fat sits right under the skin, naturally in the perfect location to keep meat moist during cooking. If you want a flavorful, juicy bird, for goodness' sake don't peel off the skin!

One of the latest new trends in the food world falls squarely in the category of everything-old-is-new-again: grass-fed beef. Pasture-raised beef has all kinds of advantages, both for you and for the animals. You may have heard that grass-fed is good for you because of its higher omega-3 content. That's true. But to get that omega-3, you have to get large cuts of meat with an exterior layer of fat (or the liver, or the bone marrow, or other "nasty bits"—see below). Compared to most grocery store beef, which comes from grain fed cows and is heavily marbled with heat-resistant saturated fat, the muscle in pastured cows is relatively lean. So when you buy a grass-fed steak, it's practically fat free and will dry out quicker during cooking than the typical grocery store steaks that you might be used to.

More Than Flavor: Fat's Synergistic Effects

Have you ever wondered why fat tastes so good? We have five well known flavor receptors. 1) Sweet, which detects carbohydrate. 2) Sour, which detects acid (acid plays a role in making nutrients more available). 3) Bitter, which detects antioxidants, some of which are also poisons. 4) Salty, which detects sodium and other minerals. And 5) Umami, the amino-acid detector described above. If we have no receptor for fat, why do we like it so much?

It's not just your imagination that fat free cookies don't taste as good as the real thing. Fat was long thought to impart flavor by way of the nose. But in 2005, French researchers blocking off study subjects' ability to smell using—you guessed it—clothespins on their noses found evidence of a receptor in the mouth that does detect fat, called CD38.[149] The subjects proved they could detect a variety of long-chain fatty acids, from saturated, to monounsaturated, to polyunsaturated, as well as potentially harmful oxidized fat. They could even discriminate between fatty acid types.[150,151] Just as Ayurvedic culinary masters indicated thousands of years ago, there may be six major flavor groups our tongue can detect.

Not only can we detect fat, just as with other flavor ligands, there is a synergistic effect. When fatty acids bind to their receptors, it affects other taste buds such that their ability to detect sour, salt, and bitter flavors is enhanced. This makes sense because many of the compounds that taste sour and bitter are fat soluble, and fat would be expected to enhance their absorption into our bodies as well. So it appears our tongues are wired to guide us toward nutritionally complex foods. Unless a food has been "doped" with MSG, other artificial flavor agents or sugar, or if our senses are dulled by chronic sugar ingestion, if something tastes delicious, it is almost guaranteed to be good for you.

Why Organic, Pasture-Raised Meat is Worth the Price

If you have a limited budget and you want to get organic, skip the low-fat fruits and vegetables and head over to the butcher aisle. Organic animal products give you more bang for your buck because they benefit from *bioconcentration*. Concentration refers to the percent of a substance present in something. *Bio*concentration is a process that results in a living organism having a higher concentration of a substance than its surrounding media.

Bioconcentration is usually used in reference to pollutants. When you spray plants with herbicides and pesticides, some get taken up into their tissues. When animals eat these plants, they also eat the pesticides and herbicides. The majority of these chemicals are fat soluble and will accumulate in fat. Since vegetables are naturally low in fat, when you buy organic vegetables, you are only avoiding a little bit of poison. When you buy organic meat, especially the fatty cuts, you're avoiding a lot.

Bioconcentration has a good side too. After all, it's what eating is all about, getting lots of good information from what you eat. Plants bioconcentrate nutrients from the soil, so that a pound of grass, for instance, has more potassium than a pound of the dirt in which it grows. Animals carry this process one step further. Their tissues bioconcentrate the minerals grasses have taken from the soil and the vitamins that grasses manufacture.

Research has shown that caribou can see which blades of grass are the most nutrient-rich and preferentially graze on those. Presumably, other herbivores also have the same ability. This suggests that organically raised animals kept in confinement will not be as healthy as those raised on large pastures. And a creature living freely in the wild should be healthiest of all. So if you hunt, or if you know a hunter who has extra, don't let this amazing resource go to waste: Eat as much of the animal as you know how!

There's one more factor making organic meat worth the price. Organically grown animals cannot (yet) legally be given antibiotics or other drugs except in case of illness. This means the farmer has to keep them healthier, which means they're healthier to eat. Nor can organically grown animals legally (at this point) be injected with growth hormones. Growth hormones have been proven capable of surviving the cooking and digestion processes. And some believe growth hormones in animal products are adding to the problems of obesity and cancer.[152] Unfortunately, as the mega-industries grow stronger, they are changing the rules to make it easier to put the word *organic* on the label. The best bet is to get friendly with your county farmers.

Cooking Meat, Rule Number Four: Make Bone Stock

More than anything else, the health of your joints depends upon the health of the collagen in your ligaments, tendons, and on the ends of your bones. Collagens are a large family of biomolecules, which include the *glycosaminoglycans,* very special molecules that help keep our joints healthy. People used to eat soup and stock made from bones all the time, and doing so supplied their bodies with the whole family of glycosaminoglycans, which used to protect people's joints. Now that few people make bone stock anymore, many of us are limping into doctors' offices for prescriptions, surgeries and, lately, recommendations to buy over-the-counter joint supplements containing glucosamine. And what is glucosamine? One of the members of the glycosaminoglycan family of joint-building molecules.

Veterinarians have been using glucosamine supplements to treat arthritic pets for decades. But physicians dismissed the practice as a waste of time, assuming that, since glucosamine is a protein, the digestive system would break it down into its component amino acids. Nobody can explain how, but studies have shown that glucosamine is somehow able to resist digestion and pass through the intestinal wall intact.[153] Once it gets into your bloodstream, "...glucosamine has a special tropism for cartilage."[154] (That's techno-speak for "somehow, it knows just where to go.") Even more amazing, glucosamine can actually stimulate the growth of new, healthy collagen and help repair damaged joints.[155] And collagen isn't just in your joints; it's in bone, and skin, and arteries, and hair, and just about everywhere in between. This means that glucosamine-rich broth is a kind of youth serum, capable of rejuvinating your body, no matter what your age. After decades of skepticism, orthopedists and rheumatologists are now embracing its use in people with arthritis, recommending it to "overcome or possibly reverse some of the degradation that occurs with injuries or disease."[156] Given these facts, it hardly seems far fetched to suggest that eating this stuff in soups and sauces from childhood makes joints stronger in the first place.

One of Luke's golfing buddies, local Kauai born and bred, didn't need convincing. As a child of a Filipino household, he ate lots of meat on the bone growing up. One day, chopping a goat leg to stir into stew, he asked his mother about the white, shiny stuff on the ends of the bones. She told him that he had the very same kind of material in his own joints. Instantly, he decided that eating that shiny cartilage would be good for his shiny cartilage. He has eaten meat on the bone ever since, making sure to chew on the ends. Now his friends are on arthritis meds, while he's surfing and golfing twice a week.

Not only do bone broths build healthy joints, the calcium and other minerals help to grow your bones. One of my patients is a charming young boy whose father is a chef. The chef is 5 foot 10 and his wife 5 foot 5. Both parents are lactose intolerant, and so, for years his dad, the chef, made bone stocks and used them as a base for making rice, mashed potatoes, soups, and reduction sauce gravies. He did this so that he and his lactose-intolerant wife would get plenty of dietary calcium. Aside from calcium, bone broth also contains glycosaminoglycans, as well as magnesium and other bone-building minerals—basically a total bone and joint building package—most of which the chef didn't know about. However, his son's DNA did. This child of average-height parents started life at normal size, but his growth chart illustrates that, over the years, he's gotten progressively taller than average. Now, at ten, his height and muscle mass are already off the chart. By the way, his teeth are straight, he doesn't need glasses, and he is the number one swimmer on his team.

Coincidence? Misleading anecdotal data? I don't think so. We all know that vitamin D and calcium are good for a child's growing bones. And as we saw in Chapter 5, it takes a whole array of vitamins and minerals to build a healthy skeleton. Cooking meat on the bone extracts all those well-known vitamins and minerals, plus the glycosaminoglycan growth factors. To have tall, strong, well-proportioned children, we're often told to get them to drink milk. And if we're talking about organic whole milk—especially raw!—I'm all for it. But if it were my kids, I'd also make sure they were getting regular helpings of home-made soups and sauces, and anything else I could think of to get them to eat more stock.

The benefits of broth consumption far outweigh the benefits of taking a pill for a couple of reasons: First, the low heat used to slowly simmer the nutrient material from bone and joint is far gentler than the destructive heat and pressure involved in the production of glucosamine tablets. Second, instead of extracting only one or two factors, broth gives you the entire complex of cartilage components—some of which have yet to be identified in the lab—plus minerals and vitamins. Broth's nutritional complexity makes it a nearly perfect bone-building joint-health-supporting package. And it's no coincidence that it tastes great. Rich, satisfying flavors convinced the father of modern French culinary science, Auguste Escoffier, that stock was an absolute kitchen essential. "Without it, nothing can be done."

Our ancestors probably discovered the magic in bones a very long time ago. In the Pacific Northwest, archeologic digs have uncovered evidence that, centuries before Escoffier, early Native Americans supplemented their winter diet of dried fish by deliberately fracturing herbivorous animal bones prior to stewing them. Not only did this release bone nutrients, it released the marrow fat and vitamins into the simmering soup. And anthropologists studying hunter-gatherers from Canada to the Kalahari find that this practice of exploiting bone and marrow nutrients was, and is, "almost ubiquitous."[157,158] While visiting a farm in New Zealand, I met a spry and engaging 80-something woman who told me about the Scottish tradition of "passing the bone." In the little village where she grew up, nothing went to waste. Cartilaginous knee joints and bony shanks were especially prized, and passed from house to house. Each family would put the bones into a pot over the stove to simmer for a night before passing them on to their neighbor until the bone was "spent." As she hiked with us over the rolling green hills of her estate, she explained that the bones were shared because she and her neighbors were convinced that "something in them was sustaining." Indeed there is. So skip the pharmacy aisle and head straight to your local butcher for bones to make your own homemade stock.

For thousands of years, people all over the world made full use of the animals they consumed, every last bit right down to the marrow and joints. You might suppose that, over all that time and all those generations, our bodies, including our joints, might grow so accustomed to those nutrients that they wouldn't grow, repair, and function normally without them. You'd be right. And what is true of bones is true of other animal parts. Over time, our genes have been programmed with the need and expectation of a steady input of familiar nutrients, some of which can only be derived from the variety meats, which include bones, joints, and *organs*.

Pillar Number 2: Organ Meat, Offal-y Good For You

Long ago, when a deer was killed then lifted on a hook to be dismembered, the hunter began by inserting a knife just below the xiphoid process at the lower end of the sternum and briskly drawing it down to the pubic bone. When properly done, the guts spilled out of the belly and naturally fell to the ground—*off fall*. In modern usage, the term offal encompasses every part of an animal except ordinary muscle meat.

If you've ever seen one of those travel shows hosted by a snarky gourmand eating strange foods in exotic locales, you might recall watching scenes of street venders in Calcutta frying brains on a skillet, or sweetmeats served in a dusty open-air eatery in Uzbekistan, and thinking, *How can they eat that?* It's all a matter of what you've grown up with. Had you been born elsewhere, you might drool at the sight of lungs on a stick just as you might now go ga-ga over a greasy corn dog. In fact, until recently, those offal meats were a big part of American dining, integrated into our diets through a wide range of dishes. Turn the cookbook pages back just a few generations and you'll find Halloweenish recipes calling for organ meats and other variety cuts alongside familiar casseroles and crumb cakes. My 1953 version of *Joy of Cooking* lists Calf Brain Fritters and ten other brainy recipes, as well as instructions for making meals from liver, kidney, tongue, heart, head, and thymus.

If you dig further back to cookbooks printed before the Industrial Revolution, you'll find ghastly instructions requiring a witch's arsenal of implements, large cauldrons and bone-splicing hatchets. From *The Ladies New Book of Cookery,* published in 1852, listed under preparation of beef, we learn the private housewife was to "take a green tongue, stick it with cloves and boil it gently for three hours." Also included are practical tips on how to estimate internal temperature without a meat thermometer: "When the eyes drop out, the pig is half done." Plus pointers on mannerly kitchen protocols:

"It is better to leave the wind-pipe on, for if it hangs out of the pot while the head is cooking, all the froth will escape through it."

Our founding fathers' wives followed recipes that made extensive use of offal meats, especially in the fall when many animals would be killed to conserve precious grass and hay for the best breeders that could repopulate the pastures again in spring. Since offal goes bad quickly, they needed to be consumed or preserved as soon as possible. The prudent housewife of the 17th, 18th, and early 19th centuries would want to make use of every last scrap and, nutritionally speaking, nothing would better prepare her family for the long winter ahead. Offal meats are rich in vitamins, especially fat-soluble vitamins, which can be stored in our own fat reserves for months. As winter wore on, and root cellars emptied, those larders of nutrients built up internally by feasting in the fall sometimes made the difference between life and death, or a successful pregnancy and one fraught with complications.

Why You Should Eat That Liver Paté

One of offal meat's most famous proponents was Adelle Davis, a biochemist who pioneered the fledgling field of nutrition in the mid 20th century. A patient of mine, who was taken to her in the 1940s on the advice of his pediatrician for help with his disabling asthma, was not simply treated. He was *cured*. Back then, there were no handheld inhalers. Every time he developed a cold or the weather changed, his mother would have to rush him to the hospital for shots of adrenaline. Davis advised his mother to send him off to school with a thermos of pureed raw cow's liver every day, which he managed to drink primarily because he wanted to avoid the emergency room. The raw cow's liver provided a spectrum of missing nutrients to calm the inflammation that triggered his asthma attacks. But it may also have done much more, ensuring his entire nervous system was wired correctly. Today, in his seventies, his reflexes are still so fast that he can trounce Luke on the tennis court.

I don't recommend you eat raw liver unless you are familiar with the source and have taken proper measures to prevent parasites.[159] But a quick

100 gm portion			
vitamin A	7*	10,602	261*
vitamin B1	0.02	0.2	0.063
vitamin B2	0.02	4.1	0.13
vitamin B6	0.07	0.91	0.2
folate	4	217	108
vitamin C	8	23	64.9
niacin	0.1	10.7	0.553
pantothenic acid	0.08	4.57	0.616
magnesium	6	20	21

Figure 2. Organ Meats v. Fruits And Vegetables: Pound for Pound There's No Comparison. In Chapter 5, we saw how terribly nourished most American women are today. One big factor is the near complete elimination of organ meats from our diets. Without these most nutrient dense of foods, it's nearly impossible to get adequate vitamins and minerals.

*Retinol equivalents. Only animal products contain true vitamin A, fruits and vegetables contain carotenoids and retinoids, which must be converted in the digestive tract. The conversion factor used has overestimated the value of fruits and vegetables by a factor of four. These data have been revised to reflect the current knowledge, but the nutrition tables on grocery store goods have not and thus exaggerate the true amount of vitamin A.

glance at the nutrition tables for liver and other variety cuts reveals why nutrition-oriented physicians might use these parts as cure-alls like Davis did; they're the *real* vitamin supplements. As she explains in her book *Let's Cook It Right*, "The liver is the storage place or the 'savings bank' of the body. If there is an excess of protein, sugar, vitamins, and any mineral except calcium and phosphorus, part of the excess is stored in the liver until it is needed....Liver is, therefore, nutritionally the most outstanding meat which can be purchased."[160] Of course, if the cow is sickly, or raised on depleted soil, the savings bank of the liver is likely depleted as well.

The following are just a few examples of the benefits of eating different variety meats. The Latin name for the retina of the eye is *macula lutea*. (Lutea is Latin for yellow.) This thick, membranous yellow layer of the eyeball is a rich source of the nutrient *lutein*, a member of the retinoid family of vitamin A precursors. Lutein supplements are now promoted as being good for prostate health and for preventing macular degeneration. The fat behind the eyeball is a rich source of vitamin A and lutein. (If you think you'd rather swallow a supplement than pop an eyeball after breakfast, remember that vitamins are heat-, light-, and oxygen-sensitive and unlikely to survive processing.) And while you're digesting the idea of eating eyeball fat, consider that the gooey juice in the eye is primarily hyaluronic acid, rich in glycosaminoglycans. You can get hyaluronic acid injected into your lips (to fill them out), your knee (as a treatment for osteoarthritis), and even your own eye (to treat certain ocular diseases) for $200 a dose (twenty one-thousandths of a gram). It's called Restylane. But you can get this useful nutrient into your body just by eating the eyes you find in your fish head soup, and the glycosaminoglycans will find their way to the parts of the body that need them most.

Brain and nervous tissues are fantastic sources of omega-3 and other brain-building fatty acids and phospholipids, and with more than 1.2 grams per 100 gram portion, they are a richer source of this vital nutrient than almost anything else.[161] Even windpipe contains stuff we don't get enough of these days—those glycosaminoglycans again. Many of my patients spend upwards of a hundred dollars a month buying supplemental nutrients that are far less potent than what our ancestors enjoyed daily, simply by including variety meats in their diet.

You may have noticed a pattern here: eating Eyes is good for your eyes. Eating joints is good for your joints. The idea that the consumption of a part of an animal's body is good for the same part of your own is an interpretation of homeopathy—meaning *like cures like*. Unfortunately, today most of these powerful "supplements" are going to waste as today's meat producers wash these rich sources of nutrition down drains in the slaughterhouse floor, or pass them off to rendering plants where heaps of rotting tissue are reprocessed into animal feeds, yellow fat, and something called "recycled meat." The good news is, since our society values them so little, if your butcher can save them for you, he'll likely sell them to you cheap. The bad news is, once we've got them, making them taste good isn't especially easy to do; it takes a little time and know-how. For adults, the reward is a powerful resistance to disease. For children, the awakening of their genetic (growth) potential brings rewards that are indescribably greater.

Pillar Number 3: Better Than Fresh, Fermentation and Sprouting

Egyptians set aside their dough until it decayed, and observed with pleasure the process that took place. **—Herodotus, 5th century BC**[162]

On a recent trip to the Bay Area where I was giving a talk on nutrition, a good friend took us out for lunch. "You're into healthy food," she said. "There's a hip new vegan restaurant we've got to try." Opening the menu felt like cracking open a history book to do your assigned reading; nothing looked appetizing. Though the menu was peppered with pop-nutrition vernacular—"living," "dynamic," "enzyme," the selections were simply awkward interpretations of familiar foods: the raw pizza, the cold burrito. Luke ordered the burrito, a compressed disc of rancid seeds laureled with a splash of fresh greens. I ordered the pizza, an identical compressed disc with a different kind of dressing on the greens. The greens were good. The disc was not. Truly living food is more dynamic than salad leaves, and more potent than a plate of compressed seeds; it's food that's been *awakened* by the process of fermentation, sprouting, or both.

Vegetarians in particular will benefit from these two potent methodologies for enhancing nutrition. Fermentation and sprouting are crucial for one simple reason: Plants didn't evolve with the idea that they should be good to eat. In fact, plants spend a great deal of energy thwarting overzealous grazers and other creatures that would gladly eat them into oblivion. Not as helpless as they may seem, plants protect their foliage, stems, seeds, roots, and to a lesser degree even their fruits, with natural insecticides and bitter toxins that make some plants unsafe for human consumption. Unless your species has evolved the physiologic means to neutralize them, a plant's various hemagglutinints, enzyme inhibitors, cyanogens, anti-vitamins, carcinogens, neurotoxins, and allergens say, "Eat at your own risk." Although I disagree, some investigators have gone so far as to suggest that "nearly all the carcinogens in the diet are of natural rather than—as widely perceived—industrial origin."[163] Sprouting and fermenting effectively deactivates many of these irritants, which explains why sprouted grains and lacto-fermented vegetables are known to be easier to digest.

Many of today's best foods were originally fermented, sprouted, or both. Take away fermentation and there's no such thing as wine. Or beer. You can forget bread, yoghurt, and cheese. Chocolate's out, since cacao nibs must sit in the sun for a week or so to let the fruit ferment around the nibs and develop the full symphony of flavor. And the same goes for coffee berries. The list of fermented foods grows surprisingly long when you throw in things like sauerkraut, pickles, ketchup and other condiments that—though now industrially mass-produced by steeping in vinegar and salt—traditionally generated their own acid preservatives during fermentation. In *The Story of Wine*, writer Hugh Johnson celebrates fermentation as a central driving force of civilization. The oldest recipe known to exist, written in cuneiform, is for a kind of beer bread. If we'd never allowed cereal grains to sprout, we would never have invented bread nourishing enough to sustain a population; for the first ten thousand years of wheat and grain cultivation, the technology to crush open the kernels did not exist.[164] And so, for the majority of human history, life-giving bread was made not with flour, but with partially germinated seeds. Unfortunately, even in places like France, people often fail to appreciate their own wild, indigenous microbes. And so many foods (cheeses, breads, wines, etc.) have had their flavors tamed by way of pasteurization, by the use of faster-acting cultures that are easier to work with, or both.

In the next two sections, we'll take a look at the battle of wills between human and vegetable, and see why traditional, low-tech methods for neutralizing plant toxins and maximizing nutrition are far more effective at producing healthy products than contemporary methods.

Fermentation, Part I: Single Cell Vitamin Factories

The human digestive system is a chimera. It's one part *us*, one trillion parts *them*. We supply the long, hollow tube that begins at our mouth and coils for a dozen meters or so inside our abdominal cavity until it ends at the rear. The microbial world populates the tube with enough bacteria and fungi to outnumber our own cells ten to one.[165] The average human colon contains over 800 species of microbiota and at least 7000 different strains.[166] 60 percent of the fecal matter you produce consists of microbial bodies. Are all these microbes just freeloaders, or do we somehow benefit from their presence?

To answer that, we need to understand something about a process called *fermentation*. My Webster's dictionary describes fermentation as an "enzymatically controlled transformation of an organic product." The key term is *transformation*. Bacteria are capable of transforming indigestible, bland, and even toxic compounds into nourishing and delicious foods. Without them, multi-celled organisms, from flies to frogs to mammals, would be unable to digest their food. With an arsenal of enzymes, microbes can break down toxins that might otherwise sicken or kill us outright, turn simple sugars into complex nutrients, make vitamins our diets might otherwise lack (such as K_2 and B_{12}), and wage chemical warfare on would-be pathogens. All we do for them is provide a warm place to work and plenty of water. From their perspective, we are the freeloaders living off their hard labor.

The obliging microbe isn't especially particular about where it lives. Requiring little more than consistent temperature, water, and a few organic materials, bacteria and fungi are equally happy whether inside our digestive tract, in a warm clay pot in the sun, an oak casket in a cave, a leather sac, or even an egg buried underground. Thousands of years ago, people learned to harness the power of these invisible "factors," which developed predictably under a certain set of conditions. That skill opened up a world of possibility, enabling us to preserve our food and create a whole new set of flavors.

Fermentation would ultimately be put to use by people around the globe, and form one of the foundational pillars of all traditional cuisine.

Though today we tend to think of bacteria and fungi in our food as unwanted enemies, usually calling them "germs," civilization owes much to these contaminants. Without yeast naturally present in the air, we never would have been able to leaven our bread, and in the 1960s, doctors discovered a dramatic example of the value of leavening. Poor Turkish families were having children with a type of dwarfism initially thought to be due to genetic mutation. When no defective gene could be identified, researchers looked to nutritional problems. It turned out that the mothers of affected children, as well as the children themselves, had low levels of zinc and other minerals. Further investigation revealed the cause of the mineral deficiency to be unleavened bread consumption.[167] Wheat, like all seeds, contains mineral-binding compounds called *phytates,* which hold minerals in stasis until conditions are right for germination. Yeast and other microbes (such as those in sourdough) contain enzymes (called *phytases*) that break down phytates in the seed, freeing the zinc, calcium, magnesium and other minerals from their chemical cages. The parents of dwarfed children were buying cheaper, unleavened bread and were also unable to afford much meat, a good source of zinc and magnesium. The unleavened bread was the last straw. Bound to phytates, the zinc and magnesium in the bread passed through undigested, leading to mineral deficiencies that prevented proper expression of the children's bone-building genes.[168] This is just one example of what happens when people buy food based on price rather than on its nutritional value. Because few people appreciate the difference between authentic food that costs more, and similar substitutes that cost less, manufacturers skip the labor-intensive fermentation steps whenever they can.

Which is why I want to tell you the truth about soy.

Some of my patients speak so proudly about how they've started eating tofu and drinking soymilk, obviously presuming that I think these things are healthy, I can hardly bear to burst their bubble. Soybeans contain chemicals called *goitrogens* and *phytoestrogens,* which disrupt thyroid and sex hormone function. The Chinese and Japanese who traditionally ate soy would soak, rinse, and then ferment the beans for extended periods, neutralizing the harmful compounds and using the fat- and protein-rich beans as a substrate for microbial action. Traditional tofu, natto, miso, and other cultured soy products are incredibly nutritious. Commercially made soymilk, tofu, and soy-based infant formulas, on the other hand, are not. Loaded with goitrogens and phytoestrogens, these foods are known to cause hypo- and hyper-thyroidism, thyroid cancer, and—particularly when consumed during infancy or pregnancy—male and female reproductive disorders.[169,170] I have helped several patients with abnormal thyroid hormone levels and menstrual irregularities return their lab results and their bodies back to normal simply by advising them to stop eating soy.

Pound for pound, fermented material will have more nutrition packed into it than the raw material it came from because, aside from acting like miniature detoxification machines, microbes add heaps of nutrients to whatever it is they're growing in. Using enzyme power, single-celled bacteria and fungi manufacture all the vitamins, amino acids, nucleic acids, fatty acids (and so on) they need from simple starting materials like sugar, starch, and cellulose. They can thrive on foods that would leave us horribly malnourished. But we are bigger than they are. When we eat yoghurt, real pickles, real sauerkraut—or any food containing living cultures—our digestive juices attack and destroy many of the little critters, exploding their fragile bodies. Many survive (and protect us, see below), but those who are digested donate all their nutritious parts to us. Though after the fermentation process is finished foods like wine and cheese no longer contain living organisms, they have been enriched by the life-forms they once housed: Wine has more antioxidants than grape juice, and cheese more protein than milk.[171] The little critters can actually make all the vitamins we need except D, and all the essential amino acids. And they have one more trick up their sleeve. As if it's not enough that they can free up minerals, preserve our food, manufacture vitamins, and clean up the nasty plant chemicals that our bodies can't handle, once inside your body, they will literally fight for your life.

Fermentation, Part II—Boost Your Immune System With Probiotics

In 1993, *E. coli* hamburgers from Jack in the Box restaurants sickened hundreds of children, killing several. Around the same time, *E. coli* outbreaks in the apple industry led to the requirement that apple juice be pasteurized. In 2006, spinach laced with manure made more people ill. In 2008, salmonella-tainted tomatoes were blamed for another outbreak—until they decided it was actually Jalapeño peppers. It seems as though there's always something yucky in our food ready to make us sick. No doubt, there are nasty microbial agents in the general food supply all the time. The question is, *Why do they make some people deathly ill while leaving the rest of us alone?*

Turns out, it has to do with our social lives. I'm not talking about the people we go to parties with, but our bacterial bosom buddies. Microbiologist Dr. Bonnie Bassler discovered that microbes have social lives too.[172] Far from behaving like mindless pre-programmed specks, they form gangs, coordinate efforts, and even scheme against other groups of bacteria. In fact, the turbulent world of micro-organisms shares all the violence and drama of a Spaghetti Western. And the microbial world operates under the same binary rubric. As far as your body's concerned, when it comes to bacteria and fungi, there really are just two kinds: good and bad.

The first group, often referred to with the umbrella term *probiotics*, is comprised of the same beneficial bacteria that preserve, detoxify, and enrich our food. These microbes are friendly and very well behaved. After all, we feed and house them, so it is in their best interest to keep us healthy. To that end, they secrete hormones that help coordinate the muscular contractions of intestinal peristalsis, while keeping a sharp look out for bad guys: the *pathogens*. Probiotics work with our immune system. If pathogens hope to gain a foothold, they have to get past the phalanx of probiotics first. While you're watching *Survivor* or *Top Chef*, microbes in your gut are making alliances and scheming against each other for control of your internal real estate.[173] Not only does the outcome of their battles determine whether or not a deadly strain of *E Coli* in your manure-tainted spinach kills you, studies have shown that live-cultured foods containing probiotics help to prevent a whole range of allergic, autoimmune, and inflammatory diseases.[174,175,176]

The people who originally mastered the art of fermenting fruits, vegetables, meats, and so on were probably seeking ways to preserve their food. Crops tend to ripen all at once. Fish swim in schools. Many game animals travel in large herds. These periodic abundances necessitated the development of effective food-preservation methods. The microbial world is so obliging that a little salt, a container, and some know-how are all you—I should say the microbes—need. Today we have simpler options for preserving our food, including canning, refrigeration, freezing, pickling (seeping in vinegar) and drying. But in terms of nutrient conservation, each pales in comparison to fermentation, which often adds new nutrients. Even your refrigerator can't keep fresh fruits and vegetables from declining in nutrient content. Vitamin C, for instance, declines so drastically in storage that refrigerated green beans lose 77% after only seven days off the vine.[177]

If you've never fermented anything, you should. With a little instruction and practice, you can make yourself the best sauerkraut you've ever tasted. And it's ridiculously easy: Shred a cabbage in the food processor. Mix with a full teaspoon of salt and a little liquid from a jar of Bubbies brand pickles (or other fermented vegetable product) and pack into a lightproof container with something heavy, like a jar full of water, sitting on top to keep the cabbage under the liquid. Cover with a towel to keep the bugs off. Wait a week or so, and eat.

Not simple enough? Okay, here's something even easier. With sprouting, you just let nature take its course.

Seeds of Change: Why Sprouted Grain Bread is Better than Whole Wheat

A lot of my patients tell me that they feel better when they cut wheat from their diet, and more kids than ever are developing celiac disease and other allergies to wheat and products made from wheat. After 10,000 years of cultivation, why the sudden change? There are plenty of potential causes, from the GMOs to the pesticides to the fact that flour is often heavily contaminated with mold toxins and allergenic proteins (insect parts and rat feces).[178] Even when organically grown, manufacturers treat wheat flour like a construction material, extruding it into geometric shapes and puffing it into crunchy cereal cushions, rendering the proteins allergenic.[179] Whether you suffer from wheat allergies or you just want to buy the healthiest bread available, bread made from sprouted wheat (or other grains) is your best bet.

Wheat seeds are called wheat berries. Like all seeds, wheat berries can be sprouted. These days, the only exposure most of us get to sprouts is at the salad bar. People used to eat sprouted stuff all the time, only they didn't let the sprouts develop as fully as those in a salad bar. Our ancestors who didn't have mills were able to acquire more nutrition from their harvests of grain than we do today with all our technological advancements simply by waiting until the germination process begins.

Why does germinating a seed first make it more nutritious? Seeds are designed to greedily hang on to their stored proteins, fats, and minerals over extended periods of time. To that end, the plant sheaths them in a hard, nearly impenetrable carapace and locks down nutrients with chemical binders that digestive enzymes can't loosen. Moistening the seeds for a few days activates the plant's own enzymes—including phytase, which digests phytates—to soften the seed, free up bound nutrients, and even create new ones by converting stored starch and fatty acids into proteins and vitamins.

Today's bread is nothing like the bread described in the Bible. The crust of a Domino's pizza and bread made by indigenous people around the world are, nutritionally speaking, as alike as a packet of chicken-flavored powder and wild grouse. Modern bread is made of flour, while ancient breads were made of ground, germinated seeds. Although some of the stone artifacts found in places like Peru, the Nile Delta, or North America may look like something you could use to grind wheat berries into dry flour, I suspect the berries were partly germinated first. Wheat berries are as hard as ball bearings. It's far easier to use seeds softened by germination. I know because I've conducted a study.

In grade school, a friend of mine returned from a visit to a Native American reservation with a set of milling stones that we just *had* to build an afternoon's drama around. We both plaited our hair in what we understood to be proper squaw fashion and walked out into her backyard to figure out how to make "genuine" Indian bread. It was 1973, when every East Coast mother walked in step with hippy trends, so naturally my friend's kitchen had plenty of wheat berries with which to experiment. Enthusiastic as we were, those tiny brown pebbles tested our patience to the breaking point, shooting laterally off the grinding stone and onto the ground until we were convinced that this methodology would fail to generate oven-ready dough by the time my mom was to pick me up. We decided to take a short cut. Back in the kitchen, her mother had a jar of lentils soaking in water, softened but not yet fully sprouted. They were smushy enough to hold still under the rolling stone. In no time, we had ourselves a small pile of greenish-yellow lentil "dough." (More of a paste, really, since lentils have no gluten). Ever since, I've been skeptical of anthropologists' claims that similar stones were used to grind wheat or other hard seeds into flour. More likely, seeds used for making bread were pre-softened by letting nature take its course.

You can soak any kind of seed you want, from kidney beans to wheat berries and more. Simply put some into a jar, cover with water, then cover with a bug-proof cloth and, in anywhere from one to four days, the seeds will start to germinate (you'll need to change the water once a day). You can tell once they've awakened because you'll see a tiny white rootlet begin to take form. That's the point at which it's ready to be used as a vitamin-rich version of an ordinary kidney bean or wheat berry. Or even easier than doing it yourself, you can buy breads made with sprouted grain in health food stores. Usually, you have to look in the freezer section because, without artificial preservatives, these breads mold quickly.

If you can't find sprouted grain breads, the next best thing is whole wheat. But when shopping for bread, be aware of a savvy marketing trick. The label on brown bread can say *wheat flour* even though they used white flour because, yes, even white flour originally came from a wheat field. The addition of caramel coloring turns the dough dark, completing the illusion that you've bought healthier, whole wheat bread. Until the food producers' lobbyists strip them of all meaning, you can feel fairly confident when the ingredients include the words *whole-wheat flour*. Or better yet, sprout some wheat berries and use them to bake your own.

Pillar Number 4: Fresh, the Benefits of Raw

Every time I give a talk about nutrition, someone in the audience will raise a hand to ask my opinion of the latest antioxidant miracle being said to have otherworldly curative properties. Maybe it's bearberry, or bee pollen, or goji, or ginseng. It could be a liquid extract, or a powder, or a pill—it doesn't really matter. The idea behind *all* antioxidant supplements on the market is the same: to give the consumer a blend of electron-trapping chemicals that help prevent the two most common causes of tissue inflammation and degenerative disease: lipid oxidation and advanced-glycation-end-product formation. (See Chapters 8 and 9.) And every time, my answer goes like this, "If you want antioxidants, skip the latest fad products and use that money to buy fresh food."

Fresh Greens: Potency that Can't be Bottled

There are so many antioxidant miracles on the market now that, if you were so inclined, you could spend an entire paycheck and barely scratch the surface. But it would be a waste of good money. What the nutraceutical industry doesn't want you to know is that there's nothing unique about any of their "unique" formulations; *all fresh fruits and vegetables* contain antioxidants, flavinoids, and other categories of chemicals used as selling points on nutraceutical packages. In fact, as they will tell you, they make their products from fresh fruits and vegetables. It's just that they use fruits and vegetables with more exotic-sounding names.

The truth is, you'll get a better blend of antioxidants simply by eating a variety of familiar greens, along with fresh herbs and spices: Sprinkle your marinara with basil and thyme, or make your own salad dressing with garlic and dill. Because supplements have been processed and certain chemicals may concentrate, supplements can have side effects. Fresh, whole foods (including raw meat and fish) universally contain a safe, balanced blend of antioxidants because all living organisms—plant and animal—use them to prevent oxygen damage. Plants are capable of manufacturing so many different kinds of antioxidants that we'll probably never catalogue even a tenth of them. Family names for some of the more common antioxidants include flavinoids, terpenes, phenolics, coumarins, and retinoids (vitamin A precursors). Since antioxidants must work as a team to be effective, where you find one, you find a lot—*but only when they're fresh.* If you want a power pack of antioxidants, you can get them cheap if you follow writer Michael Pollen's advice and grow a tray of fresh herbs out on the balcony. They tend to taste a whole lot better than a capsule of sterile dust.

Why is freshness so important when it comes to antioxidants? As much as antioxidants retard oxidation, oxygen spoils antioxidants. Antioxidants protect our tissues against oxygen damage by acting like selfless chemical heroes, throwing themselves in the line of fire to protect other chemicals from free radical and oxygen damage. Not only do antioxidants gradually lose their ability to do this over time, as oxidation inevitably occurs during storage, their potency can be neutralized through the drying and/or heating of processing. This is why a lot of foods deliver the most antioxidant punch when eaten raw.

You can taste how much nutritional power a given plant is packing: More intense flavor means more intense nutrition. Both nutrient density and flavor intensity result from a bioconcentration of vitamins, minerals, and other nutrient systems. Pungent vegetables like celery, peppers, broccoli, arugula, and garlic contain more antioxidants, vitamins, and minerals per bite than tuberous vegetables like potatoes and turnips. Remember, cooking burns up antioxidants and damages many vitamins. So the more you eat cooked foods, the more you need to balance your diet by eating fresh, uncooked, pungent-tasting herbs and vegetables.

Be aware that raw isn't always better, thanks to cellulose, the material that gives plants their stiffness and their crispy crunch. Locked within cellulose-rich cell walls, vitamins and minerals in high-cellulose plant products pass right through our omnivore's digestive system. Without heat or caustic chemicals, cellulose can only be broken down using specialized bacteria and extended gut-fermentation—something humans lack the intestinal yardage to accomplish (though they can replicate it; see section on fermentation, above). Studies show that a mere one percent of the retinoids (vitamin A precursors) in raw carrots, for instance, get absorbed.[180] But cooking (which hydrolyzes cellulose in much the same way it hydrolyzes proteins) increases that percentage to thirty.[181] Only a short list of plant parts are low enough in cellulose for our digestive enzymes to break them down without either cooking or fermenting them first, and these include fresh herbs and spices, nuts and fruits, and young, tender lettuce leaves and other leafy greens.

However we eat our veggies, raw or gently cooked, freshness is paramount. As Mrs. A. P. Hill wrote in her 1867 cookbook, "It cannot be questioned that articles originally good and wholesome derive a poisonous character from changes taking place in their own composition." Therefore, "[a] few only can be kept twelve hours without detriment." This was before refrigeration, of course. But even so, the precipitous drop in nutrition and flavor after picking—and the fact that most grocery store vegetables are grown in poor soil, picked before they're ripe, and then travel the world in cold storage, reducing nutrition and flavor further still—helps explain why so many kids won't eat their veggies.

While gaining access to many of the nutrients in plants often requires (judicious) use of heat, many animal products are so abundant in nutrients that adding thermal energy risks fusing them together. This is why we need to cook our meat so gently, and why raw meat and seafood dishes comprise a valuable part of many international diets, from sashimi in Japan to ceviche in Spain and South America to steak tartare, popular around the world. But there's one animal product we think of as fresh even though the vast majority of what we find in most grocery stores is, in reality, anything but: milk.

Fresh Dairy: Why Mess With Udder Perfection?

Milk may be the single most historically important food to human health. Not just any milk, mind you, but raw milk from healthy, free-to-roam, grass-fed cows. The difference between the milk you buy in the store, and the milk your great-great grandparents enjoyed is, unfortunately, enormous. If we lived in a country where raw milk from healthy, pastured cows were still a legal product and available as readily as, say, soda or a handgun, we'd all be taller and healthier, and I'd see fewer elderly patients with hunched backs and broken hips. If you're lucky enough to live in a state where raw milk is available in stores and you don't buy it, you are passing up a huge opportunity to improve your health immediately. If you have kids, raw milk will not only help them grow, but will also boost their immune systems so they get sick less often. And, since the cream in raw milk is an important source of brain-building fats, whole milk and other raw dairy products will also help them to learn.

It's a common misperception that milk drinking is a relatively new practice, one limited to Europeans. The reality is that our cultural—and now, our epigenetic—dependence on milk most likely originated somewhere in Africa. It is highly likely that milk consumption gave those who practiced animal husbandry such an advantage that it rapidly spread across the continent and then into Europe and Asia. With such widespread use, it's likely that to allow for optimal expression, many of our genes now require it. In those countries where people's stature most benefited from the consumption of raw milk, when raw milk is replaced with a processed alternative, their bones take the hardest hit. It's a case of the bigger they are the harder they fall. In places like Norway, Sweden, and Denmark, people now suffer from particularly high rates of osteoporosis and degenerative arthritis.[182]

Our genes have been infused with real dairy products for tens of thousands of years. Recent geologic and climatologic research reveals that between 100,000 and 10,000 years ago, the Sahara was a lush paradise of grassland. During that window of abundance, the human population exploded. To deal with the consequential depletion of wild resources, people began experiments in "proto-farming," a term coined by biologist and historian Colin Tudge to describe humanity's slow-motion leap from living in harmony with the land as hunter-gatherers to adopting the now-familiar program of altering the ecology to suit our interests. Author Thom Hartmann explains in his book *The Last Hours of Ancient Sunlight*:

> *Something important happened around 40,000 years ago: humans figured out a way to change the patterns of nature so we could get more sunlight/food than other species did. The human food supply was determined by how many deer or rabbits the local forest could support [...]. But in areas where the soil was too poor for farming or forest, supporting only scrub brush and grasses, humans discovered that ruminant (grazing animals like goats, sheep, and cows) could eat those plants that we couldn't, and could therefore convert the daily sunlight captured by the scrub and wild plants on that "useless" land into animal flesh, which we could eat.*

Or drink, as the case may be.

For millennia, much of the world's population has depended largely on milk for nutritional sustenance. However, the medical world has been ignorant of milk's nearly ubiquitous use, confused by the issue of lactose intolerance. Because Europeans have lower rates of lactose intolerance, most Western physicians presume that only European populations have historically practiced dairying. But this confusion arises in part because most Western physicians don't know very much about fermentation.

Lactose Intolerance

Lactose is the major type of sugar in milk. Nearly everyone can digest it while we're babies and dependent on our mother's milk, but many people lose the lactase enzyme in the lining of the intestine, growing lactose intolerant as they get older. Fermentation breaks down lactose, and so you don't need that enzyme as long as you only eat fermented dairy products, such as yoghurt and cheese. The reason people living in warmer climates tend to be lactose intolerant more often than Europeans stems from the fact that fermentation progresses rapidly in warmer climates. Once fermented, the potentially irritating lactose sugars are gone. A child living in a warmer climate would, after weaning, have such infrequent need for the lactase enzyme that the epigenetic librarian would simply switch the gene off. In cooler European climates, fresh milk stays fresh for hours or days, and was presumably consumed that way often enough to keep the lactase enzyme epigenetically activated throughout a person's life. If you have true lactose intolerance, as opposed to a protein allergy, you should be able to tolerate yoghurt, cheese, and cream (dairy fat contains little to no lactose—and minimal protein).

Why Most Milk is Pasteurized Today

Most of us also have heard that milk needs to be pasteurized to be safe. But we haven't heard the whole story. For perhaps thousands of years, people who gave their animals the basic, humane care they deserved survived and thrived drinking completely raw, fresh milk. The need for pasteurization was a reality when in-city dairies housed diseased cows whose hindquarters ran with rivulets of manure. Tainting milk's reputation even further, around the same time, dairymen were often infected with diphtheria, spreading the deadly bacteria through the medium of warm, protein-rich milk. But no epidemics have *ever* been traced to raw milk consumption when the cows were healthy and the humans milking them were disease free.[183] If the animal is sickly—as they invariably are when raise in crowded, nightmarish conditions—its milk should probably not be consumed at all. When that's your only choice, then, yes it ought to be cooked first to reduce risk of potentially lethal infections including undulant fever, hemolytic uremia, sepsis, and more. But it's not your only choice.

If you erase any ethical entanglement, impulse of social responsibility, nagging moral prohibition, and investment in human health, you could call milk pasteurization a good thing. In terms of volume of product output per production unit, pasteurization plays a crucial role in converting small family farms into perfectly efficient milk producers for the national brands:

cheaper feed (silage and grain instead of fresh grass and hay), more cows per square foot, more "milk" per cow. That explains why big agribusiness roots for pasteurization. But how did the rest of us get convinced?

Our fear of fresh milk can be traced to the energetic campaigning of a man named Charles North who patented the first batch-processing pasteurization machine in 1907.[184] A skilled orator and savvy businessman, he traveled small towns throughout the country creating publicity and interest in his machines by claiming to have come directly from another small town, just like theirs, where people were dying from drinking unpasteurized milk.[185] Of course, his claims were total fiction and doctors were staunchly opposed to pasteurization.[186] The facts were on their side. Unfortunately, North had something better—fear. And he milked that fear right into a small fortune. The pasteurization industry mushroomed from nonexistence to a major political presence. Today, at the University of Pennsylvania where medical professors once protested that pasteurization "should never be had recourse to,"[187] medical students are given lessons on the many health benefits of pasteurization.

Whenever I have a patient who was raised on a farm, one who looks tough and boasts how rarely they get sick, I ask them if they drank raw milk as a child. Nine times out of ten, they say yes. Every family dairyman I've talked to keeps raw milk around for their own families and happily testifies to its health benefits. Unlike meat or fruit or really any other food, milk is unique in that its one and only purpose is to nourish something else. Not only is it loaded with nutrients, it is engineered with an intricate micro-architecture that is key to enhancing digestive function while preventing the nourishing compounds from reacting with one another. Processing fundamentally alters this micro-architecture and diminishes nutritive value significantly. How much of a difference does this make? Enough that, based on their health and bone structure, I can guess with a high degree of accuracy which of my patients had access to raw milk as a child and which did not.

Since 1948, when states began passing mandatory pasteurization laws, raw milk fans have waged a bitter battle against government intervention.

During hearings in which laws requiring pasteurization have been challenged, pasteurization proponents deny any nutritional difference between pasteurized, homogenized milk and raw. But as dairy scientists point out, heat denatures proteins, and homogenization explodes the fat droplets in milk. This is significant. Even to the naked eye, there's a difference: Unlike cooked milk, the fresh product has a layer of cream floating at the top. But to fully understand how these two products differ, we need to bust out the microscope.

The Difference Between Fresh and Processed

If we put a drop of fresh milk on a slide, we see thousands of lipid droplets of varying size streaming under the cover slip and maybe a living lactobacilli or two wiggling from edge to edge. These come from the cow's udders which, when well cared for, are colonized with beneficial bacteria, as is human skin. We want good bacteria in our milk. These probiotics protect both the milk and the milk consumer from pathogens. Good bacteria accomplish this by using the same bacterial communication techniques we read about in the section on fermentation.

Using the powerful electron microscope, we can magnify milk 10,000,000 times. Now we can see casein micelles, which are amazingly complex. Imagine a mound of spaghetti and meatballs formed into a big round ball. The strands of spaghetti are made of protein (casein), and the meatballs are made of the most digestible form of calcium phosphate, called colloidal calcium phosphate, which holds the spaghetti strands together in a clump with its tiny magnetic charge. This clumping prevents sugar from reacting with and destroying milk's essential amino acids.

Each tiny globe of fat in the milk is enclosed inside a phospholipid membrane very similar to the membrane surrounding every cell in your body. The mammary gland cell that produced the fat droplet donated some of its membrane when the droplet exited the cell. This coating performs several tasks, starting in the milk duct where it prevents fat droplets from coalescing and clogging up mom's mammary passageways. The milk fat globule's lipid bilayer is studded with a variety of specialized proteins, just like the living cells in your body. Some proteins protect the globule from bacterial infection while others are tagged with short chains of sugars that may function as a signal to the intestinal cell that the contents are to be accepted without immune inspection, streamlining digestion. Still others may act as intestinal cell growth factors, encouraging and directing intestinal cells growth and function. As long as the coating surrounds the milk fat globule, the fat is easily digested, the gallbladder doesn't have to squeeze out any bile for the fat to be absorbed, the fatty acids inside the blob are isolated from the calcium in the casein micelles, and everything goes smoothly. But if calcium and fats come into contact with one another, as we'll see in a moment, milk loses much of its capacity to deliver nutrients into your body.

Let's go back to the light microscope to take a look at pasteurized, homogenized milk and identify what distinguishes it from raw. One striking difference will be the homogeneity of fat globule sizes and the absence of living bacteria. But the real damage is hiding behind all this homogeneity and is only revealed under the electron microscope. Now, we see that these fat blobs lack the sophisticated bilayer wrapping and are instead caked with minerals and tangled remnants of casein micelles. Why does it look like this? The heat of pasteurization forces the sugar to react with amino acids, denaturing the proteins and knocking the fragile colloidal calcium phosphate out of the spaghetti-and-meatballs matrix, while the denatured spaghetti strands tangle into a tight, hard knot. Homogenization squeezes the milk through tiny holes under intense pressure, destroying the architecture of the fat globules. Once the two processing steps have destroyed the natural architecture of milk, valuable nutrients react with each other with health-damaging consequences.

Processing can render milk highly irritating to the intestinal tract, and such a wide variety of chemical changes may occur that processed milk can lead to diarrhea or constipation. During processing, the nice, soft meatball of colloidal calcium phosphate fuses with the fatty acids to form a kind of milk-fat soap. This reaction, called saponification, irritates many people's GI tracts

Before Homogenization

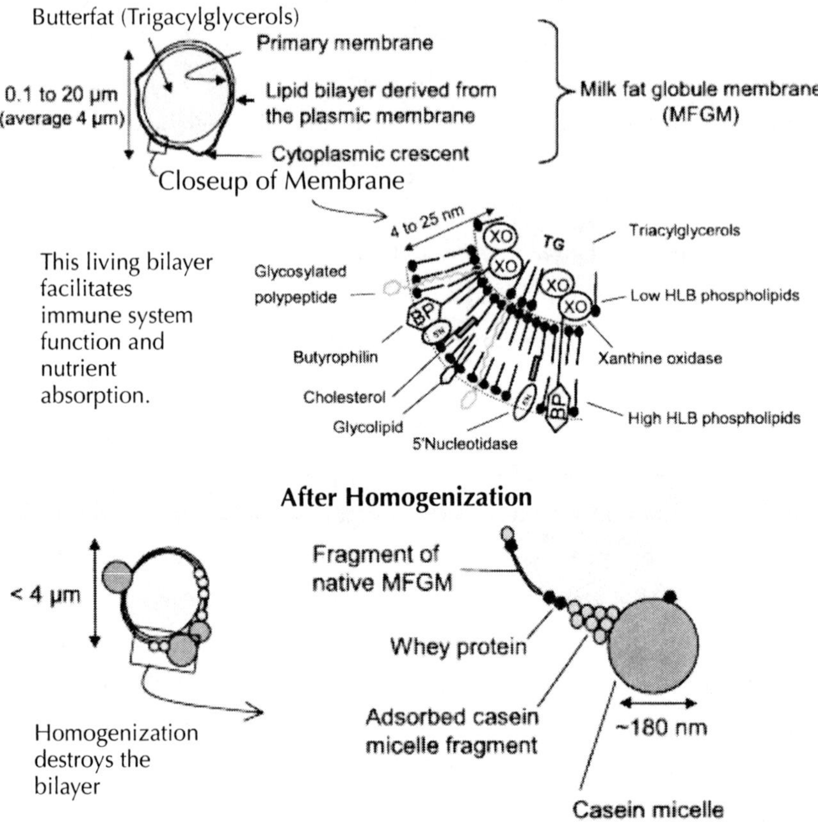

Figure 3. Effects of Processing on the Milk-fat Globule. Before homogeniztion, the lipid bilayer around a milkfat globule is identical in structure to the membrane around each one of your cells. Homogenization forces the globules, which can be up to 20 microns across, through holes less than a micron across, stripping those membranes from the majority. Pasteurization bakes the milk, caking adherent casein (milk protein) and calcium phosphate crystals against the tiny globules of fat, rendering amino acids and minerals more difficult to absorb.

From Does homogenization affect the human health properties of cows milk? Michalski MC Trends in Food Science and Technology 12 (2006) 423-437

and makes the calcium and phosphate much less bioavailable and more difficult to absorb.[188] How difficult? Food conglomerates have a lot of influence on the direction of research funding. And the dairy industry is big business. Little wonder that no studies have been funded to compare the nutritional value of raw, whole cow's milk to pasteurized head-to-head. But studies have been done on skim milk and human breast milk comparing fresh versus pasteurized, and the difference is dramatic: Processed milks contained anywhere from one half to one sixth the bioavailable minerals of the fresh products.[189,190] When fresh, the milk fat globule carries signal molecules on the surface, which help your body recognize milk as a helpful substance as opposed to, say, an invasive bacteria. Processing demolishes those handy signals and so, instead of getting a free pass into the intestinal cell, the curiously distorted signals slow the process of digestion down so much that it can lead to constipation.[191] Heat destroys amino acids, especially the fragile essential amino acids, and so pasteurized milk contains less protein than fresh.[192] But the damaged amino acids don't just disappear; they have been *glycated,* oxidized and transformed into stuff like N-carboxymethyl-lysine, malonaldehyde, and 4-hydroxynonanal—potentential allergens and pro-inflammatory irritants.[193]

And there's more. Many of the active enzymes in fresh milk designed to help streamline the digestive process have also been destroyed. Other enzymes, such as xanthine oxidase, which ordinarily protect the milk (but cause damage inside our arteries) can play stowaway within the artificially formed fat blobs and be absorbed. Normally our digestive system would chop up this enzyme and digest it. But hidden inside fat, it can be ingested whole, and may retain some of its original activity. Once in the body, xanthine oxidase can generate free radicals and lead to atherosclerosis and asthma. One more thing that makes raw milk special is the surface molecules on milk fat globule membranes, called *gangliosides*. Gangliosides inhibit harmful bacteria in the intestine. Once digested, they've been shown to stimulate neural development.[194] Homogenization strips these benefits away.

What does all this scientific data mean to you? It means that the processed milk you buy in the store is not milk, not really. If you can't find a good source of fresh, unprocessed milk, what can you do? Get the next best thing: yoghurt made from organic, whole milk. The fermentation process rejuvenates damaged proteins and makes minerals more bioavailable. A breakfast of yoghurt, fresh fruit slices, and nuts is nutritionally far superior to cold cereal and processed milk. But if you aren't ready to give up milk for breakfast, then get organic *whole* milk (not low fat), preferably from cows raised on pasture—not grain! Non-organic dairy may *seem* cheaper, but in reality you get far less nutrition for the dollar than you do with organic because at least organically raised cows produce *milk*. The stuff that comes out of malnourished cows living in cement milk-factories hardly qualifies as such. Whatever you do, avoid soymilk. The primary difference between *Yoohoo*, a junk-food beverage snack sold in your local 7-11, and the soymilk sold in the health food stores is that *Yoohoo* is flavored with chocolate.

Fresh Meat

Here in the US, white-gloved health department officials encourage us to cook our meat to death. Not because overcooked meat is tastier or more nutritious but because our meat has generally been slaughtered days or weeks ago in filthy conditions that enable pathogenic bacteria to proliferate all over the surface. Those, we must destroy with plenty of heat in order to be "safe." If you are lucky enough to travel to Asia, Africa, or India, you might want to stop at one of those restaurants that keep chickens out back. Why do they do this? Because fresh meat is part of every world cuisine and fresh meat can, when the animals are known to be healthy, safely be cooked rare. Juicy pinkness indicates the presence of far more nutrients than you can get when meat is overcooked.

In the 1930s and '40s, Dr. Frances Marion Pottenger conducted a ten-year experiment that gives us valuable insights into the potential long-term consequences of overcooking. Pottenger fed one group of cats raw meat and milk, and another group cooked meat and pasteurized milk. The all-raw cats produced ten generations of healthy and well-adjusted kittens. Not so, the cats on the cooked diet. By the end of the first generation, they started to develop degenerative diseases and became "quite lazy." The second generation developed degenerative diseases earlier in life and started losing their coordination. By the third generation, the cats had developed degenerative disease very early in life, and some were born blind and weak and died prematurely. There was an abundance of parasites and vermin in this group, and skin disease and allergies increased from an incidence of five percent in normal cats to over 90 percent in the third generation. Males became docile and females aggressive. By the fourth generation, litters were stillborn or so sickly they didn't live to reach adulthood. This research prompted pet food manufacturers to add back some of the vitamins lost during heating. Still, dried and canned pet food is nothing like the diets cats thrive on.

Pottenger's research highlights the importance of eating vitamin-rich, *fresh* meat. But if you don't have access to the quality of meat that can safely be cooked rare, then it's all the more important for you to make sure to get the freshest greens you can and eat them raw or gently cooked.

How The Four Pillars Will Make You Healthier

Whatever your age, whatever illnesses run in your family, whatever your "risk factors," however many times you've tried to lose weight, build muscle, etc., eating the foods I've described in this chapter will transform your body. And if you are planning a baby, eating Four-Pillar foods before, during, and after conception, and then feeding them to your child as he or she grows up, will allow the genes in his or her body to express in ways yours may not have.

Meat on the bone will bring enough of the glycosaminoglycan growth factors and bone-building minerals to make a child's joints strong and their bones tough, enabling them to grow tall and excel in sports. In adulthood, these same factors will keep your joints well-lubricated and prevent aging bones from crumbling. No combination of supplements has the right balance of bioavailable minerals and collagen-derived growth factors to fortify your body as effectively as meat on the bone.

Organ meats bring the vitamins and brain-building fats that can ensure children will have mental stability and an aptitude for learning, and continued consumption of these foods is the best way to guarantee that your brain cells and nerves stay healthy for the rest of your life. Because these nutrients deteriorate so rapidly, no pills can effectively encapsulate them.

Fermented foods, full of probiotics, protect the intestinal tract from invading pathogens. Since a healthier intestine is more able to take in nutrients, probiotics may prevent infections and allergic disorders from developing elsewhere in the body, reducing the need for repeated doses of antibiotics. Probiotics living in our intestine also produce all sorts of vitamins, which help to round out a diet that might otherwise be deficient. Sprouted foods enable you to enjoy your breads and breakfast porridges without consuming the empty calories that cause obesity and diabetes.

And finally, fresh foods are naturally loaded with more antioxidants than can possibly survive the processes of drying, overcooking, or being stuffed into a capsule and bottled.

This is just a brief look at the benefits imparted by the Four Pillars. People who aren't connected to any culinary tradition don't consume any of the Four Pillars as often as they should. If you build your diet on the foundation of the Four Pillars, and get regular exercise and plenty of sleep, you will immediately notice vast improvements in how you feel. Those differences will compound over the years to keep you looking young.

Two Steps to Perfect Health

The first half of this book provided information that has, I hope, convinced you that the source of incredible health and vitality is no mystery. Rather than leaving your fate in the hands of, well, fate, you can take control of your genetic destiny by feeding your body the same nutrients your ancestors depended on. There are only two steps to doing that. First, find the best ingredients grown on the richest soil in the most wholesome, sustainable manner. Second, ensure that your body can use those nutrients most efficiently by preparing the raw materials according to the Four Pillars of World Cuisine.

When I say genetic destiny, I'm talking about your future *and* your children's as well. As you remember from previous chapters, the building of a whole body from a single fertilized cell requires an optimum nutritional environment. Every event during the 9 1/2 months *in-utero* is a minor miracle requiring a wholesome, rich environment. No physiologic event is as dramatic as the transcription of epigenetic data from gametes to zygote. And therefore none is as dependent on good nutrients, or more vulnerable to the interference of toxins.

Two Ingredients to Avoid

Most people are aware of the harmful effects of chemical residues leftover from industrial farming and of the preservatives and other agents that have harmful physiologic effects. And those of us who care about our health do what we can to avoid them. These two ingredients are different. Not only does each one seem perfectly engineered to prevent our cells from functioning the way they should, they often appear as a tag-team duo, showing up in the same foods together. I'm talking about vegetable oils and sugar.

I'm not saying that all the pollutants and toxins so often talked about aren't hurting our health. They are. But because vegetable oil and sugar are so nasty and their use in processed foods so ubiquitous that they have *replaced* nutrient-rich ingredients we would otherwise eat, I place vegetable oil and sugar before all others, on the very top of my *don't eat* list.

When traditional people wanted to send the message that certain foods were dangerous (or, in some cases, too special for non-royal persons) they'd place them on a do-not-eat list. In Hawaii, these foods were *kapu*, or forbidden. If they noticed that a food led to deleterious effects in newborns, then they would be *kapu* for expectant moms. Every indigenous society honored such a list; to ignore it could spell disaster for mother or child. Coming up, we'll see why vegetable oil and sugar are the real culprits for diseases most doctors blame on chance, or—even more absurdly—on the consumption of animal products that you need to eat to be healthy. Once you learn what they do inside your body, I hope you'll put them both on the top of your family's *kapu* list.

Eight

Good Fats and Bad

How the Cholesterol Theory Created a Sickness Epidemic

If you had asked me ten years ago what causes heart disease, I would have answered, "Fat and cholesterol, of course." I felt confident in this advice because it seemed to make intuitive sense; I could picture fat accumulating inside a person's artery, gradually choking it closed like cooking grease in a pipe. Moreover, the American Medical Association, the American Heart Association, the American Diabetes Association, the American Cancer Society, the American College of Cardiologists, and other organizations endorsed the cholesterol theory of heart disease.

There was one thing about this theory, however, that had been nagging me for a long time: Why, if cholesterol is so deadly, were so many of my oldest patients enjoying excellent health after a lifetime of consuming butter, eggs, and red meat?

Recently, physicians and scientists at the center of establishment medicine have started asking similar questions in light of increasing evidence that the cholesterol issue warrants revisiting. A few nutrition scientists at the Harvard School of Public Health have gone so far as to suggest that "the low-fat campaign has been based on little scientific evidence and may have caused unintended health consequences."[195] Further, they contend that the low-fat, anti-cholesterol campaign may not only be a flop as far as fighting obesity and diabetes, it may be making both epidemics worse.

Thanks to Michael Pollan, who cites this article and others like it in his book *In Defense of Food: An Eater's Manifesto*, the reading public has witnessed cracks forming in the foundation of modern nutritional thought. As more researchers discover all manner of evidence that animal fat has health-promoting effects (such data has now been published in dozens of academic journals), the pressure is building toward a sea change in organized medicine.[196] Until that change comes, however, your doctor is unlikely to contradict the official guidelines. Only when current guidelines change to reflect better science will the average doctor's advice on nutrition cease to put patients at risk for those "unintended health consequences." It is no revelation to suggest that the cholesterol theory—and confidence in the benefits of cholesterol-lowering drugs—is now deeply entrenched in the medical system. What you likely haven't heard is that your doctor may be one of thousands across the country whose pay will be docked if she refuses to aggressively treat patients with these powerful medications.

By the end of this chapter, you may be convinced that there is little reason to fear cholesterol. My hope is that, at the very least, you will recognize that the cholesterol theory of heart disease is far from unassailable and that, when your doctor admonishes you to "get your numbers down," you need not accept this advice without objection.

The other thing I want you to understand is that a necessary outgrowth of the indictment of cholesterol is a rejection of the traditional, natural fats that have sustained humankind for thousands of generations in favor of modern, factory-made oils. Theirs is an extraordinary position, requiring extraordinary evidence—a burden they have failed to meet.

To understand how the current theory of heart disease falls short, we will begin where it all went wrong, with the man regarded by many as the hero of modern nutritional thought.

The Man Who Brought Us the Low-Fat Campaign

It's 1958. A tall, fit Ancel Keys stands before a laboratory chalkboard on a popular CBS news show entitled "The Search" to warn us of something he calls "The new American plague." Onscreen, we see a row of ten little wooden men standing on Keys' desk. He flicks five of them with his finger, knocking them over as he speaks: "You know the chief killer of Americans is cardiovascular disease. Of ten men we can expect five to get it." From that moment forward, America would turn to Keys for advice on preventing heart disease.

The father of the "diet-heart hypothesis" was not a cardiologist or even an MD. Keys had earned his PhD in the 1930s studying salt-water eels. His nutritional credentialing originated in the fact that, during WWII, the military assigned him to create the ready-to-eat meal that could be stored for years and shipped to millions of soldiers. Dr. Keys named his pocket-sized meal the K-ration, after himself. When the war was over, the Minnesota public health department hired Keys to study the problem of rising rates of heart attacks. But ego got the better of him.

At his first scientific meeting he presented the idea that, in countries where people ate more animal fat, people died of heart disease more often, suggesting a possible causative relationship. But his statistical work was so sloppy (see figure) that he was lambasted by his peers. Rather than cleaning up his act, Keys vowed vengeance: "I'll show those guys."[197] More than anything else, it seems, Keys wanted everyone to think he single-handedly discovered the cause of heart disease. And so did the country's margarine producers, who now had the perfect spokesperson. Though Keys' work failed to convince professional scientists (at least for the first decade or two), the margarine industry knew he still had a shot at convincing the man on the street. If the public thought butter and other animal fats would "clog their arteries," they might buy margarine instead.

A few years after the embarrassing performance in front of an audience capable of sniffing out misleading statistics, Keys was on TV laying out those same, misleading statistics to a trusting public. The American Heart Association, which depends on large donations of cash from the vegetable oil industry, jumped on the bandwagon with Keys. They took his sloppy statistics and ran, eventually convincing most doctors that "steak is a heart attack on a plate" and margarine made from hydrogenated vegetable oils (full of trans fat) was healthy. Within a decade, grocery store shelves were loaded with ready-to-eat foods, and Americans were buying. No longer insisting on fresh food from small farmers right in our neighborhoods, we'd been convinced that products made in distant factories were safer, healthier, and better. Funny thing is, they were also cheaper. But even Keys had his doubts about eating them.

Oops! Everything I Said About Saturated Fat Was Really About Margarine —Paraphrasing Ancel Keys, PhD

By 1961, under increasing scientific scrutiny, Keys began to waver in his support for his own (now publicly accepted) diet-heart hypothesis.[198] Scientists had pointed out Dr. Keys' misleading use of scientific terms. In public, he denounced animal fat as the culprit behind the rising rates of heart attacks. But in his laboratory and human experiments, he didn't use animal fat.[199] His subjects were fed margarine made from partially hydrogenated vegetable oil. And what was in the margarine? Trans fat—a full 48 percent! To conclude from studies that used hydrogenated vegetable oil that animal fat causes heart disease is utterly nonsensical.

Unfortunately, the public never heard the straight story. Because margarine contains saturated fat (made during the hydrogenation process that also generates trans fat), industry had the opening they needed to put an anti-saturated-fat spin on Keys' findings. Ignoring the presence of trans (and other distorted fats in margarine), spokesmen simply blamed saturated fat. And on TV, Keys equated saturated fat with animal fat, completing the deception.[200] This ingenious spin on the facts is akin to poisoning rats with strychnine-laced milk and then blaming the deaths on the milk.

The anti-saturated fat, anti-cholesterol ball was rolling along nicely, and there was so much money being made selling "healthy" low-cholesterol, low-fat processed foods, the rolling ball wasn't going to be easy to stop. All the news reports you've ever heard on the hazards of saturated fat and cholesterol have been based on studies that were performed by using hydrogenated vegetable oil full of unnatural molecules that aren't found in butter, steak, or any natural food.[201] With so much junk science saturating the

How Keys Faked It

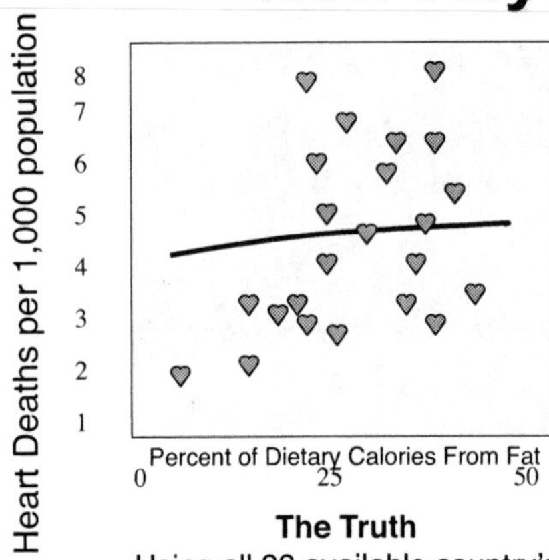

The Truth
Using all 22 available country's data, we see a poor relationship between total fat intake and heart disease

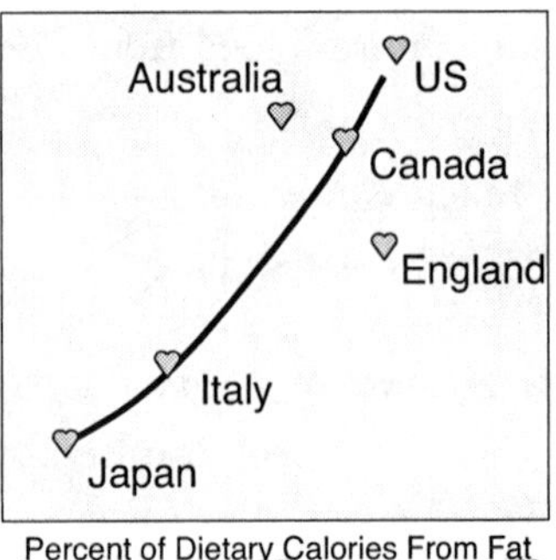

What Keys Published
Selecting six countries according to margarine use, and deleting the rest, produces a tight correlation.

Lies, Damn Lies, and Statistics. Keys blamed natural fat consumption for heart attacks. But the US, England, Canada and Australia had the highest levels of margarine consumption. Keys never mentions margarine in his famous Six-Countries Study and the deception was never exposed. Keys is still considered a hero of modern medicine.

media, professionals who give nutritional advice need to go beyond the sound bites to find the truth for themselves. While it's easy to go with the flow and tell patients to "cut out animal fat," doing so turns well-meaning healthcare practitioners into unwitting participants in an ongoing campaign to sell high profit-margin man-made substitutes for natural foods—substitutes which, in turn, make people ill.

Let's take a moment to look at some of the consequences of Dr. Keys' pet theory. Prior to his campaign, people ate far more saturated fat and cholesterol rich foods than we do today, but heart attacks were so rare they were almost unheard of.[202,203] Over the past century, as butter consumption dropped to less than one quarter of what it was (from 18 pounds per person per year to four), vegetable oil consumption went up five-fold (from eleven pounds per person per year to 59).[204,205] In 1900, heart disease was rare.[206] By 1950, heart problems were killing more men than any other disease.[207] Now, at the dawn of the second millennium, heart disease is the number one cause of death in both men and women.[208]

Natural fat consumption: down. Processed fat consumption: up. Heart disease: up—*way* up. Forget for a moment what the "experts" are saying, and ask yourself what these trends suggest to your inner statistician. The next time you go to the grocery store, see how many foods you can find that don't contain vegetable oil as an ingredient. What do you make of the fact that, while watching TV at home, you catch a 60-second health spot espousing the benefits of some low-cholesterol spread, followed by a commercial for a cholesterol drug, then another one for erectile dysfunction? What does this scenario say to the critical thinker in you?

What's been dropping us like flies is not any upsurge in saturated fat consumption, but an upsurge in consumption of *two major categories* of pro-inflammatory foods: vegetable oils (a.k.a. unnatural fats) and sugar. Cutting both from your diet will not only protect your heart, it will help protect you from *all* chronic diseases.

To help you understand why it's completely unscientific to blame natural fat for heart disease, I will appeal to your inner chemist, showing you why natural fats are beneficial. But first, I want to give you just a little bit of the history of these oils and why, though the wealthiest people (who have their own live-in chefs) rarely go near the stuff, vegetable oil has managed to work its way into nearly every product the rest of us eat every day. Food manufacturers use vegetable oils for the same reasons other manufacturers use plastic: It is easy to manipulate chemically, the public can be taught to ignore the consequences of its use and, best of all, it's cheap.

The First Bad Fat

In the late 1800s, Emperor Napoleon III offered a prize for a butter substitute to feed his army and "the lower classes."[209] The goal was a product that cost very little and wouldn't rot on extended sea voyages. After some experimentation, a chemist named Hippolyte Mege-Mourie found that squeezing slabs of tallow under pressure extracted oily elements that fused into a solid when churned together with skim milk. The dull grey material had a pearly sheen and so Mege-Mourie called it margarine, after the Greek *margarites*, meaning pearl. It didn't taste good, but it was cheap.

Not cheap enough for America, however. Raising, housing, feeding, breeding, and milking cows is an expensive enterprise compared to growing plants. By the turn of the century, chemists had found a way to reinvent the reinvented butter by starting with material nearer the bottom of the food chain: Cottonseeds. There were sacks and sacks of them lying around without much use. In fact, the tiny black seeds were hard to store because, if left alone, they would ferment and make a terrible stink. Chemists recognized that odoriferous volatiles meant the oil was reacting with oxygen, and they smelled opportunity. The reactive nature of the oil meant that it had the potential to be chemically modified for a variety of purposes and, soon enough, they found a way to spin this worthless byproduct of the textile industry into solid gold. Thus began a happy relationship between chemists, farmers, and petroleum companies that continues to this day.

To make the liquid cottonseed oil more like butter, they needed to thicken it into a solid paste. Chemistry offered two options: either tangling bunches of oil molecules together or making the individual molecules less flexible and more stackable. The first option creates a primordial form of plastic, too inedible to pass as food. So they chose the second option. They engineered a transformation of the fatty acids in the oil, ironing them almost flat with heat, pressure, and a nickel catalyst. The key to making the product appear edible was the catalyst, which prevented the molecules from tangling up into plastic. When the oils get squashed flat in this process, their double bonds change from the natural bent and flexible configuration to something stiffer. *Trans* fat was born.

We call partially hydrogenated fatty acids *trans* fat after the type of bond that holds the carbon atoms together. Naturally occurring fatty acids contain bonds in a *cis* configuration. In this configuration, fatty acids are highly flexible, which prevents crystallization (solidification), and so the molecules behave as liquids. Partial hydrogenation does two things: It irons some *cis*-configuration bonds completely flat and switches others around to *trans*. Converting a *cis* fatty acid to saturated or *trans* makes it a stiffer and more stackable molecule. This is why partially hydrogenated vegetable oils solidify like butter (which contains naturally stiff and stackable saturated fats). Cottolene was the first major brand to be successfully marketed in the US, over a century ago. It didn't taste quite like butter, but it was cheap. This process is still used to make "butter" for "the lower classes" today.

Now, most experts agree that consumption of inexpensive butter substitutes such as margarine and shortening is bad for our health. Nevertheless doctors are generally loath to recommend butter to their patients. So what do people use instead? Some of the most dangerous food products in the store.

Nature Doesn't Make Bad Fats

One of the fundamental concepts of this book is that physical beauty isn't, as it turns out, in the eye of the beholder. Beautiful living things are the manifestations of the immutable laws of natural growth, rules grounded in mathematics. These rules apply everywhere, even at the molecular level.

Biomolecules, including fatty acids, cholesterol, and DNA, typically twist into either hexagonal or pentagonal configurations to facilitate their interaction with each other and with water. Processing distorts the fatty acids in vegetable oil so that they can no longer assume the typical five- or six-sided geometry. Like Chinese finger traps, our enzymes pick up these dis-

Table 1: Good Fats and Bad

Good Fats These traditional fats can handle the heat involved in processing and cooking	**Bad Fats** These industrial-era fats cannot handle the heat involved in processing or cooking
Olive oil Peanut oil Butter (Yes, butter!) Macadamia nut oil Coconut oil Animal fats (lard, tallow) Palm oil	Canola oil Soy oil Sunflower oil Cottonseed oil Corn oil Grapeseed oil Safflower oil Non-butter spreads (including margarine and the so-called Trans-free spreads)

Table 2: Foods Loaded with Pro-Inflammatory Fat (Don't eat these)	
Margarine and Spreads	The classic "one molecule away from plastic" food that backyard animals won't eat. Very little in here other than trans fat and twisted fatty acids that are worse than trans. Don't let kids near it; it interferes with normal bone growth and sexual development.
Salad Dressing	Aside from water and vinegar, most store-bought salad dressing is pure vegetable oil plus sugar and flavoring agents.
Rice Milk	One serving contains 1 tsp vegetable oil and just under an ounce of liquefied rice. There's nothing else to this stuff—except the synthetic vitamins. We tell diabetics not to eat rice, so why would drinking it be good for anyone?
Soy Milk, Soy Cheese, Soy-based Meat Products	Processing damages the soy bean's cell membranes, releasing PUFAs which are rapidly oxidized to harmful MegaTrans fats. Whole soy beans can be part of a healthy diet.
Breakfast Cereals	Most breakfast cereals are extruded, pressed, flaked, and/or puffed. The slurry is then hardened with a coating of vegetable oil, which acts like a protective varnish that can maintain the product's shape and prevent dampness from making it soggy.
Nuts (Oily nuts only. Raw or dry roasted nuts are good for you, but read labels carefully.)	Nuts are often cooked in "peanut and/or vegetable oil." Peanut oil would be fine, but since it costs five to ten times more than vegetable oil, I doubt they use peanut. Nuts are more vitamin and amino-acid rich when eaten raw.
French Fries	Restaurants can reuse frying oil for a week or longer. These oils can turn so toxic that they are often too degraded to be recycled as biodiesel fuel.
Crackers and Chips	Many patients assume that since crackers are bland, they are healthy. (This always makes me sad. Blandness indicates an absence of nutrients.) Factory-made crackers and chips are fried in oils that can be used over and over, increasing the concentration of the worst kinds of pro-inflammatory fats: MegaTrans.
Granola	Up to half the calories in granola may come from vegetable oil.
Soft breads, buns, and most store bought muffins	I saved these for last because, though the total unnatural fat content tends to be low, most people eat a lot of these products in a typical week, and they constitute a major source of trans and especially harmful, pro-inflammatory MegaTrans fats.

torted fatty acids and then can't let them go, which hampers cellular function so profoundly it can kill your cells. And if you eat enough trans, cellular dysfunction will eventually kill you. Vegetable oils rarely kill children, but they can disrupt normal metabolism so profoundly that a child's *dynamic symmetry* is lost, and their skeletal proportions become imbalanced.

No food represents such a full spectrum of molecules—from healthy to distorted and extremely toxic—as fat. Good fats are some of the best foods you can eat. And some of the healthiest, most robust people on the planet live in cultures whose diets are highly dependent on natural fats, like animal fat. But take those good-fat foods away and replace them with foods high in refined carbohydrates and distorted fats, and the same problems we have in our country begin to crop up around the world: weight gain, heart troubles, mood disorders, other chronic diseases, newborn children exhibiting organ and facial deformation and other hallmarks of physical degeneration. So far, establishment medicine blames milk and meat. But I blame toxic, distorted fats (and sugar). Fortunately, the principle behind avoiding toxic, distorted fats is easy to remember: *Eat natural fats and avoid processed ones*. This formula works because nature doesn't make bad fat, factories do.

The seductive flavors of fat-rich foods tempt us for good reason. Unlike sugar—which offers no nutrition—a meal complete with animal fat actually helps us absorb and taste other nutrients. This is why butter makes other foods taste so delicious.[210,211,212,213] And because animal fats contains cholesterol—a natural appetite suppressant—they satisfy in a way that little else can.[214,215,216] In contrast, vegetable oils impair vitamin absorption and do little to suppress appetite, so you eat more and get less nutrition.[217]

When you worry about chemicals hidden in modern food, you might first think of MSG, pesticide residues, and contaminants, like mercury. But compared to bad fats, those are small potatoes. Of all the dietary changes attending modernization, nothing compares to what we've done with fats and oils. Over the past 100 years in the US, our fat intake has gone from largely animal-based and natural to plant-based and so unnatural that our bodies can't adapt. Thanks to Dr. Keys and his associates in industry, and now, also in the AMA, we have been tricked into questioning our own senses, convinced that our health depends on staying away from these once-prized sources of sustenance and herded into buying tasteless, processed, "neutral" vegetable oils instead. Without even realizing it, we've traded in healthy fats for toxic ones, and now it's making us sick.[218]

The Trouble With Vegetable Oil

Let me ask you something: What do you supposed would happen if, several decades ago, an unknown lipid scientist conclusively proved that an artificial fat molecule present in margarine, as well as all kinds of other products for sale in every grocery store in the country, was deadly, and was very likely causing disease, growth defects, and premature mortality. And what if that scientist had the opportunity to present this public health information to Congress? Would Congress have responded? Would their corporate supporters—companies as powerful as Unilever, Monsanto, and ADM—have recalled the millions of products containing the toxin, halted their production lines, given up their subsidies and, if necessary, torn up millions of acres of corn which (no longer devoted to the production of margarine) would no longer be needed? Would they have abandoned margarine production and gone back to making real butter, trading in the cash cow of margarine products for actual, milk-producing cows? Or, rather, would the corn product freight train roar straight through the scientist's warnings, and even pick up speed as agribusiness marketing engineers frantically shoveled disinformation into the firebox?

We don't have to guess at the answer, because there was such a scientist, and her findings were brought to Congress—back in 1977—to warn of the dangers of trans, present in hydrogenated oils. We can only presume that the wealthy politicians who learned of Dr. Mary Enig's research had little personal experience with cheap butter substitutes or the convenience foods that contain them. But the rest of us were eating plenty of the stuff and we continued to do so decades after Enig's warnings because we never heard them. Only after European countries outlawed trans fat did we finally hear that it might be bad for our health.

Why did it take the US so long to take trans fat seriously? Earlier, I mentioned that scientific discoveries that are incompatible with commercial interests have a tough time making it to the papers. Trans is just one example. Cigarette smoking, another. Asbestos, another still. And, I'm guessing that, if there's something you and your family might be eating every day that scientists already know is deadly, you'd like to know about it now, not 30 years from now. That's why I'd like to tell you the truth about vegetable oil.

Vegetable Oil Should Not Be Heated

Vegetable oils contain mostly heat-sensitive *polyunsaturated* fats. When heated, these fragile fats turn into toxic compounds including trans fat.[219] The heat sensitivity issue means that all processed vegetable oils, and all products that contain vegetable oil, necessarily contain trans fat. Canola oil degrades so rapidly that a testing company, needing to find the purest canola oil to use as a standard against which other oils could be compared, couldn't locate any canola oil even from pharmaceutical-grade manufacturers with a trans fat content lower than 1.2 percent.[220]

This means that vegetable oil, and products made from vegetable oil, contain trans fat—even when the label seems to guarantee them trans free. But because heat so readily distorts their fatty acids, vegetable oil, and products made from vegetable oil, also contain something that is worse for us than trans. Before we get to that, I'd like to take a moment to compare and contrast the various fatty acids and their ability to handle heat.

Who Can Take the Heat? Cooking-Fat Basics

For the purposes of cooking, we want to pick the kinds of fats that can take heat. On that count, saturated fats (present in butter, coconut oil, lard, and traditional fats) win hands down. Why? Because they can resist a kind of heat-related damage called *oxidation*. Thanks to their shape, saturated fats have no room for oxygen to squeeze in, and even high heat can't force these tough molecules to be more accommodating. Monounsaturated fats have room for just one oxygen molecule to sneak in. But it's not easy, so monoun-

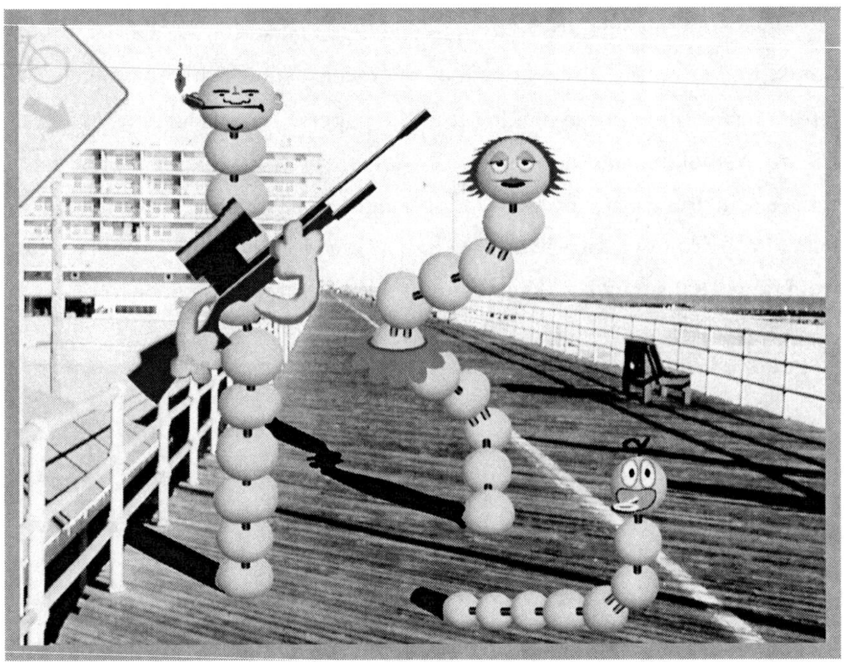

Figure 1. The Fatty Acids. Saturated Fat (left), Polyunsaturated Fat (center) and Monounsaturated Fat (right). With no double bonds, saturated fat resists oxidation and is nearly immune to free radicals. Because saturated fat can stop free radicals in their tracks, saturated fat protects other members of the fatty acid family.

saturated fat-rich olive oil is still okay to cook with. Polyunsaturated fat—now that's another story. As it turns out, having two places where oxygen can react makes reactions not twice as likely to occur, but *billions* of times more likely. This exponential increase in reactivity is true of molecules generally, not just fats. TNT (trinitrotoluene) has six places where oxygen can react, making it so reactive it's literally explosive! But we're not cooking with explosives in our frying pans, are we? Actually, in a sense we are, though on a slightly less dramatic scale. And it is those explosive oxidative reactions that we need to avoid.

The oils extracted from seeds that get processed into vegetable oils are composed primarily of polyunsaturated fatty acids, PUFAs for short. If you want to remember which type of fatty acid most readily reacts with oxygen, just remember this: *"PUFAs go Poof!"*

Biology makes use of this reactivity. Enzymes in plants and animals fuse oxygen to polyunsaturated fats on purpose to change them from one shape to another. For example, fish oil isn't anti-inflammatory per se. The human body deliberately oxidizes the PUFAs in fish oil to convert them to anti-inflammatory agents. But this mutability also means polyunsaturated fats are more capable of being accidentally altered, and thus heat is a threat to their utility.

Where Does Vegetable Oil Come From?

Vegetable oil is the lipid extracted from *corn, canola, soy, sunflower, cottonseed, safflower, rice bran* and *grapeseed*. Vegetable oil doesn't come from broccoli, and it doesn't equate to a serving of greens. It is found in almost all ready-made foods, from granola and squishy-soft baked goods, to rice milk and soymilk, to vegetarian cheese and meat substitutes, to frozen meals and side dishes, even salad dressings that say olive oil on the front. I once purchased a package of dried blueberries only to discover, after I brought it home and read the label, that they were coated with vegetable oil.

There's a reason these oils are particularly temperature sensitive. Seeds stay dormant over the cold winter. But come spring thaw, the heat-sensitive PUFAs wake up in response to warming, facilitating germination.[221] To protect the PUFAs from damage as the ground warms and the sun's rays beat down on them, the plant has loaded its seeds with antioxidants. Unfortunately, refining these oils ultimately destroys both healthy PUFAs and their complementary antioxidants, converting them into distorted, unhealthy molecules. So what was healthy in the seed isn't healthy in the bottle.

Canola Oil: Just Another Vegetable Oil

When I advise my patients to avoid vegetable oils, they often tell me that they only use canola oil, as if it were somehow exempt. I can't blame them for thinking this; the canola industry goes to great lengths to present their product as heart healthy, and the American Heart Association plays right along. They claim that canola oil is rich in anti-inflammatory omega-3 essential fats. And there's a grain—I should say *seed*—of truth to that claim. There's just one problem: omega-3 is a PUFA, which means it is easily distorted when exposed to heat. And since the omega-3 in the canola seeds has *three* places for oxygen to react, it's really, really reactive. Canola oil still in the seed may indeed be full of omega-3, but factory-processed canola oil, *even organic expeller pressed,* contains mutated, oxidized, heat-damaged versions of once-healthy fats.[222] If we could somehow get canola oil out of the seed without exposing it to heat, it would be good for us. But nobody can.

Well, that's not entirely true. In the old days, flax and rapeseed (a relative of canola) were gently extracted in the home using a small wedge press. Over the course of a day, the wedge would be tapped into the press a little further until, ever so slowly, the golden oil would start to drip, fresh and full of natural antioxidants and vitamins. These oils were *not* used to fry food, and therefore never exposed to damaging heat. If you aren't up for installing a wedge press in your kitchen, a few small enterprises can provide flax, hemp, and other healthy omega-3 rich oils—none of which should ever be used for cooking.

"*Stop The Presses!*" Oil Seeds Plead, "*You're Squeezing Me Too Hard!*"

If we took a stethoscope and placed it to the side of a giant factory press as it applied more and more intense heat and pressure to a batch of tiny oil seeds, we might very well hear the following: "Ouch!" Or words to that effect. The muffled cries that follow would indicate that, rather than being treated like little ambassadors of a heart-healthy diet, they were being processed and refined like so much motor oil. In fact, one of the initial steps involves the use of hexane, a component of gasoline. If you were to get up close and catch the stench of the initial extract, you might never imagine it could be cleaned up. Making these stinky oils palatable requires a degree in chemical engineering; it takes twenty or so additional stages to bleach and deodorize the dark, gunky muck. So-called health products contain "expeller pressed" oil, which only means they didn't use hexane gas. Organic, expeller-pressed oil has gone through all the other steps.

Olive, palm and other oils that are good for us (see Table 1) have mostly saturated and monounsaturated fatty acids, which are not so fragile. They are also easily extracted at low temperatures. Vegetable oils come out less readily, and are more prone to side-reactions that polymerize and mutate the fat molecules. So getting them out creates a witches' brew of toxic lipids, only some of which will be removed. The rest, you eat.

Chemical analysis shows that even bottles of organic, expeller-pressed canola oil contain as much as five percent trans fats, plus cyclic hydrocarbons (carcinogens) and oxyphytosterols (highly damaging to arteries).[223] Of course, natural fats are all okay before they're processed and refined, so there's no harm in eating corn, soybeans, sunflower and other tasty seeds.

Inflammation and Free Radicals

Maybe five percent trans (and other mutant fats) doesn't sound that scary. The real trouble is not so much that there's bad fat in the bottles (and other products). The real trouble has to do with the fact that after you eat these distorted, mutated fatty acids, they can reproduce inside you.

Imagine a zombie movie, filmed at the molecular level, except the mutant fattys don't stumble through your bloodstream in slow motion. Using *free radicals* (defined in the next section), mutated PUFAs convert normal fatty acids into fellow ghouls at the rate of billions per second. I call this conversion-on-contact *the Zombie effect* because, as every horror-movie connoisseur knows, when a zombie bites you, you become one of *them*. When a throng of molecular miscreants starts hacking away at your cells, things can really get scary. Their ability to damage normal PUFAs makes this class of oxidized PUFAs more dangerous than the trans fat we've all heard about on the news. Since they're a lot like trans, only worse, I call them *MegaTrans*.

There are many technical names for MegaTrans, including peroxidized fats, lipoxygenases, oxidized fat, lipid peroxides, lipid hydroperoxides, and a few others. Think of them all as different gangs of bad fats. While some of these toxic fats are in the trans configuration and others aren't, that's not the

Normal Heart

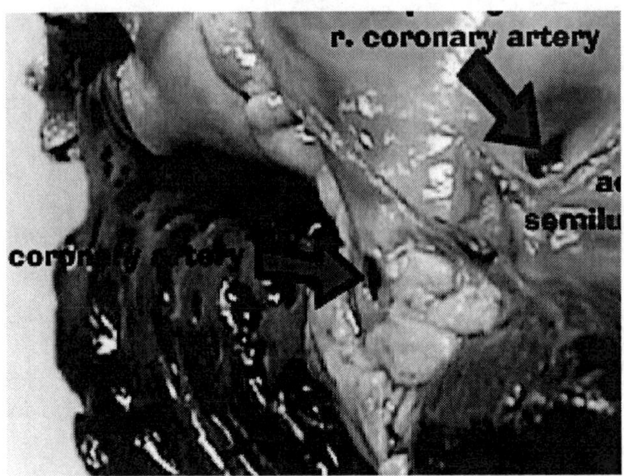

Figure 2. Healthy Hearts are Smooth, Glistening, and Clean. The upper right corner of the picture shows the inner lining of the aorta where the arteries supplying the heart muscle itself branch off, the top arrow points to the right coronary artery. Compare this to figure 3.

point. The point is these toxic fats are all gangsters with one thing in common: They're really bad for you. They contaminate all foods with trans fat and, in fact, all foods made from vegetable oils. They're bad because they lead to the formation of free radicals, which not only turn normal polyunsaturated fatty acids into mutants; free radicals can damage almost any part of your body: cell membranes, chromosomes, other fats—you name it.

The Reason Vegetable Oil Inflames Your Arteries

Free radicals are high-energy electrons that are involved in every known disease. They behave like molecular radiation, burning everything with which they come into contact, inside your body or out.

In the frying pan, MegaTrans reacts with oxygen to generate one free radical after another. Frying in vegetable oils doesn't so much cook your foods as blast them with free radicals—fusing molecules together to make

French Fried Heart

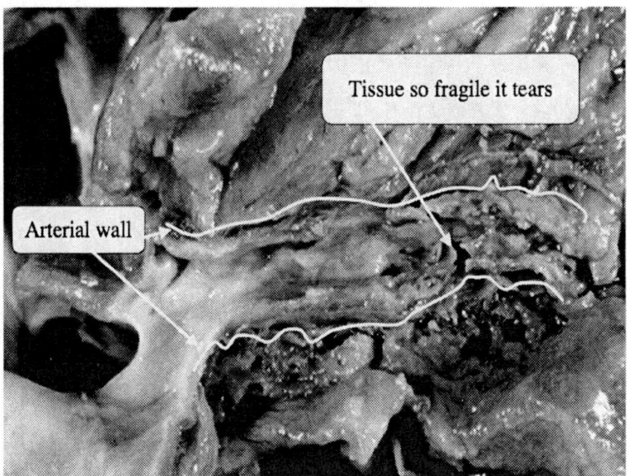

Figure 3. Heart Attack Victim. When arterial linings are coated with MegaTrans fat, free radical cascades literally fry living tissue. Here, the artery and surrounding heart muscle are greasy and fragile, much like crispy fried food. Compare this to Figure 2.

the material solid. Chemists call this series of reactions a *free radical cascade*. Free radical cascades damage normal PUFAs, turning them into ugly molecular ghouls (the Zombie effect). Just a little MegaTrans in the bottle of canola oil can become a lot of MegaTrans after you—or the cereal/donut/frozen dinner manufacturers—cook with it. On the plus side, free radical cascades make your food extremely crispy. (Free radical cascades also happen to play a role in the polymerization reactions that make plastic solid. This is probably the origin of the well intentioned, but not strictly scientific, assertion that "margarine is one molecule away from plastic.") On the minus side, free radical cascades make your arteries extremely crispy. They will also damage other bodily tissues, which can generate *inflammation*, a kind of chemical chaos that interferes with normal metabolic function.

Traditional cooking methods often make nutrients more bioavailable and are, for that reason, anti-inflammatory. Cooking with vegetable oil, on the other hand, destroys complex nutrients. So aside from the fact that foods cooked in vegetable oil will deposit loads of Zombie fats into your tissues where they can, with little provocation, blast your tissues with free radicals, foods cooked with vegetable oils will also carry fewer vitamins and antioxidants than foods cooked using traditional methods and better oils.

Free radicals can fry your arteries and, as I suggested earlier, eating foods fried in vegetable oil may very well precipitate a heart attack. But something happens before you have a full-blown heart attack: Your arteries stop responding to normal body stresses. It's called abnormal *endothelial function*. And there's a test for that.

How Your Doctor Can Tell If You Have French-Fried Arteries: ED and Endothelial Function

In 1999, a team of lipid scientists in New Zealand wanted to see what eating deep-fried food does to our arteries in the short term. They planned to feed subjects french fries and then test them to see if their blood vessels were still able to regulate blood flow normally (this ability is called endothelial function). The test is performed by slipping the patient's arm into a blood pressure cuff, then squeezing it to cut off the blood flow for a few minutes. Normally, on releasing the cuff again, the oxygen-starved arteries open wider so blood can come rushing back in, just like you would suck in more air after holding your breath for a while. This dilation response depends on the *endothelial* cells lining the blood vessels, which have to be healthy enough to generate the *nitric oxide* that makes arteries dilate. If endothelial cells can't make nitric oxide, or if the nitric oxide they make gets destroyed too soon, a person's circulatory system can't work correctly.

Male sexual function depends on healthy endothelial function, for reasons that pertain to arterial dilation and the obvious tissue expansion facilitated by such dilation. What may be less obvious is, if a person has ED (erectile dysfunction), they (most likely) have endothelial dysfunction, meaning their health problems extend beyond the bedroom. Specialized centers can perform an endothelial function test on anyone. This easy test tells your doctor how healthy your arteries are and how readily they can deliver blood in

Vegetable Oil: Good Mother, Bad Babies

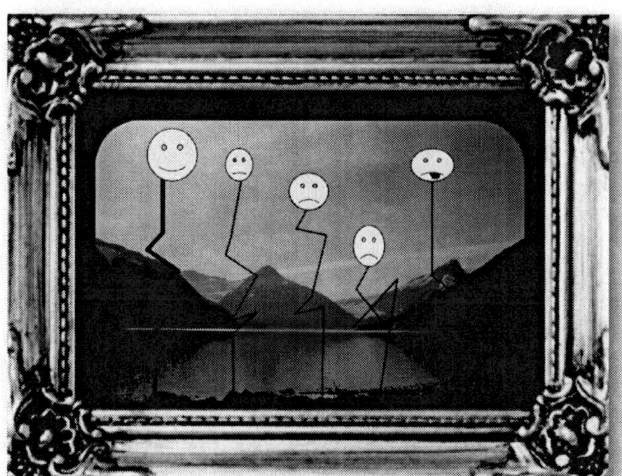

Figure 4. Normal PUFA (Left) and Heat-Damaged Offspring (Vacationing in North America). This is the family of fats found in margarine, spreads, and vegetable oils. The mother of the family is linoleic acid, an essential fatty acid of the omega-6 family. Notice her symmetry; she is the only natural fat in this picture. On the right, giving us the raspberry, is the most well known of the distorted fatty acids, trans fat. In the middle, are other distorted fats. Notice their asymmetric, almost random shapes. These are most plentiful in used frying oils. Omega-3 fats in canola and fish oils can also serve as the parent molecule for a similar-looking family of heat-damaged fats.

response to exercise or other activities.

The scientists in New Zealand acquired week-old frying oil from a typical restaurant (rich in MegaTrans), and made one more batch of fries. Four hours after study subjects ate the fries, they slipped their arms into blood pressure cuffs to test their endothelial function. The effect of the oil was unmistakable. Before the fries, the subjects' arteries had dilated normally, opening seven percent wider. Afterwards, there was almost no dilation—barely one percent.[224] (Is week-old frying oil commonly used? While the law requires that fryer oil be replaced weekly, I know one restaurant owner who told me of a new oil that extends this time to two weeks or even longer.[225])

What this test tells us is that after eating food fried in vegetable oil, your blood vessels won't work right. You may feel lethargic. Men may suffer from temporary ED. As the authors point out, exercising after a fast food meal will

How Can Something So Bad Taste So Good?

If fast-food fries and other crispy treats are so awful, why would nature allow them to tempt our tongues so tantalizingly?

Fast-food flavors are not real. Were they not doped with MSG, sugar, and other chemicals, you'd realize how flat those curly fries and meat nuggets taste. They're crispy, yes, but they lack flavor complexity. What happened? Processing and cooking with vegetable oil destroys complex nutrients and deadens flavors. (Flavor ligands become fused, rendering them either unrecognizable or too large to fit into your taste bud receptors.) You can get all the tangy, zesty, savoryness that you love in fast food from traditional cooking methods that enhance food flavors naturally by making nutrients more bioavailable.

also stress your heart.[226] Why? MegaTrans free radicals attack the nitric oxide signal that arteries send when they sense oxygen levels are low. Without that signal, your muscles don't get the oxygen they need. The most active muscles will be the most affected—and your heart is always active.

Men with ED have sick endothelial cells that can't generate normal amounts of nitric oxide. Viagra works by helping sick endothelial cells in the penile arteries generate nitric oxide as if they were healthy. Nasty frying oil temporarily inhibits that ability. You could call it anti-Viagra. But listen up boys: if you keep eating foods made with vegetable oil (especially if you also eat too much sugar), you'll damage those endothelial cells so much that even Viagra won't work any more.

The New Zealand study was performed on young people with healthy arteries, but what might happen to a person whose arteries are older, or already damaged? After reading the study, I started asking patients admitted to the hospital for heart attacks what they'd eaten last. So far, *everyone* has told me they ate something fried in vegetable oil. One Japanese man had eaten fried fish, which goes to show you: The use of vegetable oil can turn an otherwise healthy meal into a 911 emergency. That winded feeling you get when you try to exercise may be a sign that you are just out of shape. But it may mean that MegaTrans has already damaged your arteries.

The Best Test for Arterial Damage

An endothelial function test will tell you something about the health of your arteries. But there's an easier way to determine whether or not they've been damaged. If you've been eating vegetable oil and sugar-rich foods, you can be certain they have. Some people want proof, of course. It's like spending money; some of us know when we've been spending more cash than we're bringing in, and others of us have to look at that bank statement to confirm the bad news. So if you can't get an endothelial function test, but you still want to test the condition of your blood vessels, there are several other things you can do.

One is to have your doctor check your fasting blood sugar level. If it's 89 or higher, you may have *prediabetes,* a condition in which your cell membranes have become too rigid to take in glucose as fast as they normally could. (This often leads to insulin resistance and "full blown" diabetes.) And what makes cell membranes stiff? MegaTrans-instigated free radical damage, nutrient deficiency, and sugar. It's also not a bad idea to check your blood pressure. Normal levels range from 80-120 over 50-75. Higher than 130/80 (while relaxed) can indicate abnormal endothelial function. You can also get a test of your liver enzymes. Elevated liver enzymes occur when MegaTrans explosions damage liver cells. Finally, you can get a cholesterol test. But interpreting the test correctly requires some knowledge of the way fats circulate through your body, a physiologic function I call *The Lipid Cycle.*

How I Interpret Cholesterol Levels: Introducing the Lipid Cycle

The idea that fat clogs up our arteries the way it clogs up the pipe under the kitchen sink creates a powerful image. But it's wrong. You can eat all the fat and cholesterol you want, and none of it will get into your arteries without first being wrapped inside a special layer of protein. These special proteins suspend all the fats inside them in the solution of our bloodstream, and this is what prevents dietary fat from clogging our arteries. The resulting little blobs of fat wrapped in protein are called *lipoproteins.*

You've heard of LDL and HDL? Those are two types of lipoproteins.

Lipoproteins: Superheroes of Lipid Circulation

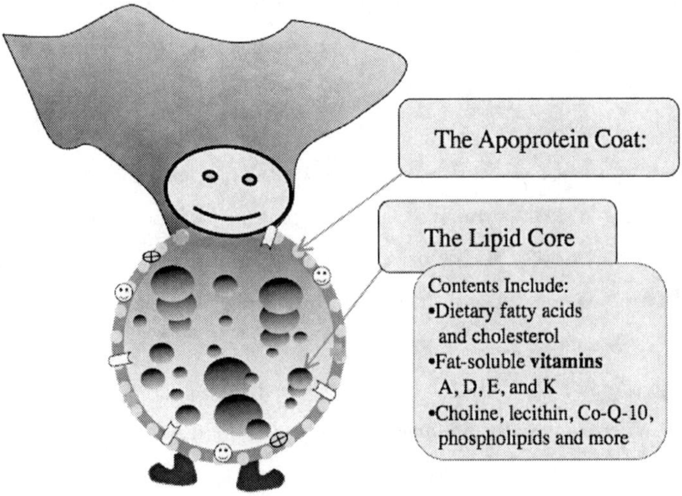

The Apoprotein Coat:

The Lipid Core

Contents Include:
•Dietary fatty acids and cholesterol
•Fat-soluble **vitamins** A, D, E, and K
•Choline, lecithin, Co-Q-10, phospholipids and more

Figure 5. Lipoproteins Carry Fat-soluble Nutrients in the Bloodstream. Lipoproteins have two essential parts, like an M&M: an outer coating (made of proteins called apoproteins), and soft, yummy insides (made of fat, called the lipid core).

Lipoproteins are designed like M&Ms: just as the candy's coating prevents the chocolate inside it from getting all over your hands, the protein coat enables lipoproteins to circulate throughout your body without getting their messy insides smeared on your arterial walls. Of course, lipoproteins don't carry chocolate. If your diet is healthy, your lipoproteins are full of essential fats, vitamins—all kinds of good stuff. If you eat bad fat, your lipoproteins carry bad fat too, and that can make the whole fat circulation system break down. When the fat circulation system breaks down, people's cholesterol numbers get out of whack. HDL may go down, while LDL and triglycerides may go up. Let's take a closer look.

How the Lipid Cycle is Supposed to Work

If you eat like the average American, somewhere around forty percent of your dietary calories probably come from fats (in my case, it's more like 70

Lipoproteins: The Nitty Gritty

A lipoprotein is a particle made of fat (lipid) that's been wrapped with a protein coat (hence, lipo-protein). Some lipoproteins are big, and some are small. The big ones are generally lower in density than the small ones because they carry so much buoyant fat. Some of the big ones are called LDL, for low-density lipoprotein. And some of the smaller ones are called HDL, for high-density lipoprotein. Sound bite science has us calling HDL "good" and LDL "bad," but these terms are misleading. Both LDL and HDL help deliver vitamins and essential fatty acids to our tissues. Though it may contain bad fats, no lipoprotein is inherently bad. Furthermore, lipoproteins exist in a wide variety of densities (their particular density depending how much protein they contain), and their densities vary as they circulate throughout the body during their life cycle. The binary designations of "high" and "low" density are arbitrary and only add to the confusion. Calling LDL and HDL bad and good *cholesterol* doesn't make sense either, because lipoproteins aren't cholesterol. They are protein-encased particles that contain cholesterol *and all sorts of other kinds of fats*—many of which are vitamins and other essential materials. Lipoproteins distribute all these materials to tissues in need. Without enough of these tiny nutrient couriers in circulation, our tissues would starve.

percent). As we've seen, the job of the lipoproteins is to make sure all that nutrition gets distributed correctly. Lipoproteins contain some cholesterol, but mostly they contain triglycerides, other fatty nutrients (like lecithin, choline, essential fatty acids, and phospholipids), varying amounts of fat-soluble vitamins, and retinoids—all wrapped inside a protein coat.

After your food is broken down by enzymes in the intestine, the fat and most other nutrients get absorbed into intestinal cells (called *enterocytes*). Here, fat and fat-soluble nutrients are prepared for circulation through the bloodstream. Since fat particles won't dissolve in blood, the intestinal cells wrap these tiny balls of fatty nutrients in a protein coat. Lipoproteins made in the intestine are called *chylomicrons*. Other tissues that participate in the lipid cycle make other types of lipoproteins, all with the same general design: a blob of fat wrapped in protein.

Cells that make lipoproteins don't throw just any old protein coating over the fats, kick the little particle out into circulation and say, "Good luck!" The cells of our bodies must be able to recognize lipoproteins as sources of fatty nutrients. So the protein coating (made of *apoproteins*) also serves as a kind of barcode describing the particle's origin and contents. When released

Cholesterol Numbers: The Nitty Gritty

Your cholesterol profile contains *four* different numbers: total cholesterol, LDL, HDL, and a triglyceride value. The two numbers I'm most interested in are the triglyceride and HDL levels. HDL should be over 45 in men and over 50 in women (I've seen it as high as 108.) I like to see LDL less than three times the HDL value. This ratio, together with triglyceride levels less than 150, tell me a person's fat-distribution system, lipoproteins, and diet are healthy. I don't worry about a high *total* cholesterol number if the *ratio* of LDL to HDL is within an acceptable range. On the other hand, if triglycerides are above 150 and/or HDL level below 40, it's very likely that your lipoprotein cycle is disrupted.

into circulation, the wonderfully designed apoproteins also function like little handles, enabling hungry cells to grab the lipoprotein particle as it floats by.

As with any package delivery service, the accuracy of this labeling system is critical to the success of the whole delivery process. If anything were to damage the label (we'll return to this idea soon), the lipoprotein would fail to carry out its function, and the whole system would be thrown out of whack.

After the packaged lipoprotein leaves an intestinal cell, it travels through the bloodstream for several hours, completing many circuits. As it floats along, it deposits its fatty nutrients into the tissues that need them most.

Hungry tissues get fed by signaling endothelial cells lining their smallest blood vessels to place special proteins on their surface, which act like tiny fishing rods set to snag lipoproteins as they float by. Once snagged, the particle may unload some of its payload into the endothelial cell or, alternatively, the endothelial cell may open up a tunnel-like structure right through its center to allow the lipoprotein to pass from the bloodstream, through the endothelial cell, and directly into the hungry tissues.

Hours after a meal, the amount of fat in circulation drops as lipoproteins either exit the circulation or give up their fat and shrink (gradually increasing in *density* as they travel). Eventually, the liver picks up the shrunken, high-density remnants and sorts through the contents to recycle anything useful while discarding any waste. Unwanted or damaged fats exit by way of the bile system back into the intestinal tract for disposal.

The lipid cycle can take any of several different routes. Fats can enter the circulation by way of the intestine (as chylomicrons) or by way of the liver, or even by way of the skin. There are actually multiple points of entry. Even the brain may participate. Fats can exit the cycle by being transported into a hungry cell, or by being exported out of the body through the liver's bile system.

The liver is like a transfer station. It sorts through the incoming lipoproteins to separate the good fats from the bad. When it has collected enough good fats, the liver fashions its own lipoproteins (called VLDL, for Very LDL), complete with new identifying labels, and sends them back into the bloodstream again. These particles go through another arm of the cycle, following the same series of steps, delivering cargo piecemeal or transporting to a final destination intact. Those particles that deliver cargo piecemeal eventually get small enough to be picked up by the liver again, where they will be disassembled and their fats either discarded or recycled once more.

One loop of the lipid cycle starts in the intestine and distributes lipids you just ate. Another starts in the liver and distributes lipoproteins your liver made. And a third loop starts in the *periphery*—that is, the rest of the body—and distributes lipoproteins made by the skin, brain, and other organs. Each of the three sources (intestine, liver, and periphery) manufactures its own brand of lipoproteins complete with its own proprietary labels.

When everything works properly, your arteries stay wide-open, pretty pink, and clean. But when fats don't get delivered properly, they pile up in the bloodstream, damaging epithelial cells and giving arteries a yellowish, irregular, lumpy appearance that is conspicuously unhealthy (see Figure 3).

Obviously, this intricate and ancient internal postal system is amazing and complex. And I don't mean to imply, by describing it to you, that I know everything about the way it works. I don't. But let me tell you a secret: neither do the drug manufacturers who tell us we need to get our LDL numbers down, and they have just the pill to do it. As with any system of the body, you don't need to fully understand it to be able to disrupt it with powerful chemicals, which is exactly what cholesterol-lowering drugs do.

How Bad Diet Damages Lipoproteins and Causes Arterial Disease

To understand how diet affects HDL, LDL, and triglyceride levels, imagine a six-year-old girl traveling back and forth across the country by plane between the homes of her divorced mom and dad. Suppose that this young child is traveling unchaperoned and carries an identification tag on a string around her neck displaying her name, the addresses of both parents, and contact information. If the receiving parent wasn't at the airport, this tag would enable airport officials to know who she was, where she was coming from, and where she needed to go. But if the tag were to get damaged so that

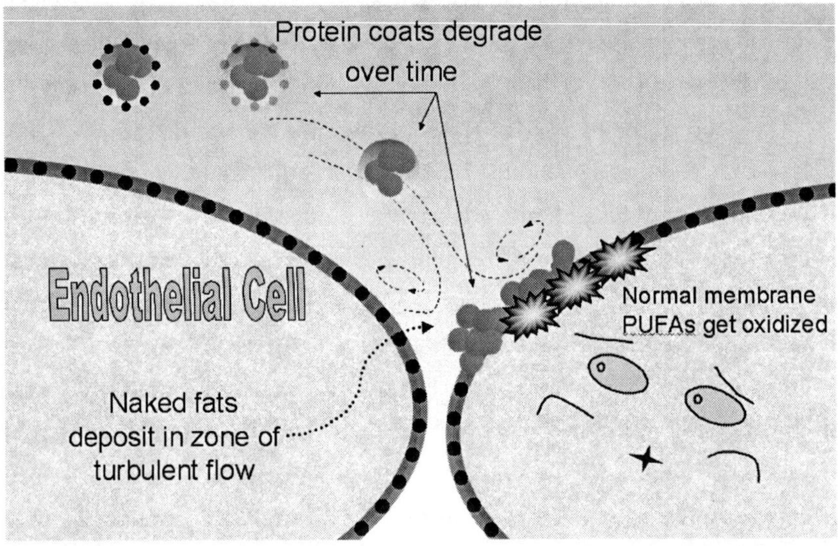

Figure 6. Fatty Streak: How Atherosclerosis Begins. The endothelial cell on the right is worried because bad fats from degraded lipoproteins are landing on his outer membrane where they incite free radical cascades that can interfere with normal cell metabolism or even kill the cell, see Figure 7. Once the endothelial cells are damaged or destroyed, bad fats can seep directly into the tissue below, where they can attract white blood cells into the arterial wall. This is the earliest stage of atherosclerosis, called the "fatty streak."

the words became unintelligible, it wouldn't do any good, and she'd be lost.

If your lipoprotein particles have their labels damaged, they can get lost too. Like vagrant children hopelessly tugging the shirtsleeves of every stranger they see, lipoproteins missing proper identification are given the cold shoulder from cells unable to recognize them. These orphaned lipoproteins float aimlessly through the bloodstream, begin to disintegrate, and ultimately collect onto the lining of your arteries (see Figure 6) where they may cause problems.

What damages lipoprotein labels? One of the most important factors appears to be sugar. As I'll discuss in the next chapter, sugar adheres to things by a process called *glycation*. Over time, this stiffens cell membranes, leading to prediabetes and consistently elevated blood sugar levels. Whenever blood sugar levels are high, it creates an opportunity for sugar to gum

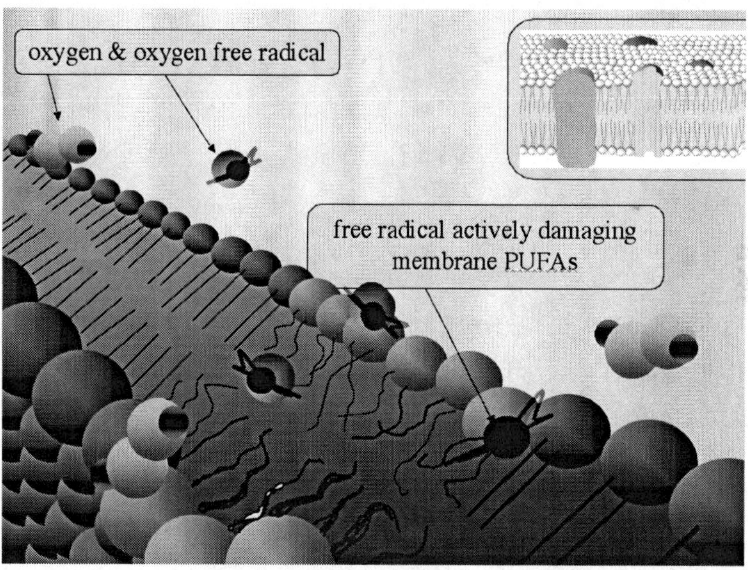

Figure 7. How Free Radicals Damage Membranes. This is a close up view of a cell membrane under attack. This particular section of membrane is composed of PUFAs. (The insert in the upper right is a cross section of the same membrane.) As the free radicals (black) cascade through the membrane, its PUFAs get mangled and distorted. The hormone receptors and nutrient channels in this part of the membrane will no longer function, putting the entire cell at risk.

up the protein labels on your lipoprotein particles. And that's a problem.

In 1988, researchers working in Lyon, France discovered that when the labels on HDL particles got jammed up with sugar, they simply fell off.[227] The study was done in a test tube, where the denuded HDL particles adhered to the glass. In your body, the naked fat would be exposed to blood. That's no good, and I'll explain why below. Let me first point out that one of the common findings in diabetic patients is a low HDL level. One possible explanation is that the excessive sugar in their blood has knocked the coats off their HDL, and the naked particles have fallen out of circulation.

And what about LDL? In 1990, another experiment investigated what sugar does to LDL. This time, the labels didn't fall off, but rather became so deranged as to be illegible and unrecognizable to hungry cells.[228] As a result, glycated LDL particles stay in circulation too long, which would explain why some diabetics have high LDL levels: With so many undeliverable LDL packages floating around, they just start adding up.[229,230] (When LDL levels are high because of glycation, then high LDL is a problem, as we'll see.)

Most diabetics have high triglyceride levels. Triglyceride is not a lipoprotein. Like cholesterol, it is a component of all lipoproteins. Triglycerides are carried in both LDL and HDL particles. But the vast majority of triglyceride is carried by chylomicrons (the lipoprotein particles your gut makes right after a meal) and *very low-density lipoproteins* (VLDL), which your liver makes from recycled fats. These plump nutrient carriers want to deliver their cargo into your hungry cells. But, like all lipoproteins, they can't do the job all alone. They need a special enzyme—think of it as a dock-worker—to pick the fatty acids up and carry them into the cell. A study done in 1990 showed that sugar interferes with this process.[231] So if you have high blood sugar, that sugar may shred the lipoprotein coats beyond recognition, or simply rip them off the particles' backs. If the particles ever do make it to a cellular dock, sugar keeps them from completing the delivery. With so many barriers to getting nutrition into hungry cells, it's no wonder people with diabetes feel hungry all the time.

As you can see, there is plenty of evidence that sugar can gum up, jam, or simply confuse the otherwise perfectly orchestrated choreography of fat and nutrient delivery that is the lipid cycle. Inevitably, this leads to a lot of misdirected—and, as far as the body is concerned, missing—cargo. How much of a problem is this? That depends on what kind of material has gone missing. If a shipping company misplaced a few thousand baby bottles, the authorities could tell the HazMat units to stay home. If, on the other hand, they lost a couple pounds of high-grade uranium, there would be cause for concern. In your body, one of the most dangerous things a lipoprotein can carry is oxidized, pro-inflammatory fat—MegaTrans. When that gets spilled inside your arteries, your body calls on its own HazMat unit.[232] But in prediabetics and diabetics, so much bad fat is released (either all at once or over time) that the cleanup crews can't keep up and arteries wind up getting injured by free radical cascades and, literally, fried (see Figure 3).

Sugar and vegetable oil combine forces to destroy arteries. First, sugar blocks lipoproteins from getting to their destination, forcing them to dump their cargo into your arteries. Second, the explosive, MegaTrans-rich vegetable oil cargo coats arteries with a toxic goo. If you want to keep your arteries healthy, you'll want to know what that toxic goo does. Let's take a look.

Atherosclerosis: How Bad Fats Lead to Heart Attacks and Strokes

When fat coats your arteries, it does not automatically cause a heart attack or stroke. If the fats are in any way useful, the endothelial cell may simply absorb them. However, if your diet is high in vegetable oil, then the fallen lipoprotein particles are useless debris, polluting every avenue, side street and back alley of your circulatory system.

Then again, the damage wrought by MegaTrans is nothing as peaceful as litter quietly blowing through the streets. At a molecular level, it's more like Darth Vader's evil forces strafing the surface of Yoda's home planet with white-hot streams of free radicals. Large swaths of the cell membrane are scorched as Zombie-fats spawn and free radicals propagate across the surface, incinerating everything they touch—ion channels, sugar transporters,

A Play-By-Play Pictorial of a Heart Attack (Or Stroke)

Figure 8 (A-I) Degraded lipoproteins drop out of circulation, landing on the lining of your blood vessels where they attract a cleanup crew of white blood cells. But sometimes, during the cleanup procedure, oxygen ignites a free radical reaction so large that the underlying collagen is exposed to flowing blood. Whenever collagen contacts blood, clots form. If the clot is large enough to disrupt arterial flow, it may cause a heart attack, stroke, or venous thrombosis (a blood clot in your leg).

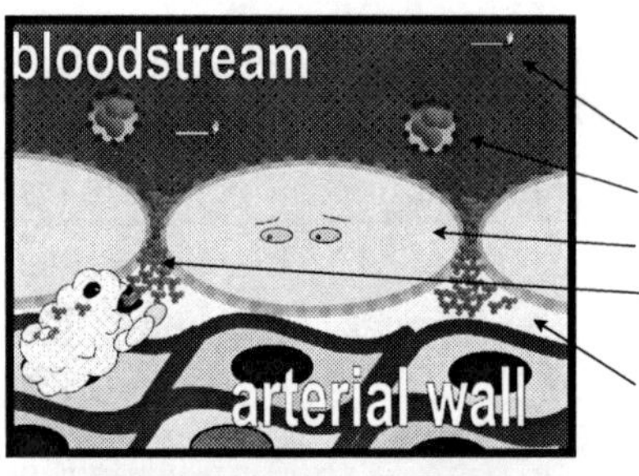

A) Degraded Lipoprotein Contents Attract a White Blood Cell.

- **Oxygen**
- **Lipoprotein**
- **Endothelial cell**
- **Degraded Lipoprotein Contents (MegaTrans Fat)**
- **Collagen layer of the arterial wall**

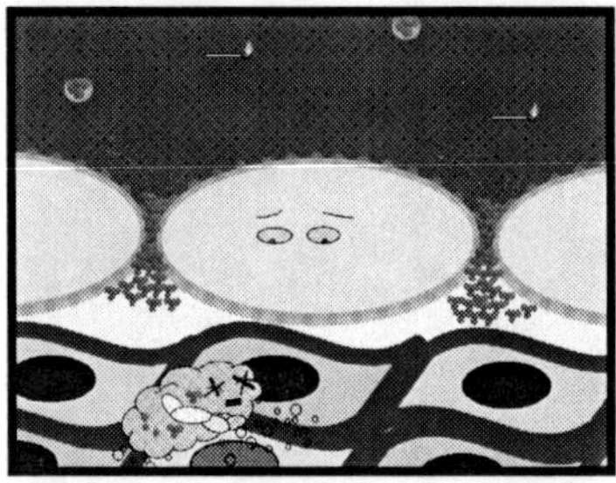

B) MegaTrans Kills the White Blood Cell. The white blood cell does its job by ingesting lipoprotein detritus, including MegaTrans. This overwhelms the white blood cell. Pro-inflammatory enzymes leak from its body into the tissue that supports the arterial wall, weakening it.

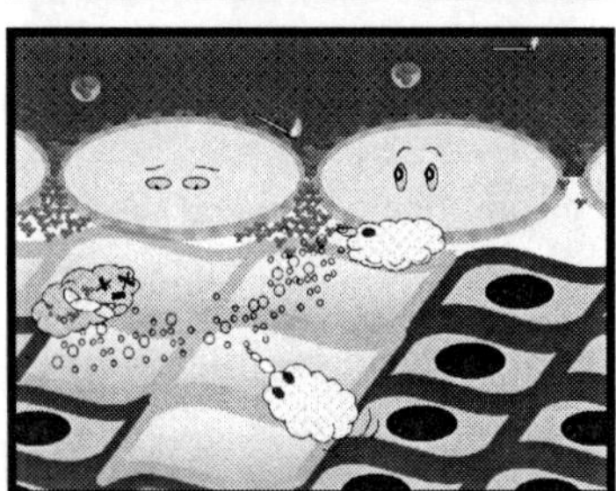

C) Inflammation Attracts More White Blood Cells. The dying white blood cell sends out pro-inflammatory *chemokines*, chemical signals that summon white blood cells from the surrounding tissue. Meanwhile, the leaking pro-inflammatory enzymes continue chewing through collagen, creating a soft area in the arterial wall. This is *unstable* plaque (see text).

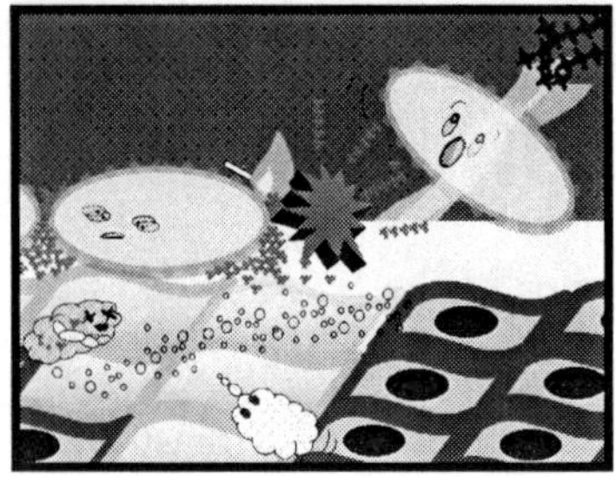

D) Oxygen Reacts Explosively With MegaTrans. Oxygen molecules and MegaTrans molecules with identical spin states meet, react, and explode. This dislodges an endothelial cell, exposing the underlying collagen layer. Thin wisps of collagen dangle into the bloodstream where they attract platelets. The dislodged endothelial cell knows there is more trouble ahead.

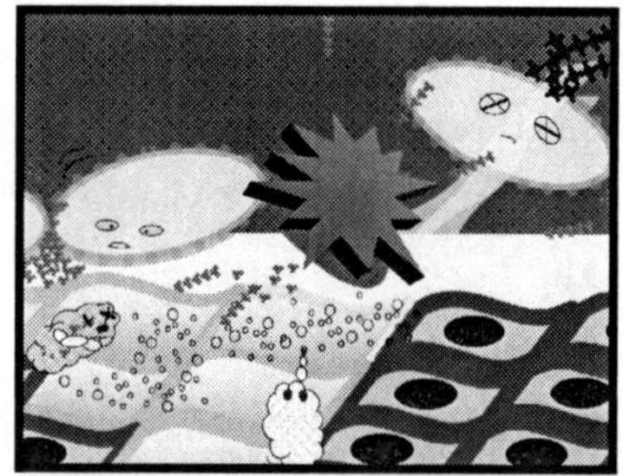

E) The Free Radical Reaction Continues. After detonating, the free radical cascade spawns more and more MegaTrans, many of which match the spin state of ordinary oxygen present in abundance in the bloodstream. As the reaction grows in strength and the explosion becomes more powerful, the collagen layer is further damaged and weakened

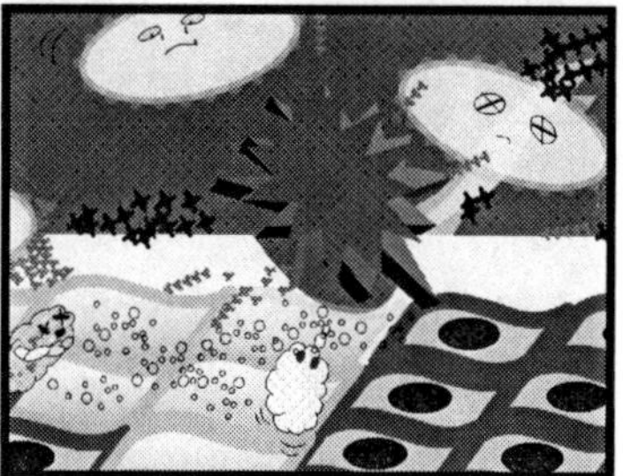

F) A Race Against Time. The inflammatory reaction has triggered the gathering white blood cells to release collagen-destroying enzymes. Now, platelets must coat the collagen layer before the enzymes so weaken the supporting arterial wall collagen that the pressure in the artery creates a tear.

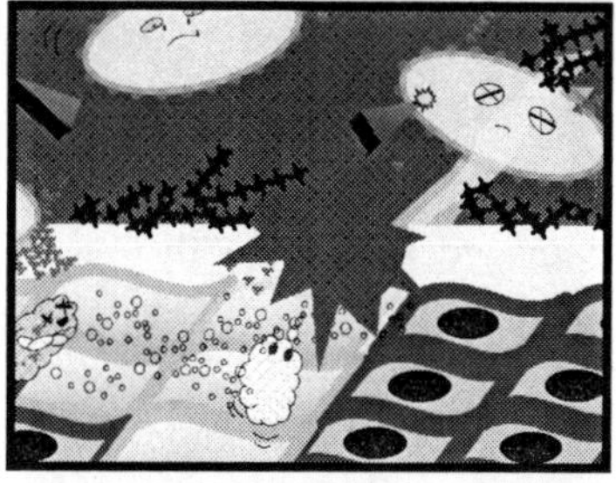

G) Worst Case Scenario. If a tear forms, the mixture of pro-inflammatory chemicals generated by the gathering white blood cells would be exposed to flowing blood in the artery, creating an enormous clot. If this is an artery in the brain, the result would be a stroke. If in the heart, a heart attack. Let's hope the platelets can clot the area off in time.

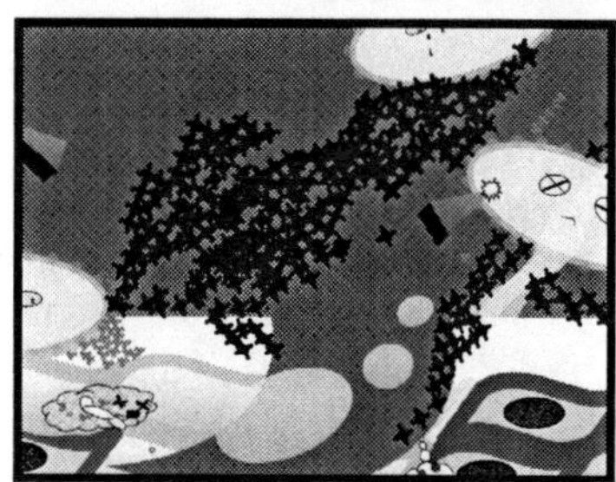

H) The Tipping Point. Today is not a good day for this person's blood vessel. The unstable plaque has ruptured into the bloodstream, and the pro-inflammatory mixture will now generate a sizable clot, shown in the next frame.

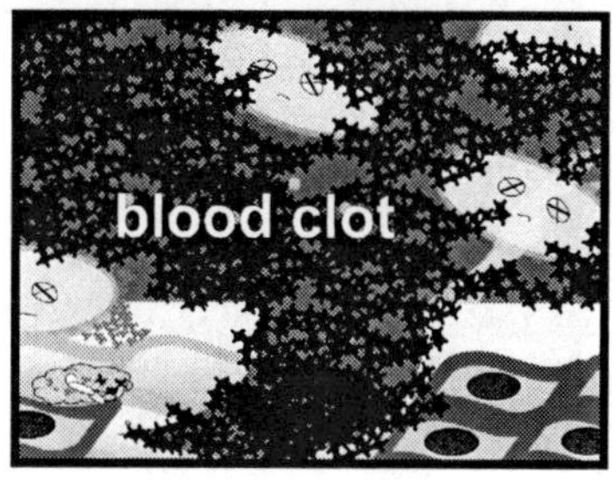

I) Deadly Or Not? There is no test that can see if your arteries contain *unstable* plaque that can lead to this kind of clot. The commonly performed angiogram only shows narrowing that results from buildup of thick, older plaque. Stable plaque has been hardened with a matrix of calcium, proteins, and cholesterol and is therefore unlikely to rupture.

hormone receptors. This disables, and ultimately destroys, functional cells. This is how free radicals fry arteries. Over the years, the damage can become so advanced that it is visible to the naked eye. It looks a lot like fried chicken skin.

And it's about as crispy and weak as fried chicken skin too, and tears more easily than the unfried version. Free radical chain reactions have weakened the underlying collagen scaffolding and polymerized the arterial walls into a kind of crunchy protein plastic. Now the artery can easily rupture and bleed.[233] If blood ever contacts collagen directly it will clot, plugging up the artery. And that's how you get a heart attack or a stroke. So it's a blood clot, *not fat*, that shuts off the flow of blood. That's why ER doctors treat heart attacks and strokes with clot busters, not fat busters.

What does plaque have to do with any of this? Think like your body. Your arteries are under continued attack from MegaTrans and sugar. Although your entire vascular tree is being damaged, some sections are getting fried so badly, they are in danger of rupture. Your body tries to repair badly damaged sections with a patch made of protein, calcium, and cholesterol. Most of these patches do just fine, holding the arterial section together for

Fat Versus Oil: What's the Difference?

Lipid is a generic term for both fats and oils. If the lipid is *solid* at room temperature, it's called fat. If it's *liquid*, it's oil. Butter is solid, so it's called a fat. In general, lipids made of stiff, inflexible saturated fats are solid and those made of fluid, flexible unsaturated fats are liquid. However, to describe butter (and other animal fat) as "saturated fat" is not strictly correct, because some fatty acids in butter are not saturated.

All storage fats (as opposed to fats in cell membranes and other actively functioning fats) exist in a chemical assemblage called a *triglyceride*. A *tri*glyceride is made with *three* fatty acids which dangle like keys from a chain made out of glycerol, to which each of the fatty acids are bound. The fatty acids can be any combination of saturated, monounsaturated, and polyunsaturated. Butter carries more saturated fatty acids in its triglyceride chains than vegetable oil, but not all are saturated fat. If they were, butter would be as stiff and solid as wax. Vegetable oil actually contains saturated fatty acids, but not as many as butter. The different blends of saturated and unsaturated combine to generate the final melting point of the fat.

the rest of your life. But just as with arterial tissue, patches can be weakened. And when they are, they can bust open, bleed, and clot.

The stable plaque can grow so thick that it will narrow a section of an artery enough to be visible on an angiogram. A cardiologist will typically point a finger at a picture of the narrowed section, tell you how you are a ticking time bomb, and schedule you for bypass surgery or stenting. But that one, thick plaque is not the real problem. If you have such a thick, stable plaque that it's visible on an angiogram, it's a sure thing that your entire vascular tree has been damaged, and there's really no way to tell where you might develop a clot. If I had my way, instead of hearing "You need surgery to save your life," people would hear "You need to get off vegetable oil and sugar immediately. But if you're unwilling to do that, then I'll need to crack your chest open and replace as many of these damaged arteries as I can with cleaner blood vessels from somewhere else in your body."

How Fast Food Causes Birth Defects

Eating vegetable oil doesn't just mess up your arteries. Those disruptive free radicals can interfere with just about everything a cell might need to do, leading to just about any disease you can name.[234,235]

At no point in our life cycle is this disruption more devastating than while we're developing in the womb. In 2006, when researchers tested the blood of mothers whose babies were born with congenital spinal and heart defects, they found evidence of oxidative stress,[236,237] exactly what you would expect to find in someone eating lots of vegetable oil. In 2007, an article in *Genes to Cells* showed how oxidative stress can disrupt hormone production and interfere with hormonal responses, suggesting that women who consume vegetable oil while pregnant are increasing their child's risk of all kinds of growth deformities and disease.[238] So if you are pregnant or plan on getting pregnant, banish vegetable oil and foods containing vegetable oil from your kitchen, and get the stuff out of your life.

Genetic Experimentation—On You

You may have noticed the various cut-off levels over the years to identify people at "high risk" of a heart attack. Years ago, if your total cholesterol was 300 or less, your doctor would have said you were fine. Soon, that number was lowered to 200. Now people also watch their LDL, "safe" levels of which have been lowered from 200 to 160, to 130, to 100, and now 80. Currently, the average person's LDL level is still about what it's always been, around 120-130[239]. The controversial 2001 revision of the cholesterol guidelines means nearly half of the US population can now be labeled "high risk." And drug companies are raking it in. According to Harvard's Dr. John Abramson and former New England Journal of Medicine editor Dr. Jerome Kassirer, the reason our medical leadership plays along, unflinchingly insisting that there's no potential harm from pushing these numbers so low, may stem from financial conflicts of interest.[240,241]

So what's a good number? As I've said, I like to see LDL less than three times the HDL value. If it's higher, you may have prediabetes and fat-encrusted arteries. Keep in mind the really important number is your fasting blood sugar level—and we'll learn more about that in the next chapter.

The war against cholesterol is not without casualties. Women with the lowest cholesterol levels have five times the rates of premature births as women with higher levels. Even when carried to term, babies of mothers with low cholesterol are born smaller, with abnormally small brains.[242] Remember, epigenetic alterations can accumulate over generations. So when these small-brained babies have babies of their own, while on low-cholesterol diets themselves, it's anybody's guess what the outcome of this ongoing experiment will be.

Now that you know what I think of Public Enemy Number One, let me tell you what I think about its conspirator, Public Enemy Number Two—sugar.

Nine

Sickly Sweet

How Carbohydrate-Rich Diets Block Metabolic Function

If you've just finished Chapter 8 and are coming to grips with the fact that vegetable oil is in so many foods that save you time in the kitchen, and you're now wondering how on Earth you'll manage without them, then brace yourself. You are about to be advised to get rid of sugar—even the sugar you didn't realize you were eating. But take heart. Processed foods made with vegetable oils are also the foods typically loaded with sugar, so cutting vegetable oil automatically helps you to cut sugar intake. And keep in mind that, by cutting out these two deadly toxins, you'll be allowing your genes to operate as they should and immunizing yourself against chronic disease. Once you get rid of vegetable oil and sugar, and start on the Four Pillars, everything you eat will help keep you young, slim, smart, and beautiful. Even if you really love sweet stuff, cutting your sugar intake way down isn't a big deal. I did it, and life's been easier now that I'm free of all those cravings, energy swings, and addictions. And I can taste the sweetness in foods that my palate couldn't detect before. The only truly difficult part of getting sugar out of my life was the first step, accepting the fact that, because of my own chronic ailment, I had no choice.

A Sticky Mess

On August 5, 2002, I finished a cup of coffee sweetened with homemade caramel sauce and set off on a mission to retrieve a species of Hawaiian fern.

The hike into the hills on the south side of Kauai took me up a steep grade through mud and three-foot grass that wound itself around the wheel of my wheelbarrow. When my knee started hurting, I figured it would get better later, as it always had. I was wrong. Way wrong. The pain would continue to get worse over the ensuing months and then worse still after a desperate surgery. Soon, I could barely make the journey from the parking lot into the grocery store, and it was a struggle just making it through my workday. Eventually, we discovered that a virus had taken residence in the fluid inside my knee. I had to make a choice: either tame my cravings for sweets or give up any hope of recovery.

How could sugar cause such a serious and unusual problem? What I had learned in medical school was that sugar was energy that could be "burned off" by exercise. Besides, the one nutrition course I took made it clear that my body's main enemy was cholesterol, not sugar and other carbs. Fortunately, Luke suspected otherwise. One day he handed me a newsletter he'd gotten from a friend and pointed to an article that said "1/2 teaspoon of sugar puts white blood cells to sleep for four hours." The article was missing a few experimental details; there was no description of whether the study was done in a lab culture dish or in living subjects. Though I tend to be wary of articles missing those kinds of facts, it did prompt me to do a little research of my own. I started looking into the effects of sugar on living cells, and what I found was horrifying.

Of course, we need sugar in our bloodstream just to stay alive. Glucose is the primary fuel for most of the cells of the body. But things go awry when you eat more than your body can deal with. Because sugar—in high concentration—is a rarity in nature, the human metabolism is simply not prepared for exposure to the 200 plus pounds the average American now consumes yearly.[243] Times were, only the wealthy could indulge in sweets made with refined sugar. Now, sugar is a mainstay of the modern diet.

After my (long-overdue) review of the literature on sugar's effects on body biochemistry, I found that the consequences of excess sugar consumption are disastrous, especially in childhood. As sugar seeps into your tissues,

Exercise and Sugar

If you are a competitive athlete or if your job involves heavy labor, your muscles act like sugar sponges, sopping the stuff from your bloodstream before the levels get dangerously high. But don't think, like I did, that exercise enables you to get away with eating junk. For one thing, that junk destroys your collagen (see Chapter 11). It also forces you to store fat. Even as a college-level cross-country runner burning thousands of calories during two-hour daily training sessions, my dorm-food diet was so low in nutrients that, in spite of all the exercise, I actually developed one of the earliest signs of diabetes, called *trunkal obesity*.

While far from fat at 5 foot 4 and 125 pounds, my waistline was surprisingly unflattering. Underneath rock-hard abs (I also did hundreds of sit ups a day) my intestines were coated in *omental* fat, a very unhealthy form of fat that develops in everyone eating low-nutrient, high-carb, high trans-fat, high vegetable oil diets. This gave me a classic "apple-shaped" figure even though I wasn't overweight. At age 35, when I started eating better, I finally lost that omental fat and developed a more feminine waistline. (I also grew an inch taller!)

it coats the surface of cell membranes, with life-changing consequences. As a young girl, I would often sneak away to the corner candy store or munch on handfuls of the chocolate chips I would sometimes find hidden in the kitchen pantry, stressing my body's connective tissues already weakened by my low-fat, low-cholesterol, no-meat-on-the-bone diet. And the sugar encrusting my cells interfered with hormone receptor function, disrupting the complex series of physiologic developments scheduled to take place during puberty. As a result, I had no idea what all the fuss over boys was about until shortly after I went off to college.

Sugar Changes How Our Hormones Work

You may have heard that, on average, we gain ten pounds a decade after the age of 35; women, in particular, start reporting that they can't eat like they used to. This phenomenon may be directly related to the biochemical effects of sugar binding to hormone receptors, jamming them, and rendering us insensitive to the hormone *insulin*. Once you are insulin resistant, blood sugar levels rise higher still, leading to diabetes and all its related disorders, including weight gain, circulatory and sexual dysfunction. For the same reasons sugar jams hormone signals, it also clogs nutrient channels, weakening bone and muscle and slowing neural communication, which can impair mood and memory and lead to dementia. While all this is going on, sugar stiffens the collagen in your tendons, joints, and skin, causing arthritis and premature wrinkling, while interfering with the production of new collagen throughout your entire body. And because sugar changes the surface markers your white blood cells need to distinguish between indigenous cells from invaders, it opens the door to cancer and infection.

How does sugar do all this?

Glycation: The Reason Sugar is Bad for You

Ever notice how licked lollipops and half-chewed taffy have a tacky feeling? Sugar feels sticky because, once dissolved in water, it reacts with proteins on the surface of your skin to form easily breakable chemical bonds. When you pull your fingers apart and feel the sticky resistance, you're feeling the tug of those bonds being broken. The process by which sugar sticks to stuff is called *glycation*. Glycation reactions are reversible, but with enough heat or time, the temporary bonds becomes permanent due to oxidation reactions. The products of these later oxidation reactions are called *advanced glycation end products*, or AGEs. And that's a useful acronym, because AGEs make you *age* unnaturally fast.

When you toast bread, oxidation reactions generate AGEs in the proteins and sugars present in wheat. These AGEs change the bread from soft, pliable, and pale to hard, stiff, and brown because the proteins and sugars form cross-links that stiffen the bread. The same thing happens inside your body as AGEs cross-link normally mobile proteins. This hardens your cells and tissues, making them brittle and stiff. Fortunately, at normal blood sugar levels, the reactions occur so slowly that cleanup crews of white blood cells keep them under control by breaking them down. The kidney cleans these

AGEs from the blood and excretes them from the body. It is these waste chemicals that give urine its characteristic yellow color.

The clinical implications of having your tissues hardened by sugar-protein cross-links are vast and far-reaching. Cross-links turn the semi-permeable surfaces of arteries into impervious walls, preventing nutrients from exiting the bloodstream. When trapped nutrients can't escape your bloodstream, where do you think they end up? Lining your arteries. As we saw in Chapter 7, when lipoproteins deposit on the arterial lining, they attract white blood cells, and can cause blood clots and/or atherosclerotic plaques. A few cross-links on your white blood cells slows them down, making infections more likely and more serious, enabling nascent cancer cells to grow under the radar unchallenged. Are your joints creaking and stiff? AGEs can form in them too. AGEs (primarily from high blood sugar) are one of two major biochemical phenomena that make us look and feel old (the other being free radicals, primarily from vegetable oils). To get a better idea of how AGEs impair normal body functions, let's take a close-up look.

How Sugar Affects Your Circulatory System

Far from being a hollow tube where blood components randomly bump about, blood vessels are busy places where coordinated events take place in parallel with each other thousands of times per second. Guided only by the thermodynamics of their own design, the biologic materials in your blood perform acrobatics as perfectly choreographed as a Las Vegas circus act. This concerted effort between teams of biological chemicals is what makes a muscle contract, a sweat gland produce sweat, and your brain translate optic nerve input into a recognizable face. But when too much sugar creates cross-links between moving parts, *all* cellular activity is impaired. Let's take a look at just three cell types in your circulation—white blood cells, the blood vessel lining cells (called *endothelial* cells), and red blood cells—to see how sugar cross-links make it impossible for them to do their jobs.

Pushed by the currents of blood, circulating white blood cells travel over the lining of the blood vessels by rolling along like little tumbleweeds. When responding to the call of tissues in trouble, white blood cells must exit the bloodstream. How do they know where to go? Inflammatory chemical messages from the affected tissue seep through intercellular spaces to reach the endothelial cells lining the bloodstream. Those cells then put up little flags on their surface telling white blood cells to exit the blood vessel. The white blood cells magically transform from rolling blobs into flat, flowing amoeba-like creatures, and wriggle through tiny spaces between endothelial cells into the troubled tissues below. All this is basic physiology. But our knowledge of the biochemistry of sugar helps us understand how glycation reactions between sugar and protein can cross-link the endothelial cells, blocking those

Quantity Over Quality

Earlier in the book, we talked about the need to revise the way we think about food. Rather than "building blocks" made of carbs, fat, and protein, food is more akin to a language comprised of, and ultimately communicating with, complex dynamic living systems. That life-giving complexity is getting hard to come by.

As the remaining environment is polluted, used up, or replaced with human development, the unavoidable mathematics dictate a ratio of less complexity per capita. The more obvious outcome of this is the fact that it's becoming increasingly difficult for individuals to surround themselves with nature in their daily lives. Though less obvious, the very same process is taking place on our dinner plates.

A whole wild salmon, liver from a free-range grass-fed calf, and a pint of unpasteurized cream from pastured cows all share in common the fact that they are highly complex living systems. And each communicates to our cells the conditions of the complex micro-ecology from which those animals fed. What they also share is that they each require a large section of healthy earth or sea to produce. At the opposite side of the spectrum is carbohydrate. This relatively simple food, lacking in complexity, has the advantage of needing very little space to produce, and that space need not be pristine. Needless to say, it's cheap. As world resources shrink, economics increasingly necessitates that people consume more carbs, which is to say, sugar. The process represents a simple trade off between human population size and individual health—quantity over quality. These days, much attention is devoted to access to healthcare. But the real health issue is access to nature, primarily by way of real, healthy food.

tiny spaces, and prevent white blood cells from getting to where they're needed. And it follows that the more cross-links you have, the more your immune function is impaired.

AGEs are a primary reason diabetics develop circulatory problems. Over the life of a red blood cell (three months or so), the protein-rich red cell sops up sugar like a sponge, growing stiff and bloated. One of the jobs of the spleen is to test the quality of red blood cells in circulation. It does this by making them pass through a maze of gradually narrowing corridors. Any cell too puffed up with sugar gets destroyed. But when sugar levels are high all the time, the spleen can't remove all the bloated cells from circulation, so they wind up clogging tiny capillaries. This is why diabetics go blind and develop numbness and infections in their feet. What's true of white, red and endothelial cells is true of every cell in your body. If sugar so drastically impairs the function of cells that are already fully formed, imagine what it might do to cells that are still developing.

How Sugar Causes Birth Defects

In Chapter 5, we discussed fetal alcohol syndrome, the term given for the constellation of congenital abnormalities attributable to maternal alcohol consumption. The well-known version of this syndrome is called fetal alcohol *effects*. This describes the less profound, and therefore less noticeable, affects of maternal alcohol consumption at (presumably) more moderate levels. Since most mothers would like to do all they can to avoid birth defects, they usually follow their doctor's advice to avoid alcohol altogether. I think doctors should apply the same kind of reasoning when it comes to the consumption of sugar.

It is an accepted medical reality that if you have diabetes you run up to ten times the risk of having a child with a major birth defect, including major facial anomalies like cleft palate. Uncontrolled diabetes has been shown to have "a profound effect on embryogenesis, organogenesis, and fetal and neonatal growth."[244] The most conscientious doctors, therefore, tell their diabetic patients hoping to get pregnant to get their diabetes under control first.

But what about those women who are borderline diabetic, insulin resistant and hyperglycemic?

In my opinion, just as doctors now prohibit even moderate drinking in pregnancy, I think it's time to take sugar consumption seriously as well. As we'll see below, tens of millions of Americans, including many expectant mothers, suffer from diabetic complications and don't know it. We know that *major* birth defects are more common in diabetics, but what about lesser growth anomalies like those of fetal alcohol effects or second sibling syndrome? Could the cross-linking effects of a high-sugar, high-carb diet likewise impair the full development of facial features?

Given all we know about the disastrous effects of sugar on our cells, there's reason to believe the answer is *yes*. A few cells sticking together at key points in embryologic development is very likely to disrupt and distort the development of a growing baby. This is why I counsel *all* my pregnant patients to reduce their sugar intake as much as possible. If they want something sweet, they'll have to wait for the perfect smile on their baby's face.

How Eating Sugar Causes Type II Diabetes

Every cell needs a constant supply of glucose, so it must be readily available. The pancreas, a sock-shaped gland tucked behind the stomach, keeps sugar levels between about 70 and 85 mg/dl all the time. But a blast of sugar from a Big Gulp, a giant cookie, or spongy soft piece of cake, can overload the pancreatic control systems, and soak your tissues in sticky sugar long enough to form a mess of AGEs, which will need to be cleaned up. If the clean up isn't finished before your next treat, cell membranes are so full of cross-links that they are slow to respond to insulin, and sugar levels rise higher. This enables more cross-links to form than before, and so the cells respond even more poorly to insulin. This is the vicious cycle that so many people get trapped in, as, eventually fasting sugar levels rise above 90 (or 100, depending on the doctor), and a person is diagnosed with elevated blood sugar levels (or prediabetes), and finally as levels continue to rise, with diabetes.

Since so many people with blood sugar problems have parents with the same condition, they naturally assume it's hereditary, and therefore inevitable. But that's not the case. If anything is being passed from parent to child here, it's bad eating habits. If you can take control of your habits, you can escape the vicious cycle, normalize your blood sugar, and even cure diabetes.

Experts Recommend Treating Prediabetes as Diabetes

You may know that diabetes increases your risk of having a heart attack. What you may not have heard is that more moderate versions of elevated blood sugar are dangerous as well. A study done in 2007 showed that people whose fasting sugar was even the *slightest* bit above normal (currently defined as 100mg/dl) when admitted to the hospital with a heart attack were up to *five times more likely to die* in the next year than heart attack victims whose levels were normal.[245] These people with elevated blood sugar weren't given a diagnosis of diabetes. Instead, they were told they had "impaired fasting glucose." What that diagnosis typically means to the patient is that—since they don't have "diabetes"—they're in the clear.

But here's the truth: all the things that frighten us when we hear our doctor say the word diabetes—kidney failure, blindness, stroke, amputation, heart attack, etc.—apply to impaired fasting glucose as well.[246] People with "impaired fasting glucose," or "glucose intolerance," or "insulin resistance," or "prediabetes," or even the slightest elevation of fasting blood sugar levels, should be warned that they are at risk for all the complications associated with diabetes. If it were up to me, we'd put all of it under the umbrella of diabetes. But whatever you call it, if your blood sugar's elevated, take that as a big red flag telling you that it's time to cut your sugar (and vegetable oil) intake dramatically.

So exactly how high is too high?

89 And 100: Two Numbers that May Save Your Life

Many experts have suggested that the threshold at which we diagnose diabetes (it's now 125 mg/dl) should, in light of all this evidence, be revised down. I agree. When I first started practicing medicine, I used the cutoff that everyone else used: 125. But since I've been in Hawaii, where high blood sugar levels are common, I've noticed something remarkable. Once people's fasting levels reach 89, they tend to start gaining weight. And because high blood sugar disrupts the lipid cycle, some even develop atherosclerosis. If you have a fasting level of 89 or higher, you may be on the threshold of being sucked into the vicious cycle that leads to overt diabetes. In my practice, I check fasting sugar levels on anyone who has any kind of symptom attributable to diabetes or who is simply overweight. If the level is 89 or higher, I recommend that they permanently cut their total intake of carbohydrates (including sugars) down to 100 grams a day or less.

Maybe it seems as though I'm being overly strict about sugar. To put the issue into perspective, realize that two hundred years ago, refined sugar was a costly commodity traded in tiny portions, like pepper. As you'd expect, sugar-related health problems were confined to the wealthy.[247,248] Today, thanks to cheap energy and labor—and sugar from beets and corn—diseases attributable to sugar have been made available to all.

Hypoglycemia is a commonly recognized problem of low blood sugar. But it may also be the earliest sign that a person is on their way to developing insulin resistance. The symptoms of hypoglycemia include feeling tired, hungry, shaky, or nauseated before lunch or dinner. These feelings come from adrenaline, which helps the liver pump out more sugar but also makes us shaky, nauseous, even panicky. Because sufferers often figure that their symptoms are due to "low" sugar, they often self-medicate by eating more sugar which, as we'll see next, only makes the problem worse.

True Tales of Sugar-holics

Sugar-Induced "Spells"

Meet Mary, a nurse who worked in my office until a few years ago. Always on top of her game, she double-checked the charts to make sure we doctors didn't overlook any records. To stay alert, she would eat something sweet several times a day. Not candy, mind you. Just the "healthy" stuff, fruit and energy bars. She was fit, exercised regularly, and kept her weight down. Over the years, however, she began to notice some shaking in her hands when she was hungry. But she could make it stop by having another sweet snack, which she would keep stashed away in a special section of her purse. When she hit menopause, those hunger spells suddenly morphed into something more frightening. One day, when the surgeon she was assisting asked for the 4-0 suture, Mary just stared into space, unresponsive and confused. She remained in a fog for about two minutes before snapping out of it. To make sure it would never happen again, she decided to eat something sweet a little more often. Later, when her blood was tested, the doctor told her everything was fine. If anything, he said, her fasting sugar levels were on the low side.

"It's my hypoglycemia," Mary told me. I told her that she was *causing* hypoglycemia by eating sweets and blunting her response to hormones so that the body produced more and more to get the same response. Neither of us was expecting what came next.

A few months later, Mary blacked out at the wheel and drove off the road into a ditch. Luckily, nobody was hurt. In the hospital, the neurologist said those spells she'd been having were seizures and put her on anti-seizure medication. But the medication made her drowsy and she didn't want to take it, so she came to me looking for an alternative.

As any menopausal woman knows, fluctuating hormone levels can cause irritability. This was part of Mary's problem. Rising and falling estrogen and progesterone were affecting her brain and causing anxiety. But that wasn't the only issue. The big problem was the foil-wrapped snack hiding in her purse. Years of the habit had soaked her tissues in extra glucose often enough to generate cross-links too numerous to clean up. Since her cellular response to insulin was just a little delayed, her pancreas would keep releasing more. Of course, her response to glucagon—the hormone that tells the liver to release sugar—was sluggish as well. Imagine an airline pilot trying to trim a plane whose response to the controls is delayed by ten seconds or so. As her sugar levels dropped below 60, Mary's brain was deprived of glucose, triggering a stress response from the adrenal glands. They would in turn release *adrenaline* which, like glucagon, instructs the liver to release stored glucose. Adrenaline also affects the nervous system, causing anxiety, shakiness, and even nausea. Rising and falling sugar, estrogen, and progesterone in combination with mixed signals from high levels of insulin, glucagon, and occasional bursts of adrenaline ultimately caused a short circuit in the brain that resulted in a seizure. Once a short circuit like this develops, it makes it easier to have another seizure. So taking her off the seizure medication, as she wanted me to do, could be risky.

I suggested a compromise. I recommended that she follow a strict low-carb diet, which we reviewed. I also lowered her medication a bit, monitoring her blood to ensure we were still in the therapeutic range. I cautioned that if she were ever to lapse from the diet she would need to raise the dose of medication again. After some initial difficulty taming her ferocious sweet tooth, Mary has now been following the diet and been seizure free on a low dose of medication for five years.

Is this a happy ending? I suppose. She is, after all, less dependent on seizure medication than if had she continued her high-sugar diet. Had she continued, even the full dose of medication may not have been able to prevent the seizures completely. But here's the other side of the coin: From what I've learned about sugar and its affects on human health, it's not altogether unlikely that suffusing her bloodstream with toxic levels of glucose over a period of years may have been a sufficient cause of her seizure disorder. In other words, take the energy bar out of her purse ten years ago, and Mary might never have had any need for seizure medication, *ever*. Does this make me want to grab energy drinks, energy bars, and fruit juice out of people's hands? You bet. Not just because sugar causes illness, but because sugar-induced problems pull otherwise healthy people into a medical system that loses revenue when people are healthy. It needs them—meaning you—to be sick. That's why I'm giving you all the details. Hospitals, clinics, and much of the medical industry depends on keeping you in the dark. But genes depend on you to learn the truth about what it takes to eat right.

"I Don't Want Heart Surgery"

Gary is a scuba instructor. His job requires him to be ready to take action whenever one of the tourists on his boat gets into trouble. When he started feeling a fluttering in his chest, he needed to nail down exactly what was happening and do something to stop it. Though he could navigate the Hawaiian currents with his eyes closed, he had no idea how to navigate the medical system. So like many people, instead of starting with a visit to his primary care doctor, he went straight to the emergency room.

The ER doctor couldn't diagnose the source of Gary's problem because, when he went in, everything was fine. The ER doctor ordered a few tests, including blood tests and an EKG, all of which turned out normal. Just to be thorough, the ER doc sent Gary to his primary care doc to get a referral to a cardiologist, who did still more tests. All normal. Just to be sure, the cardiologist wanted an angiogram. If that test showed anything out of the ordinary, like a slight narrowing of an artery, the patient would be nudged into position as a candidate for a major procedure—a stent, or even heart surgery.

This is when Gary came in to see me. His regular doctor was on vacation, and he was too anxious too wait.

"I don't want heart surgery," he said. I told him that, since I don't do heart surgery, he'd come to the right place. I looked over his records and only one element of his entire history caught my attention, his fasting sugar level. It was 92. Though generally considered "normal," I see this number as high because, as I mentioned earlier, anything *over* 88 (89 or higher) seems to invite problems. I wasn't surprised to find his sugar was a bit high. I'd noticed that his heels were slightly calloused, and I've found that patients with high sugar levels often develop a dry callous on their heels.

The chest fluttering Gary described is termed a *palpitation*. Palpitations are disturbances in the heart rhythm which, in my experience, occur more often in people who eat lots of sugar. Just as with seizure disorders, sugar-induced surges in hormone and energy levels irritate the nerves. In his case, the swings disturbed the nerves surrounding his heart. I asked Gary to tell me about his diet and discovered he was a classic sugar-holic. A sweet cereal for breakfast, a Snickers bar at 10 a.m. to buoy him through his morning lull, then a sandwich for lunch, followed by another Snickers. Oh, and don't forget the fruit juice and soda. It was a routine he'd followed for years but now, at 39, it was catching up with him. Whenever his sugar levels dropped, the palpitations started.

I told him that if he wanted to avoid palpitations, he would need to cut his sugar in half, minimum. And to make clear the seriousness of his predicament, I also told him that his high fasting glucose was a bellwether sign that he was on the verge of losing his sensitivity to hormones—all hormones, including testosterone. Testosterone helps men (and women, by the way) maintain libido. But when you gum up testosterone receptors on the surface of cells, they don't respond to signals as readily. When, at the same time, you're gumming up the cells lining the blood vessels, the vessels can't dilate and fill up with blood. What we have here is a recipe for ED.

For Gary, this warning struck home, so to speak. I explained that if he wanted to avoid diabetic complications, including ED, it would be best for him to cut sugar out altogether. And that's what he did. Within a couple weeks, he was seeing all kinds of improvements, and so was his girlfriend. He traded in sugar for something even sweeter, and sugar-induced palpitations for a better kind.

Gary didn't need heart surgery. He needed a sugar-ectomy. Had he gotten his angiogram, there's a fair chance that the cardiologist would have found something of interest. A tiny anomaly, a narrow spot on the dye-shadow, something—anything—to convert this healthy, fit, life-loving person into a cardiac case. And once that happens, as the side effects and complications from pills and procedures begin to pile up, once you are dependent on one or more medications for the rest of your life, once a healthy heart is refashioned into a living carrying case for the latest piece of medical gadgetry, you're in. And good luck finding the door. In Gary's case, as with millions of Americans, the passage into the medical labyrinth, from which so many people never return, is encrusted in sugar.

Cutting Cholesterol Medications by Cutting Sugar

Jane was a thin, suntanned, enthusiastic tennis player with a total cholesterol of 260 and LDL of 170. A nurse, she was well indoctrinated with a fear of cholesterol. She assumed that because her father had a heart attack, her diet was low in cholesterol, and she exercised fastidiously, her cholesterol levels were "due to genetics." She also knew that cholesterol medications might cause muscle aches that would affect her tennis game. Still, she was so terrified of high cholesterol that she was willing to take the chance and came to me for a prescription.

Naturally, she was surprised when I said that first she needed to get a fasting blood sugar test. Now that you've read about the lipoprotein cycle in Chapter 8, you shouldn't be surprised. Blood sugar affects numerous physiologic functions, even those you might assume have nothing to do with sugar, like cholesterol.

Too much sugar can make your LDL levels go up. If you've been reading carefully, in addition to the mechanisms we talked about in Chapter 8, you also know that, when sugar cross-links capillaries, they get stiff. One of the reasons capillaries must remain flexible is so that they can allow the passage of LDL and other lipoproteins to underlying tissues (see Figure 1). When sugar cross-links make capillaries stiff, these channels can't open fast enough, if at all. As a result, the blocked-off LDL is forced to stay in circulation longer, and LDL serum levels rise. Most of the cholesterol in circulation is manufactured by your body, so if your endothelial cells aren't working right, no matter how much you restrict your cholesterol intake, it's nearly impossible to bring your serum cholesterol down—unless you cut your sugar intake or, alternatively, get on a cholesterol-lowering drug.

Jane agreed to cut her sugar, and her LDL soon plummeted to 120 which, given her HDL of 85, was just fine. Jane's high LDL had nothing to do with family history and everything to do with her sugar intake. She didn't

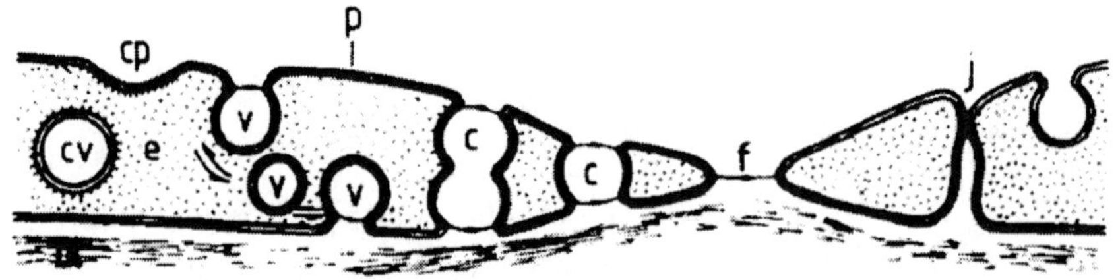

Figure 1. Endothelial Cell in Cross Section Showing Nutrient Transportation Options. An endothelial cell lining the artery must have lots of pores through which bulky lipoproteins can migrate from the bloodstream to hungry cells below. See how the membrane opens up? (The vessicle "V" and channel "C" allow the passage of lipoproteins.) Nutrient transportation would be reduced if high glucose concentrations were to generate cell membrane cross-linking. P=Membrane facing Plasma. CP=Coated Pit. CV=Coated Vessicle. F=Fenestration. J=Junction

From: Cellular Aspects Of Transcapillary Exchange. Physiological Reviews. Vol 63, No. 4, Oct 1983. Nicolae Simionescu.

need a medication, she just needed to identify the hidden sources of sugar in her diet and avoid them.

The Sugar Headache

Susan's headaches were awful. As she described them, they felt like a hot blade had been plunged through her right eye. For 20 years, she'd been told that she had migraines and was given all kinds of migraine treatments, with little effect. Quite often, there was nothing she could do but wake up her husband in the middle of the night to drive her to the ER for intravenous painkillers. Without warning, another agonizing series of headaches would materialize, tear her life apart for days or even weeks, and then just as suddenly disappear.

When I saw her, I told her a couple things she was surprised to hear. One was that these weren't migraines. They were cluster headaches, which would respond to an entirely different kind of therapy: breathing from an oxygen tank.

The second surprise was that she might be able to mitigate or even cure her headaches permanently by—you guessed it—cutting out sugar. I told her about sugar's effects on nerves and how adrenaline and other hormone fluctuations are so irritating to the brain that they can cause pain or, in extreme cases, seizures. Cluster headache sufferers are often addicted to sugar, eating sweets throughout the entire day. By the middle of the night, their blood sugar levels have bottomed out and hormones are swinging wildly to compensate. On some nights, this wakes them up with screaming pain. For any pain sufferer, cutting back on sugar is a great first move. Combined with a little exercise, cutting sugar could very well prevent Susan's headaches altogether.

Saying it is one thing. Doing it's another. "I don't eat that much sugar," Susan insisted. Very few people say otherwise. It could be true, or it could be the reflexive addict's denial. I remember responding the same way to my husband back when I was downing more than a quarter cup of sugar a day, which I admitted to Susan. We talked about her diet and, as it turned out, we both came to realize that she was in fact eating lots and lots of sugar. That's the good news. My advice to dump sugar, unfortunately, didn't take, and the habit won out. When the headaches came, she treated them successfully by reaching under her bed and breathing in the oxygen. When the oxygen wasn't enough, she headed to the ER for relief.

Whenever one of my patients goes to the ER, I get a little note. One day, it occurred to me that I hadn't gotten a note for a while about Susan. I thought maybe she'd moved, until she came in to see me for a physical. I asked her how her headaches were doing. She said she read somewhere that cutting sugar out of her diet might help her headaches and she hadn't had a single one since she'd changed her habits. She was very proud of the fact that she'd even resisted cake at her own birthday party.

Cutting sugar to treat headaches? Who would have thunk it? Sometimes people need to take ownership of information in their own way, and that's just fine with me. What matters is that she came around and decided to notify the cookie monster on her back that its free meal ticket had been revoked.

In all these medical cases, you may have noticed a theme emerging. Sugar wreaks havoc with the entire nervous system, so much so that one of the first things I ask about when someone comes in with a nervous disorder is their sugar intake. But it's not just nervous system disorders like anxiety, heart palpitations, and pain that make me think of sugar addiction. It's also recurring infections, joint problems, and allergic disorders like eczema, hives, and runny noses, and more.

Susan's story, like mine, shows us that people can be in denial about their sugar intake even while suffering horribly from its effects. The forces of denial overwhelm the forces of reason, preventing us from seeing what we are doing to ourselves. And who among us is sober enough to break sugar addicts from their spell? We are a nation of sugar addicts, surrounded by fellow sugar addicts raising sugar-addicted kids, with constant access to cheap and powerfully addicting sugar. The addict's cravings go way beyond wanting the sweet taste. Long-term sugar abuse actually rewires the human brain, until we are all—in a very real sense—*cuckoo* for Cocoa Puffs.

This is Your Brain on Sugar

Imagine you're a space alien doing research on the most potent drugs in the solar system. You've already written reports on cocaine, opium, alcohol, and nicotine. But on planet Earth, there's one more refined substance that seems to dwarf them all. There are few places where this substance isn't imported and included with almost everything the residents eat and drink. It's the first thing they ingest in the morning and the last they use at night. It's the centerpiece of celebration. Overweight children and Hollywood movie directors carry plastic receptacles filled with colorful drinkable versions of the stuff as though they need it like air. And although, at some level, they know it's killing them, they just won't stop.

Your report will show that the acreage and energy dedicated to the extraction, refinement, and export of this drug rivals that of criminalized compounds. It takes 1000 pounds of water to produce one pound of crude drug from cane and days of heating and refining to produce fine granules of sale-

Study Shows Sugar More Addicting Than Cocaine

Sugar has the edge over other addictive compounds thanks to the fact that it tastes better than most drugs. A study on rats entitled "Intense Sweetness Surpasses Cocaine Reward" found that between cocaine and sugar, sugar was more addicting. Their conclusion warns: "In most mammals, including rats and humans, sweet receptors evolved in ancestral environments poor in sugars and are thus not adapted to high concentrations of sweet [compounds]. The supranormal stimulation of these receptors by sugar-rich diets, such as those now widely available in modern societies, would generate a supranormal reward signal in the brain, with the potential to override self-control mechanisms and thus to lead to addiction."

Intense Sweetness Surpasses Cocaine Reward. Lenoir M. PLoS ONE. 2007; 2(8): e698.

able product. A quick study of planetary history shows that this substance has been so highly prized that it has functioned as currency for trade, and its flavor, "sweet," has earned it a greater presence in the lyrics of popular music than any other drug.

The subject of your report is, of course, sugar.

Sugar is the ultimate gateway drug. We now have research showing that exposure to sugar early in life has lasting effects on the brain that can make us more prone to developing chemical dependencies. When researchers gave young rats a steady supply of chocolate Ensure, they found "daily consumption alters striatal enkephalin gene expression." In other words, the study rats were programmed to consume substances that stimulate their opiate receptors.[249] Sugar acts as a powerful epigenetic instructor, telling your child's genes to construct a brain with a built-in hankering for drugs.

As Michael Pollan points out in *The Botany of Desire*, by producing chemistry desirable to humans, certain plants have domesticated us, turning people into pawns in their Darwinian battle to rule the landscape. Like THC in marijuana, the sugar in fruit and sugarcane entices humans, and other animals, to spread the plant's DNA. But this relationship is taken to dangerous extremes as refined sugar commands us to reorder the surface of the planet; millions of acres of tropical rainforest are burned every year to sustain the ongoing habit of a growing population. We work for corn too. Each step in the production of high-fructose corn syrup is a giant leap forward in corn's domination of the planet. Sugar-producing plants like corn, cane, beets, berries, and mangoes give us a legal high every bit as addictive as a hit of crack cocaine, though less intoxicating. What I am arguing, however, is that sugar's hold on us is more dangerous than any illegal substance because its effects are subtler and more pervasive.

If a child were given a dose of heroin, the chemical would trigger a flurry of neural activity in the pleasure centers of his brain. Sugar, whether in juice, pureed pears, or infant formula, results in the very same kinds of responses "via the release of endogenous opiates triggered by sweet taste[.]"[250] And if you regularly give kids sugar-rich commercial juices, sweet cereals, or daily cookies and candy, you're inadvertently playing the role of "enabler." Though sugar doesn't actually contain opiates like heroin, it affects us in very much the same way because it makes us release our own *endogenous opiates.*

The effect is powerful enough for solutions of sugar to work as a pain reliever. In a common practice, called "sucrose analgesia," nurses give a sip of sugar water to infants to calm them during heel sticks, injections, and other painful procedures newborns routinely undergo. It works well and has the benefit of reducing fussiness for up to a week after the procedures.[251]

In 2002, a group of neonatal nurses at several intensive care units throughout hospitals in Montreal, Canada wondered if there might be a downside to this common practice. Specifically they worried about the effect on the babies' developing brains. In spite of the convenient benefits, the nurses were granted permission to give half the babies in their study plain water, while the other half got sugar water. They found that infants who got sugar in their first seven days of life suffered neurologic effects that were still measurable when the study ended, eleven weeks later. "[H]igher number of doses of sucrose predicted lower scores on motor development and vigor, and alertness and orientation…and higher NBRS [NeuroBiological Risk Score, a reflection of processes deleterious to brain development]."[252]

What does this study indicate? Little nips of sugar water given to alleviate pain impair a baby's cognitive development.

How could sugar have such powerful effects? As I mentioned earlier, sugar induces endogenous opiate release. The study authors postulate that repeated artificially induced stimulation of the immature brain with endogenous opiates interferes with normal development of alertness and arousal systems, so much so that babies who got the most sugar became lethargic. Endogenous opiates normally play a role in making us feel okay *after* something bad happens to us. The authors suggest that using sugar to induce the brain to release endogenous opiates *during* trauma prevents the brain from developing strategies to deal with pain normally. Why do they lose cognitive ability too? That question has yet to be answered.

Life is full of stresses and trials. Normally, we deal with them and move on. But studies like this suggest that, when we offer kids sweet treats as an incentive to settle down, we're rewiring their brains, potentially preventing them from learning normal, healthy, and more socially appropriate coping strategies than screaming for a box of juice. I have personally spoken with several child psychologists who feel that discipline among children is fast on the decline. For whatever reason, more and more adults seem unable to control their kids. My feeling is that if you start loading kids with sugar as a way of controlling behavior, you are not only training them to rely on external chemicals to feel good, you are training them to manipulate you to provide them with their fix. Sorry Willy Wonka, but my patients who've taken their kids off sugar tell me they can't believe what a better, more balanced, healthier family life they now have.

Sugar Damages Brain Cells, Making it Harder to Learn

Those at the other end of life's journey should know that research into the origin of Alzheimer's dementia implicates not genetic mutation, but sugar.

As we'll see in the next chapter, your body is constantly growing and responding to signals. And every part of you is swimming with chemicals

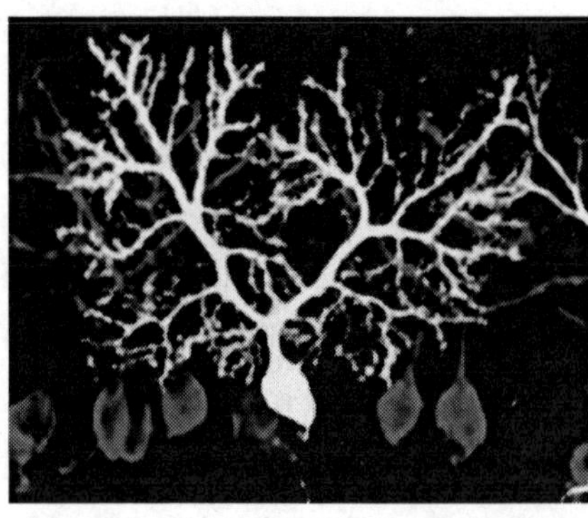
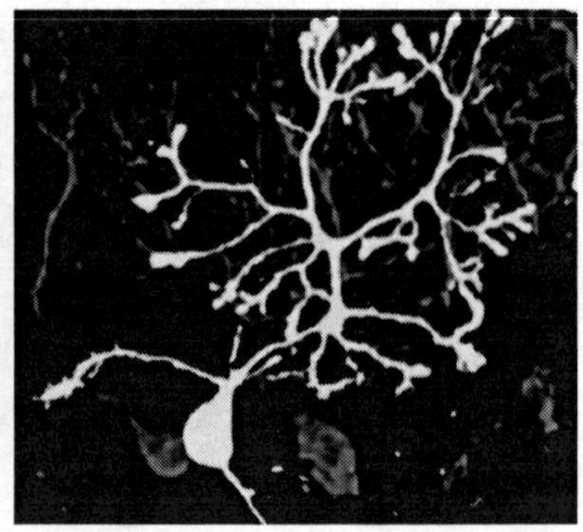

Figure 2. High-Sugar Diets May Lead to Dementia. On the left is a normal brain cell, called a purkinje cell. On the right, a purkinje cell that exhibits the reduced branching seen in demented brains. Since insulin is necessary for normal brain cell health, insulin resistance (a result of high-sugar diets) may cause similar brain cell changes.

From: Proc Natl Acad Sci U S A. 2006 February 7; 103(6): 1924–1929.

directing growth and cellular change, including your brain. When a brain is overloaded with sugar, you can see the effects on its cells.

Normally, a single brain cell looks a lot like a tree, with thousands of bifurcating branches, called *dendrites*. Dendrites on one brain cell reach out to dendrites on other brain cells to exchange the chemicals that enable us to remember, think, and experience emotions. Not surprisingly, intelligence roughly correlates with the number of branches in the brain's neural trees.

What makes the nerve cell grow more branches? It turns out that hormones do. The brain is constantly bathed in hormones that stimulate growth. Take away the hormones, and nerve cells branches die back.[253] In a way, growth factors act like dendritic Miracle Grow; the more growth factors you get, the more vigorous your brain cells can grow and the better you can think. One of the earliest stages of Alzheimer's dementia is the loss of these branches, a process called *dendritic pruning*.[254] It's likely that sugar-induced cross-linking gumming up brain cell membranes is at least part of the problem. As with any cell membrane, cross-links reduce hormone sensitivity. Less receptivity means your brain cells can't respond to growth factors. Less response means fewer branches, which mean fewer connections. It seems that sugar can act as a brain cell defoliant, changing the physical structure of your brain over the years and ultimately, for some, resulting in dementia. So if you've ever wondered why the Kool-Aid guy is always busting through walls, consider how much sugar he's drinking. He probably forgot how to use a door.

Dulling Your Senses

A study done in Iraq on sweet taste habituation showed that the more sugar we eat, the less we taste it, and the less we taste it, the more we eat. In Iraq, sweetened tea accounts for the majority of sugar consumption in all age groups. Researchers offered people four cups of tea with increasing concentrations of sugar. In rural areas, where sugar was scarce, almost nobody wanted the sweetest tea, only 0.3 percent. But among those who lived in the city for ten years or more, 100 percent preferred the sweetest tea on offer. The longer they'd lived in the city, the more sugar they wanted in their tea. The researchers asked everybody how much sugar they normally consumed, and then gave them another test to determine at what levels their taste buds could detect the presence of sugar. They found that the more sugar people tended to consume, the less they were able to taste it. Sugar had literally dulled their senses.[255]

I've done a similar experiment on my own. Using my own funding, I researched the effects of sugar on an unwitting subject—myself. For nearly a decade, I poured homemade caramel sauce into my coffee, each dose containing a quarter-cup of sugar. Luke (the experimental control) tried it once. After one taste, his eyes flew open wide, and he suggested I must be part insect. "You cannot possibly be drinking this every day," he insisted. I knew it was a lot of sugar, but no more than other people used. Like other junkies, I was rationalizing, and I ignored the advice to cut down. And that's what wore down my immune system so completely that a virus was able to take up residence in my knee. After a year or so of not being able to walk or get very much exercise, I decided maybe I should cut my sugar intake.

Gradually, I cut back. First one-eighth cup, then half of that, and then just a tablespoon or two. As I did, over the course of months, I noticed my knee slowly getting better. But as an addict, I chalked it up to coincidence.

How I Got Off Sugar and Changed My Life

Finally, I went on a trip and couldn't bring my caramel sauce, so I made do with just cream and milk in my coffee. To my surprise, it actually tasted fine. In fact, the cream tasted sweet. The next day, I noticed my knee was better than it had been in years. Recovering addicts often speak of moments of epiphany, or clarity, a moment when something finally clicks. Well, for me, the fact that I could enjoy the taste of coffee with milk and cream and *no sugar* meant that I really could do just fine without my little fix. And maybe, just maybe, my knee was improving because I was off the sugar. I'd had to step away from my habit, literally, to be removed enough from my daily routines and rituals in order to see the light. Now, as a recovered addict, I can better appreciate what my sugar-addicted patients are going through. I'm not just their doctor, I'm their sponsor.

From that day onward, I've never added sugar to my coffee. I've not had any soda or juice, I don't eat candy or cookies. I eat very little fruit. And I've cut out most starchy foods (for reasons described below). Not only has my knee recovered, the extra fifteen pounds I had on my waist since college melted away. Now I have absolutely no desire for anything sweet—except chocolate (I *am* human). But the chocolate I choose, Dagoba, is 89 percent cacao, hardly any sugar and no cheap fats. I have one-tenth of a bar three days a week, chopped fine and sprinkled over whipped cream (no sugar) as a topping for my coffee. I never thought I'd be the kind of person who passed on dessert. But now, not only am I freed of sugar cravings, my taste buds are rejuvenated. I can taste the natural sweetness in milk and cream. Even vegetables, like a raw carrot, now taste as sweet as candy. I eat as much as I ever did but weigh ten pounds less and spend less time feeling hungry. I wish I knew ten years ago how easy getting trim could be.

The Sugar Shell Game

Drug abusers say they don't have to look far to find their drug; the drug finds them. That's certainly true of sugar. The more people get wise about sugar and try to cut it out of their diet, the more manufacturers—the world's most successful drug pushers—sneak it into their products.

The problem is made all the worse by the fact that we've come to equate low-fat with healthy. Or, I should say, we've been taught to equate low-fat with healthy. But low-fat foods don't taste so great, so to make up for missing flavors from absent fat, manufacturers simply add sugar, and more sugar, and more. I'm looking at a can of Pediasure, which pediatricians frequently recommend over milk. The first ingredient is water. Guess what the second ingredient is? Sugar, accounting for 108 grams per liter.[256] Whole milk, by comparison, has 8 grams of sugar per liter.

Denying kids healthy fat often drives them to sugar. When Luke was growing up, he spent a lot of time at his grandparents' who were, like many people, on a low-fat kick. Everything in their fridge was low-fat—skim milk, low-fat yoghurt, no-fat dressing. By 4 o'clock, Luke and his siblings were tearing the place apart looking for fatty foods, anything with fat in it. And

Table 1. Sugar's Pseudonyms

Evaporated Cane Juice	Malt	Maple Syrup
Corn Syrup	Malt Syrup	Brown Rice Syrup
Corn Sweeteners	Barley Malt Syrup	Beet Juice
High Fructose Corn Syrup	Barley Malt Extract	Muscovato
Crystalline Fructose	Maltose	Succanat
Fructose	Maltodextrin	Turbinado Sugar
Sucrose	Dextrose	Invert Sugar

All of these are molecules of glucose and/or fructose and/or maltose and/or dextrose monosaccharides either alone, or bonded to one of the other two monosaccarides. All are converted to glucose or glycerine when you eat them. Glycerine forces your liver into fat-making mode for the same reason as fructose does (see text).

they found it, hidden in the cupboard in the form of Ding Dongs. On top of the fridge, in the Twinkies box. Out in the breezeway, on the wooden swing, behind the pillow, in the half-eaten package of Oreo cookies that Grandpa forgot to put back. Luke's grandparents were only trying to do the right thing, but they couldn't have set things up better to drive their grandkids not just to toxic, artificial fats but to massive doses of sugar. For this reason, weaning kids off sugar should be done in concert with providing plenty of healthy fats.

Luke's experience happened a good 30 years ago. Since then, we've learned something about how too much sugar can be a real problem. Still, avoiding sugar can be harder than you think because of what I call the Sugar Shell Game. You cut out Twinkies, but there's sugar in the salad dressing. You pass on the office cupcake, but there's sugar in the store-bought sushi. You decide to give up soda, but your "100 percent orange juice" is doped with corn syrup. (Some FDA officials suspect that many fruit juices claiming to be 100 percent natural juice are in fact sweetened with high-fructose corn syrup.[257] Fruit naturally contains fructose, so if manufacturers added more, how could anyone prove it?)

Packing In The Calories: Sugar Versus Fat

Dieters are typically encouraged to choose low-fat based on the idea that each spoonful of a low-fat product, say yoghurt or a mocha cappuccino, will have fewer calories. This fails to consider the fact that manufacturers make low-fat taste more palatable by adding sugar. Far more sugar will dissolve into water than you might assume, and so the unsuspecting dieter often swallows a load of unexpected calories. Concentrated syrups like the kind used in low-fat foods contain more calories than cream or butter: While a dry teaspoon of granulated sugar has 16.8 calories, less than butter's 33.3, when dissolved into water, freely moving sugar molecules pack together to occupy one-fifth the space, so concentrated syrups can contain up to 95 calories per teaspoon.

*From Inquiry In Action website; inquiryinaction.org/Inv4.html. Investigation 4: Dissolving solids, liquids, and gasses. (475 gm sugar in 100 gm water.)

Sweeteners are some of the cheapest ingredients around. So as the American palate is desensitized to sugar, supermarket foods undergo a kind of sweetness inflation, a race between manufacturers to hide more sugar in their products than the competition. What do you think kids want more, plain milk or chocolate? Plain shredded wheat or the frosted kind? Ice water with a twist of lime or a liter of Mountain Dew? The inevitable product of this arms race is the "energy drink," a twelve-ounce atom bomb of sugar, carbohydrates, and caffeine—everything the addict needs but the syringe.

Another way of hiding sugar is by simply calling it something else. Let's take a peek at the label of a popular brand of Raisin Bran Crunch to see just how much extra sugar they sneak in. Ingredients: "Whole Wheat, Rice, Sugar, Raisins [mostly sugar], Wheat Bran, High Fructose Corn Syrup [more sugar], Whole Oats, Glycerin, Brown Sugar [obviously sugar], Corn Syrup [still more sugar], Salt, Barley Malt Syrup [yes that's sugar], Partially Hydrogenated Soybean and/or Cottonseed Oil, Almonds, Modified Corn Starch, Cinnamon, Honey [full of sugar], Nonfat Dry Milk, Natural And Artificial Flavor, Polyglycerol Esters of Mono- and Diglycerides, Niacinamide, Zinc Oxide, Reduced Iron, Malt Flavoring [also sugar], [and a few artificial vitamins.]" (Table 1 shows other alternative names for sugar.)

Calorie-wise, almost half of what's in the box is sugar. What makes up the other half? Carbohydrates. Remember, I said manufacturers play the sugar shell game. If they can't sell you sugar, they'll happily sell you the next best thing, dirt-cheap carbs. Pasta lovers aren't going to want to hear this but, *as far as your body is concerned*, carbohydrates *are* sugar. That's right, one of the most abundant sources of sugar doesn't taste sweet.

Sugar, Sugar Everywhere

We live in a world of sugar. The single most common organic molecule on Earth is *glucose*, a kind of sugar. But unlike the candy garden in Willy Wonka's factory, we can't just eat anything we see. To humans, most of the world's glucose is not edible. It's trapped in a structural carbohydrate, called *cellulose*, which makes wood hard and leaves resilient. But another kind of carbohydrate called *starch* is digestible. Plants use starch to store energy and they reconvert it back to sugar when needed. The human digestive system can also convert starch into sugar, and every time we eat starch, it does. This is why, as far as your body is concerned, starch and sugar are almost the same.

Simple or Complex? Same Difference!

Everyone knows what a sugar high is. You eat a couple pieces of cake, and the next thing you know you're bouncing off the walls. And what happens afterwards? Your energy level plummets and you feel lethargic. If it's really bad, you feel like you're getting the shakes. The temptation is to treat these withdrawal symptoms with more sugar.

Sound familiar? Withdrawing from a sugar binge can feel a lot like withdrawing from a lot of other drugs, like alcohol. And we often treat it with the same homeopathic cure, a little hair of the dog. Of course, there are

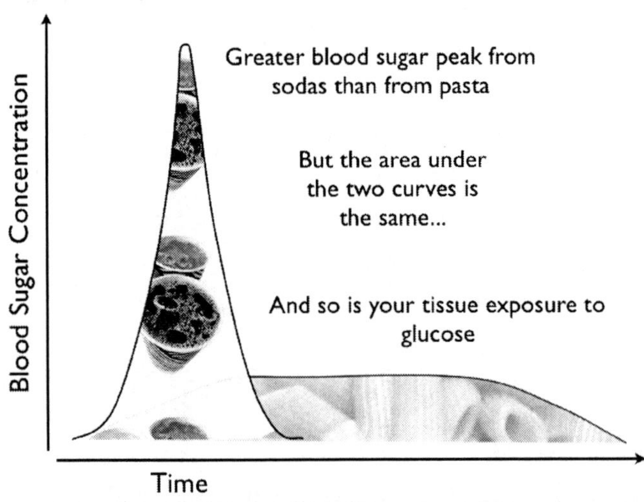

Figure 3. Area Under The Curve. In your bloodstream, complex carbs and simple carbs are all sugar. Complex carbs take more time to be absorbed, but they stay in the bloodstream longer, and have the same potential to cause AGE-related tissue damage.

other options. To avoid hangovers, you could drink less or none at all. Or, alternatively, you could avoid the spikes and valleys by maintaining a more constant blood alcohol level. You could modulate your dose by drinking more often, starting first thing in the morning. It would really be convenient if you could find some kind of a "complex" form of alcohol, one that takes time for the intestine to break down so that four or five drinks, downed all at once, could provide a nice, steady buzz for the rest of the day. If there were such an alcohol, no doubt we'd call it the "good" alcohol, the one preferred by all health-conscious alcoholics to avoid ever waking up with a hangover again.

Sugar is a "simple" carb. String a bunch of sugars together and you've got starch, a "complex" carb. There's much ado about complex carbs being healthier than sugars but, nutritionally, there's no difference whatsoever. The only difference between simple and complex carbs is how quickly they get into your bloodstream. So if you have diabetes or are just trying to avoid sugar swings, understand that when dietitians encourage choosing complex carbs for breakfast, it's very much as if they're telling a binge drinker to pace himself and get started first thing in the morning.

When you're eating pasta or a cracker, you don't feel as though you're doing anything naughty, because it doesn't taste sweet, like candy. But the molecules that make up starch *are* naughty; they're sugar. And once in your bloodstream, they'll be up to no good. Starch is like a chain gang which, when bound together in a long molecule (too long to fit into your taste buds) won't cause any harm. But if you let a cracker sit on your tongue long enough—or get broken down by digestion—the starch molecules turn into the very same sugar that you know is bad for your body.

If you've ever sat down and finished off a box of crackers, you've essentially just eaten a box of sugar. This stems from the fact that there's a big difference between ingesting and absorbing nutrients. You can swallow a small marble and say you've eaten it, but you'll never absorb it. Technically, eating refers only to the act of swallowing, whereas absorption refers to the act of bringing chemicals into your body. The point is, whether you *eat* sugar or starch, your body winds up *absorbing* sugar.

When we're talking carbs and sugar, we need to define our terms clearly. All carbs are composed of individual sugar molecules, called *monosaccharides*. Table sugar is made from glucose and fructose monosaccharides bound together into a *di*saccharide called sucrose. Mono- and disaccharides are simple carbohydrates, a.k.a. sugars. If more monosaccharide units are added to the chain, the name changes to *oligo*saccharide, *oligo* meaning few. Starches have hundreds of monosaccharide units connected together and are called "complex."

Foods like bread, pasta, potatoes, and rice are little more than containers for sugar. A seven-ounce serving of cooked spaghetti is converted into the amount of sugar contained in four 12-ounce cans of Pepsi. Unlike Pepsi, the pasta has been fortified with iron and a few vitamins. The starchy parts of plants also carry small amounts of protein and minerals, but white flour and white rice have had most of that removed. Whether the rice and bread are white or brown, whether the starch is in the form of breakfast cereal or tortilla chips, pasta or pancakes, complex or simple, you're mostly eating sugar.

The Four Pillar foods tend to have fewer carbs than their modernized counterparts. For instance, a slice of sprouted-grain bread has 70 calories. A same size slice of regular wheat bread has 110. This is because during the process of sprouting the seed converts its storage starch into nutrients. Seeds can do this easily. Our bodies can't.

I am not a big fan of breaking foods into carbs, protein, and all that. But because starchy, empty-calorie foods fill so many shelves in the store, it's one category we have to be aware of. I advise my patients with diabetes, or those who want to lose weight, that they should keep their *total* average carbohydrate intake under 100 grams per day. That means one small bowl of pasta, *or* four pieces of bread, *or* two apples, and that's it. If you are eating plenty of foods from the Four Pillars, exercising regularly, and are not worried about weight, then you can eat all the carbs you want.

Fruit Sugar

Another big source of sugar that surprises many people is sweet, sugary fruit. We've heard time and again we should "eat fruits and vegetables," as though the two are equivalent. But they're not. Vegetables contain a higher nutrient-to-energy ratio than fruit. Even fruits with decent nutrient content—like wild blueberries—are *full* of sugar. When you eat citrus, you're getting a wallop of sugar with very little nutrient thrown in. That's why, for most people, eating one apple-sized portion of fruit per day is plenty. With all that sugar, fruit just doesn't make the grade as a health food. As I tell my patients, fruit is a more natural alternative to a candy bar. And fruit juice, which lacks fiber and many of the antioxidants, is little better than soda.

People often protest the idea that fruit should be consumed in limited amounts. "At least it's *natural* sugar!" they say. Sure, but all sugar is natural. Sugar cane is natural. So is the corn from which high fructose corn syrup is made. The difference between sugar in fruit and sugar in high-fructose corn syrup (or confectioner's powder or granulated sugar) is that the former is still in its source material and the latter has been refined out of the source material and is devoid of other nutrients. And yes, that makes fruit a little better than sugar, but it's nothing to get worked up about. Though fruits do contain fiber, minerals, tannins and other flavinoids, which can function as antioxidants, sweet fruit is mostly sugar. *What about honey?* Same idea—mostly sugar and very little of anything else. Vitamin C happens to be a type of sugar we can't make and need to eat, and one orange a day gives us most of what we need. But then again, so does a green pepper (technically, a fruit), but without all the unneeded, damaging sugar.

To make matters worse for fruit lovers, fructose kicks your liver into fat-storage mode. Some believe the explosive growth of fructose consumption in the form of high fructose corn syrup may be responsible for the increased incidence of a condition called *fatty liver*. So although nutritionists and doctors will still insist that fruit sugar is better than sucrose, others aren't so sure. But everyone agrees we're all eating a lot more sugar than we should.

Can People Survive on Fruit?

Fruitarians, sometimes called fructarians, are a subset of vegetarians. Some people consider themselves fruitarians if at least half of their diet is fruit, while others go whole hog—if they'll forgive the expression—eating nothing but fruit. There are many explanations for choosing this lifestyle, from biblical references to anecdotal evidence of health benefits. The most popular seems to be that, since we are related to monkeys and other fruit-eating primates, living on fruit is only natural.

It's important to remember that many primates, including monkeys, supplement their diet with other foods like leaves, bark, bugs, nuts, and sometimes meat—even, on occasion, flesh of smaller primates. Some animals can get away with eating lots of sweet fruit because their big, rounded bellies contain digestive systems specifically designed for that purpose. The digestive tracts of orangutans, birds, and other fruit eaters are specialized to ferment the simple nutrients into more complex ones, enabling them to get far more nutrition from fruit than you could.

Is High-Fructose Corn Syrup Worse Than Table Sugar?

What is high fructose corn syrup? Is it really more likely to make you fat or give you diabetes than table sugar, honey, or any other sweetener?

Corn actually contains almost no fructose. It contains starch (a "complex" carb). Corn syrup manufacture begins with enzymatic break down of corn starch into its unit sugar molecule, glucose (this breakdown occurs in your GI tract during the digestion of any starch). Then, another enzyme converts glucose into fructose, to create high fructose corn syrup (HFCS). The fructose in HFCS is identical to the fructose that occurs naturally. What's different is that the rest of the fruit (or grain) nutrients are missing.

Before the explosion of the HFCS industry in 1978, fruit and grain (wheat, rice, oat, barley, etc.) products were the primary source of fructose. Now, grain and fruit consumption is down, and though we consume far more HFCS, our total fructose consumption has only increased by one percent. Fructose, therefore, cannot logically be blamed for today's obesity and diabetes epidemic. The root of today's obesity has more to do with the fact that total caloric intake has increased by 18 percent, and total carbohydrate intake has increased a whopping 41 percent over 1978 levels.

Animals that live on fruit or other sugary foods don't absorb very much sugar into their bloodstreams. The way their digestive tracts are organized enables these specialists to first ferment carbohydrates inside special chambers where bacteria, yeast, and other microbes grow, multiply, and manufacture vitamins, amino acids, and other nutrients (for their own use). These probiotic microbes ferment the sugar-rich fruits into a slurry teeming with life-supporting nutrients. By the time the slurry reaches a point along the digestive tract where absorption can take place, it has been transformed into something far more complex. The process is very similar to that employed by grass-eating animals to ferment high-cellulose foods into a more nutritious product. If our digestive tracts were designed like a gorilla's, we could eat a lot more fruit. But since we'd need a longer intestine to do it, we'd be carrying around gorilla-sized tummies as well.

Eat Like a Grownup!

When I was four or five, I thought of "kid foods" as things like cupcakes, peanut butter and jelly sandwiches with Wonder Bread, cereal—especially Cap'n Crunch!—and lots and lots of noodles. When the grownups went out to eat by themselves, I imagined they were eating things like liver, strange pates, smelly cheese, and thick meaty stews. In my imagination, they probably didn't even have dessert.

What I didn't know was that, since the 1980s, the USDA has promoted practically nonstop consumption of sugar for everyone, recommending that 60 percent of our daily calories come from carbohydrate-rich foods. So, it turns out, most of the adults in my life were eating kid foods too. Today, with all the finger foods, cookies, snacks, treats, and sugar everywhere, we might as well be having a non-stop birthday party. Little wonder, then, so many people are struggling with their weight. In the next chapter, you'll see that eating like a grownup can not only make you healthier, it makes getting (or staying) slim as easy as pie.

Ten

Beyond Calories

Using Food as a Language to Achieve Ideal Body Weight

In medical school I was taught a simple formula: Calories consumed minus calories burned equals weight gained or lost. Then, as a resident treating my own patients, I'd sit down with people who wanted to lose weight and lay out the formula for their benefit.

Then things got complicated. Time and time again I'd hear, *I don't understand it, Doc. I don't eat anything all day. I work out. But I'm still gaining! There must be something wrong with me. Can you check a thyroid level?* I would, but the results were always normal. I'd try suggesting that they might have been consuming more calories than they realized, pointing out that eating on the go—while driving home for instance—is still eating. But many times, patients really seemed to defy the formula. They'd eat little, go to the gym and take walks around the block, and yet the pudge refused to budge. Was it just their metabolism? Or could the energy-balance formula be flawed?

Turns out, weight gain and loss isn't so much about energy as it is about *information*. As you've read in the preceding chapters, food is far more than fuel; it's a language that programs every function of your cells. If you've been gaining weight, it's because you are eating foods and doing activities that, in essence, tell your body to pack on the pounds. You know how a few clever words can convince you to do things that, in retrospect, seem foolish? Our bodies can be convinced to do things we wish they wouldn't, too. It all depends on what we eat, and the kind of *messages* our food contains. Foods with the right messages immediately start making us healthy because our bodies are continually responding to what we do—and foods with the wrong messages can act immediately too. The Four Pillar foods instruct your body to do its very best, and once you start eating them, better health will come automatically.

To see just how powerfully the chemicals in our food—and not their calorie content—influence our cellular decisions, let's take a look at two different kinds of fats. Essential fatty acids omega-3 and -6 are nearly identical to the chemists who draw them on their chalkboards. But to our cells, they are as opposite as night and day.

Energy Versus Information: Why Calories Don't Count

In 1995, a journalist named Jo Robinson struck up a chance conversation with a scientist examining a biologic process called *apoptosis*, a kind of cell suicide in which a damaged cell recognizes that it is more likely to be harmful than useful and dutifully takes itself apart. Using catheter tubes to feed cancerous tumors growing in rats directly, he'd discovered that while injecting omega-3 slowed and even reversed growth, injecting omega-6 accelerated growth four-fold. These fatty acids contain essentially equivalent caloric energy, so why should one make cells divide and another bring cell division to a grinding halt?

Clearly, the process of growth is regulated by something other than calories. To Robinson, this research suggested something startling—not about growth in general but about the underlying cause of cancer: *A fatty acid imbalance might set us up for cancer*. She asked the scientist what kinds of foods contain omega-6 and -3. He explained, "Omega-3 comes from things like eggs, cold-water fatty fish, and plants people don't eat anymore, like flax." The growth-promoting omega-6 fatty acids, on the other hand, are hard to avoid as they are prevalent in corn, soy, animals fed these grains, and the vegetable oils inside just about every package on the food store shelves.

Robinson relived that moment in the lab as I sat with her in her home overlooking the Puget Sound, and a mix of inspiration and determination came over her face. "I knew what I had to do," she said. Together with Artemis Simopolous, she went on to write the best-selling book *The Omega Diet,* which introduced the world to essential fats and filled a huge gap in conventional nutrition education. Her book explains that in the Paleolithic era we ate roughly ten times more omega-3 than we do now, and far less omega-6. That shift in consumption has created a nationwide dietary imbalance that exacerbates numerous inflammatory diseases, including cancer, arthritis, and obesity.

Dozens of researchers have since built careers describing how omega-3 helps prevent all manner of disease. Just a little more of this one essential fat can help every cell in your body function better. That's great news. But while a lot of attention has been focused on specific benefits of omega-3, our discoveries about omega-3 and -6 tell us something more: Our cells are extremely sensitive to the specific nature of the chemical messages we send them every time we eat. By altering the blends of nutrients (or toxins) in our food, we can actually control whether our cells function normally, or convert to fat, or turn cancerous. The nutrients and chemicals we consume in effect *tell* our cells what to do—when to divide, which protein to manufacture, and even what type of cell to become.[258]

Our omega-3 and -6 ratio problem is just one of many dietary imbalances which together send a barrage of mixed-up signals to our cells, telling our bodies to store fat and lose muscle and bone—all the stuff we don't want them to do. What's key to being healthy, then, is eating foods that send the right messages. Once we appreciate how common foods convince our cells to behave in ways that make us sick, we can understand why so many of us struggle with something as fundamental as maintaining optimum bodyweight. So the Deep Nutrition formula for weight loss is simple: *Get rid of inflammation that blocks cellular communication, and eat foods that enable you to convert fat cells into healthier tissues.*

Of course, there's more to health than a healthy diet. Sleep and physical activity generate other chemicals that help your body know what you are expecting of it. So in order to reshape your body and achieve maximum health, your regimen *must* include eating real food, resting properly, reducing stress, and doing the right kinds of exercise. The rest of this chapter will take you step-by-step through what you need to do to make the most of your body's amazing potential for change.

Step 1: Appreciate What Fat Does for You

You'll never get on *Baywatch* without body fat, and I'm not just talking about Pam Anderson's most obvious assets. A twenty-year-old's face has far more fat around the eyes, lips, and chin than that of a seventy-year-old. Well-placed fat makes people look young. And, truth is, we can't be healthy without it. Aside from acting as simple mechanical insulation and cushioning, body fat generates chemicals required for sexual development and reproduction, immune defense, blood clotting, circadian rhythm, and even mood and concentration.[259,260,261] Life without any adipose tissue would be very difficult indeed. Paradoxically, not enough and too much fat tissue cause many of the same problems: "Fatless mice are prone to insulin insensitivity, glucose intolerance, hyperphagia, weight gain, fatty liver, and high triglyceride [levels]."[262] Just like fat mice.

Most of us, of course, are trying to slim down. If you've gone on a diet without achieving the body-changing results you had hoped for, chances are you've never been given the full story on fat, its function, and the steps you can take to control it. The more we understand the reasons our bodies create and retain fat, the better we can understand how to turn unwanted fat into something better.

The wonderful news is that fat cells, like all cells, are always ready to follow our instructions on what to do next. Those instructions come primarily from physical activity and the foods we eat. Contrary to popular belief, fat cells are *not* forever. But the strategy is not to "melt the pounds away" by starving, or sweating them out into the ether. As with the tumor cells that killed themselves when omega-3 was added, you can command your fat cells, by way of certain chemical signals, to do what you want.

Why Supplements Won't Work

So what are those chemical signals? That's the question that a multi-billion dollar industry has been obsessing over for decades.

In 1995, researchers working with a breed of grossly overweight mice discovered that the breed lacked a chemical called *leptin*. Biotech companies immediately saw dollar signs, investing heavily in leptin research. They even patented the gene. Shortly after its discovery, leptin was found to suppress appetite and fat cell division. Leptin researchers thought they'd stumbled onto a goldmine.

They had, but it was fool's gold. Obesity isn't a simple matter of leptin deficiency; it's a complex problem of multiple imbalances. It soon became clear that overweight people are not only leptin deficient; they are also leptin *resistant*. Their bodies are unable to hear the signal leptin sends, so giving them more leptin wouldn't help. Worse, one potential side effect of leptin supplementation includes breast cancer.[263] And so, as quickly as it came, the leptin gold rush was over. The rise and fall of leptin is emblematic of our misplaced faith in technologic fixes for biologic problems. The real solution will come not from technology, but biology—in the form of healthy food.

After learning that obese people were leptin resistant, the researchers missed an opportunity. If they'd recognized that leptin resistance might indicate that signals were being blocked, they might have asked a crucial question: *What might be blocking them?* We've already hinted at it in earlier chapters: a kind of chemical static that interferes with normal metabolic processes called *inflammation.*

Step 2: Rid Your Body of Inflammation

Pro-Inflammatory Foods: What Not to Eat

Inflammation is a huge buzzword in the nutrition world these days. You can find inflammation indices, lists of anti-inflammatory and pro-inflammatory foods, and anti-inflammation menu plans. And there are plenty of supplements claiming to be anti-inflammatory. Why is inflammation so bad?

Inflammation is disruptive. It can block chemical signals required for normal, healthy cellular growth. Inflammation also tends to generate its own signals that tell our bodies to store fat. You could say that healthy foods will educate your cells so they'll grow up to be useful members of your physiology, while pro-inflammatory foods trick individual cells into doing things that are dangerous for the body as a whole. The tendency for processed foods to cause inflammation is one big reason we have to go beyond the calorie content listed on a package to understand how the foods we eat will make us gain or lose weight. Instead of focusing on calories, if we look at the *signals* different meals generate, we can readily understand why processed foods make us build fat and the Four Pillars help us to lose it.

Distorted Fats Damage Enzymes and Lead to Cellular Death

If you've read Chapter 8, you know that heating vegetable oils leads to the formation of oxidized and distorted fats called MegaTrans, and that these two groups of fats can generate free radicals, which are pro-inflammatory. You also know that saturated fat helps you resist free radical damage, and therefore resist inflammation. So you already know two factors other than calories that influence how fats affect your health. As we'll see, distorted fats like trans and MegaTrans can also make you gain weight.

Distorted fats are pro-inflammatory because of their unnatural shapes; they act like a booby trap for your enzymes. An enzyme called delta-9 desaturase mistakes trans fat for saturated fat and picks it up. But now that enzyme's in real trouble. There's a kink in the trans molecule that acts like a barb, so that once it goes in to the enzyme, it won't come out. Another enzyme called delta-6 desaturase thinks trans fat looks like an omega-3 or omega-6 fatty acid, so it picks it up and runs into the same problem: Once it touches trans, it can't let go. Trans fat in your diet effectively deactivates many of your delta-6 and delta-9 fat-metabolizing enzymes. With enough of these enzymes shut down, your cells can no longer metabolize normal,

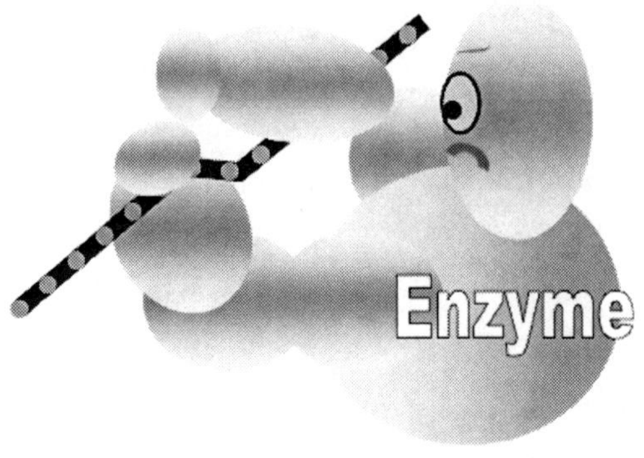

Figure 1. Pro-Inflammatory Fats Prevent Weight Loss. This poor enzyme has picked up a molecule of trans fat and now he can't let go. Abnormally shaped fatty acids knock key enzymes out of action. Without these enzymes, the body cannot act on the message to burn fat or build muscle—no matter how much you exercise.

healthy fatty acids fast enough, and at high levels they can be toxic.[264]

When free fatty acids build up in the liver, you get a condition called *fatty liver*, which can be diagnosed with an ultrasound test. Fatty liver turns on fat-building enzymes in the liver and elsewhere, which can lead to toxic levels of free fatty acids inside a cell.[265,266] Even in the early stages of fatty liver, people lose control of their weight as so many of their body tissues are forced (by malfunctioning enzymes) to convert sugar (and carbs) into fat.[267,268] Low-calorie diets don't cure fatty liver. What a person with fatty liver needs to do is rehabilitate their liver, and Four Pillar foods can do that.

Free fatty acids within liver and other cells may become toxic simply because too many can get "underfoot" (like kid's toys) and end up disturbing normal cellular activity. In muscle cells, for example, free fatty acids can interfere with the assembly of internal supports, called *microtubules*, that enable muscle cells to contract.[269] With too much free fatty acid polluting a muscle cell, the microtubules cannot be properly constructed. And so they break apart. As fat continues to build up and internal supports break down, the cell enters a state of decay called *lipoapoptosis*.[270] Lipoapoptosis kills healthy cells, leads to inflammation, immune disorders, and the buildup of additional fat.[271]

The more distorted fat you eat, the more inflammation you're fighting against. Trans fat reduces your ability to metabolize the saturated *and* essential fatty acids that you need to be healthy, so eating trans fat can initiate a vicious cycle. The Nurses' Health Study showed that a mere *two* percent increase in trans fat consumption correlated with a *40* percent increase in insulin resistance and diabetes.[272] Once you develop diabetes, your metabolism is deeply committed to converting as many calories as it can into fat. Given the power of unnatural fat to disturb metabolism, it's no wonder the advice to avoid healthy, natural fat sets us up to fail.

To successfully avoid eating oxidized fats, you must avoid all foods containing vegetable oils. As I described in Chapter 7, vegetable oils are high in *polyunsaturated* fats, which are particularly prone to oxidation and readily deformed into the collection of distorted fatty acids I call MegaTrans. And, as explained in Chapter 7, saturated fat resists oxidation. So much so that, in the body, it can help check inflammation before it gets too far out of control. So eating foods like butter, cream, and coconut oil can protect against some of the worse effects of oxidation and actually help you lose weight.

Dr. Atkins focused on saturated fat for his popular low-carb diet because he noticed eating it helped people lose weight. He didn't know about the anti-inflammatory effects of saturated fat. He just knew what worked. But without knowing exactly *why* it worked, he couldn't go so far as to advise people to avoid pro-inflammatory vegetable oils. Because of the prevailing view that saturated fat is harmful and vegetable oils beneficial, physicians and nutritionists running weight-loss organizations—from South Beach, to Lindora, to Weight Watchers—wrongly advise people to avoid saturated fat and encourage the consumption of unhealthy vegetable oils. Without the full story, people who try these kinds of weight loss programs may enjoy temporary success but in the long term are likely to run aground.

To Avoid Inflammation, Keep Total Daily Sugar Intake Under 100 Grams

High fructose corn syrup can make it practically impossible for you to normalize your weight. We've all heard that when bears need to fatten up for winter, they eat berries. It turns out that fructose sugar (in fruit, fruit juice, soda, and more) sends especially powerful fat-building signals by switching on liver enzymes for converting sugars to fat. Since most of the food you eat gets sent to the liver first, eating fructose effectively traps dietary carbohydrates in your liver and converts them to fat, preventing them from ever making it to muscle tissue where they could be burned during exercise.

So fructose-containing foods can make you pack on the pounds, but there's really no sugar that's *good* for you. As we saw in Chapter 9, sugar sticks to things. A sugar coating on your cells (in the form of AGEs) blocks hormone signals. This blocking ability is *disruptive,* and so sugar itself (when consumed in high levels) is pro-inflammatory. Excess dietary sugar disrupts hormonal signals for building muscle, for instance. You'll see below that the process of converting fat to muscle involves all kinds of hormone signals, and sugar-induced AGEs can block them all.

Because carbohydrates in your food are converted into sugars, a diet high in pastas, breads, and so on, is inherently pro-inflammatory as well. Worse, these starchy foods are so bereft of vitamins and other antioxidants that building a diet around them can make it hard for your body to control oxidation reactions once they start. This puts you deeper into a pro-inflammatory state.

For all these reasons, I tell my patients who are having difficulty shedding the pounds to keep their total carbohydrate intake to less than 100 grams per day (this total includes sugars and "complex" carbs like starches).

Of course calories do play some role in all this. That's why it's good to be aware that sugar dissolves in water so well that a teaspoon of sugary syrup can contain *up to four times* the calories as a teaspoon of granulated sugar. This means fat-free cookies can pack more fat-producing power than regular cookies. It also explains why those who have the toughest time loosing weight often have kitchens full of fat-free products.

Step 3: Learn Where Fat Comes From—And Where it Goes

Fat Grows from Stem Cells

You've probably heard of *stem cells,* immature cells derived from embryos with the potential to grow replacement parts for any organ. These are the cells you've seen researchers use to grow ears on the back of mice. Many believe stem cells hold the cure for Alzheimer's, Parkinson's, and a host of other currently incurable diseases, and someday they may. But if you want to reshape your body, harnessing stem cell versatility can help you achieve that goal today.

One of the most frustrating things about fat is its ability to seemingly appear from nowhere. It's really coming from stem cells.[273] When you eat sugar, starch, and trans fat without exercising your body will churn out new fat cells like a termite queen producing eggs. When stem cells turn into fat cells and grow plumper, you grow plumper too.

One reason diets fail is that cutting back on calories without changing any other habits sends precisely the wrong message. The body presumes that the relative scarcity of food, in combination with little activity, must mean food has become so scarce you've given up looking for more. If it has the slightest chance to store surplus energy as fat, the panicked body reasons it had better do so. Under these circumstances, stem cells stand at the ready to convert themselves into more energy-storing fat cells. Frightening our stem cells into turning into fat cells is exactly the wrong thing to do. Instead, we should capitalize on the stem cell's protean nature and convince it to turn into a kind of cell we want.

Like what, you say? Like muscle, blood vessel, nerve and bone. What's even more remarkable than stem cell versatility is the fact that grown-up fat cells seem capable of changing their identity almost as readily as stem cells can. That means you don't need to starve to get rid of all that flab; it can be *transformed* into the healthy tissues of a brand new beautiful you.

Fat Can Transform Back into Stem Cells, and Other Types of Cells

You might find this hard to believe, but fat cells require constant attention to maintain their girth. Many people who have tried to improve their looks by having fat injected into their lips and cheeks have seen their enhancement melt away when the transplanted fat cells refused to flourish in their new locations. When researchers investigated this phenomenon, they found that not only had the once-plump cells slimmed down to fusiform slivers, some had changed into an entirely different type of cell, called a *fibrocyte*, the type of cell most prevalent in the tissues into which the fat cells had been injected.[274] Apparently, fibrocytes surrounding the transplanted fat cells refused to make the introduced cells feel at home (by producing the necessary fat-sustaining hormones). Without these hormones, the receptors and enzymes that enable fat cells to do their thing—ingest sugar and fat and grow pudgy—began to shut down. Shrinking under the peer pressure of a hormonally cold shoulder, the unwelcome guests simply conformed to the rules of the neighborhood and reinvented themselves as fibrocytes.

You may be able to coerce fat cells into becoming just about anything you want. Fat tissue belongs to a class of body material called connective tissue, which collectively includes collagen, bone, muscle, blood, and associated cells. Some cell biologists now believe that one type of connective tissue cell permanently retains its ability to transform into another cell type whenever chemical signals instruct it to do so. So muscle cells can become fat cells; fat can become bone; and then a bone cell can change back to a fat cell again. This process is termed *trans*differentiation. (See Figure 2). As I'll discuss later, there is evidence that the potential for transdifferentiation may even extend across *all* tissue types.[275,276,277,278]

All this suggests that a fat cell on your thigh today might once have been a muscle, bone, or skin cell, living someplace else in your body. But why, you may wonder, would any cell decide to pack its bags and head to an entirely

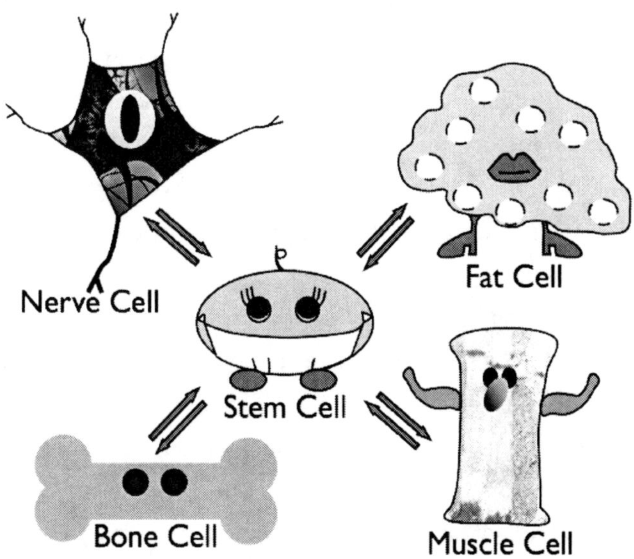

Figure 2. The Right Signals Can Turn Fat Cells Into Muscle, Bone, or Nerve. A metabolic process called transdifferentiation can make fat cells leave your adipose tissue and migrate to become new muscle, bone, and even brain cells. You can control stem cell growth by eating right and exercising, and that includes exercising your brain. (See text for supporting references.)

new location? It would if it received a chemical memo saying that its service in its current tissue is no longer required, and that it should head to its new assignment in the fat department.

So if some fat cells were once cells in preferable kinds of tissues, how can we order them to go back? One of the most effective ways to send that kind of message is with exercise. According to Dr. Robert Lustig, Professor of Pediatric Endocrinology at University of California, San Francisco, the reason exercise treats obesity *is not* because it "burns" calories. "That's ridiculous," he says. "Twenty minutes of jogging is one chocolate chip cookie. I mean you can't do it. One Big Mac requires three hours of vigorous exercise to burn off. That's not the reason exercise is important."[279] Exercise is important because it generates signals to transdifferentiate your fat.

Exercise works at least three ways: 1) It increases insulin sensitivity, so you need less insulin to get sugar out of the bloodstream. This allows your insulin levels to drop, which tells your fat cells to slow down the conversion of sugar into more fat. 2) It reduces the stress hormone cortisol. Cortisol packs fat around organs (as opposed to under the skin) where it produces lots of pro-inflammatory chemicals, which in turn tell the body to produce still more fat. And 3) Exercise makes blood sugar levels drop, and with it the potential for AGEs and the sugar-induced inflammation that blocks healthy body-building signals.

So if our body simply recycles cells from one tissue type to another, how does weight ever go down? Once fat cells store energy, they guard it jealously, reluctant to give it up. But when you convert fat to muscle, you rev up your metabolism, which drains fat cells. What's more, fat cells can undergo the same kind of cellular suicide that tumor cells can, called apoptosis.

This discovery that so many cellular transformations are occurring has unsettled the medical community, which must now abandon the old notion of a cell as something created to be a lifelong member of one particular cellular species. This model grossly underestimates the cell's protean nature. Just as genes change in reaction to what we eat, think, and do, cells change their internal construction too, *de*differentiating from a mature phase back into the immature, *pluripotent* stage of cell life. And then, from the pluripotent stage, they can be instructed to *re*differentiate back into the original, or even be recruited into another type of tissue altogether. The culture medium scientists use for inducing all those cellular transformations is not an alien brew of unnatural chemicals, but rather a full complement of vitamins, amino acids, and sugar, plus different mixtures of naturally occurring growth factors and hormones that a healthy young body normally manufactures. The readiness and completeness with which cells respond to such instructions suggests that these conversions are an integral aspect of healthy physiologic function.[280]

How Fat Cells Change

Nearly every step of the fat cell self-improvement program has been replicated in the lab. Though no one knows exactly how it functions in the body, it might go something like this: First, an individual fat cell loses much, or all, of its lipid stores. Then the shriveled fat cell gets a signal to *de*differentiate into a more mobile cell type, one that is chemically indistinguishable from a stem cell. The cell exits the fat tissue by way of the bloodstream and, once in circulation, is directed to go wherever growth is occurring—a muscle, say. Upon arrival, the cell attaches to the wall of a tiny blood vessel and waits for the stimulus to migrate into the muscle tissue itself. Once it gets the right signal, it moves inside the matrix of the new tissue and *re*differentiates to match the other cell types in its new location. Whatever the exact sequence of cell reassignment, the abilities of the magical morphing cell suggest that our body is composed not of cellular specialists, but of generalists, ready to be retrained and reassigned at a moment's notice. And that's encouraging news because it tells us that, if we know what we're doing, our best health may still be ahead of us.

Why Moderation, Small Portions, and Starvation Diets Fail

Moderation, as a program for healthy eating, made perfect sense 200 years ago when crops were grown organically on healthy topsoil, and the worst chemical monstrosities of the food industry were yet to be invented. Back then, there were no such things as Twinkies, curly fries, high fructose corn syrup, or trans fat. Today, few places remain on this planet where people flavor food with homemade broths instead of with MSG, where they still ferment vegetables and meats instead of storing them in the fridge, where they eat every part of the animal instead of just a few cuts. In places like this, "everything in moderation" would actually work. But in the world of modern, processed foods, "everything in moderation" is a recipe for a moderate level of health, which these days is hardly something you want to aim for.

Another kind of "moderation" is moderating the volume of food consumed, i.e. calorie restriction. You might think that calorie restriction might convince fat cells that they're no longer needed, and lead to apoptosis. On calorie restriction diets, fat cells shrink but they rarely disappear. For the most part, as soon as the calories return so does the fat inside the cells. Why?

Table 1: Factors That Make You Build Fat	
Omega-6 fatty acids	Converted into arachidonic acid (AA), which makes fat cells divide. Stress, sleep deprivation, and obesity generate more AA.
Insulin	Increases fat cell numbers. Signs that you may have abnormal levels of insulin are dark patches of skin in creases and under your arms, and central obesity—fat that tends to collect around the waist and under the chin. Irregular periods may also indicate abnormal insulin levels.
Sugars	Increase insulin levels. Increase triglyceride production in the liver. Trigger fat cells to "wake up" and start making fat from sugar in the bloodstream.
Thiazolidinediones (A diabetes medication)	Stimulates fat cell division. Increases fat storage. These were originally thought to be weight loss pills based on a ridiculously optimistic analysis of their effects on cell metabolism. Now we realize they exacerbate insulin resistance in the long term, and have been associated with a higher rate of heart attacks. If you are on this medication, ask your doctor if there is an alternative.
Glucocorticoids	Stimulate fat cell division. The body makes glucocorticoids all the time, but levels rise during stress and sleep deprivation.
Unnatural (MegaTrans) Fats	Promote free radical formation, cell membrane damage, and inflammation—all of which lead to the deposition of omental and submandibular fat while intercepting healthy cell-building signals.

It appears the body is cautious and, like any good manager, resists taking drastic action—like firing a cell permanently—until it has darn good reason.

The reluctance of your body to permit fat cells to undergo apoptosis means that if you never exercise *properly* (see below), though you restrict your calories, your fat tissues never receive the chemical memo that more cells are needed in another department, and so the fat cells stay put. As long as fat cells are fat cells, they have no choice but to try to pack on more fat and will do so at any opportunity. What's more, as the body converts fat cells into muscle cells there's little net loss of mass, which would explain why

Table 2: Factors That Eliminate Fat	
Exercise	Reduces insulin and corticosteroid levels as well as levels of many other less well known pro-inflammatory and fat-promoting chemicals.
Sleep	Reduces corticosteroid levels, increases levels of immune system chemicals that reduce inflammation.
Tumor Necrosis Factor Alpha	Reduces fat cell number. Produced during sleep, and in response to infection and cancer growth.
Retinoids	Reduce fat cell number. Reduce appetite. Retinoids include vitamin A from animal fat and organ meats, and vitamin A precursors (called *carotenoids*) from vegetables.
Leptin	Reduces fat cell number.
Cholesterols (Cholesterol actually represents a whole family of molecules)	Reduces appetite. Studies have shown that plant sterols and stanols effectively reduce appetite. What are plant sterols and stanols? Cholesterol that plants make. Bile acids also contain cholesterol. When secreted into the small intestine after a meal, they signal the body that you've had enough to eat. Unfortunately, nobody can get funding to study any potential benefit of cholesterol. But you can try this simple experiment yourself: Day One: eat two eggs cooked in 2 Tbsp butter for breakfast and see if you're hungry by lunch. Day Two: eat one cup of granola in one cup of skim milk and see if you're hungry by lunch. Both have about 500 calories.

people who start exercise programs don't notice weight loss right away.

Many doctors and diet gurus argue that calorie restriction works. Just look at prisoners who've been starved for months or even years. Their energy expenditure was higher than their energy intake so, *ipso facto*, the coal furnace model of physiology (the one I condemned at the opening of this chapter) holds. It's basic thermodynamics, they argue. And to an extent, they're right; there's no cheating physics. But if you're trying to reshape your body simply by reducing portion size, then realize that you're basing your dietary program on what you've seen the human body do under extreme, long-term, incredibly unhealthy starvation conditions.

Earlier, we talked about how calorie restriction without exercise tells your body to convert stem cells into fat cells as soon as you start eating again. And the body doesn't just wait patiently. It cranks up your appetite to prod you into increasing your food-seeking efforts while readying fat cells you already have to receive any forthcoming bounty. When you finally do eat a full meal, your body rushes the energy into storage—hence the typical yo-yo cycle of weight loss and rapid gain with small portion diets.

For as long as you manage to deal with your hunger, your body is forced to start using up fat cells—just as you'd hoped—but will also mine other tissues for vitamins, minerals, and essential fats. These tissues can include brain, connective tissue, and muscle. Of course, since muscle burns calories all by itself, once you start losing muscle it becomes harder to lose weight. The lesson here is that hunger is not the way to reshape your body. Here in Hawaii, the surfers have a saying: *Never fight the ocean.* If you want an athletic, svelte, attractive figure, then don't fight your body. Call a truce by eating foods from the Four Pillars, exercising, cutting stress, and getting a full night's sleep.

Inflammation Makes Fat Invasive, Like Cancer

Now that you know all kinds of body tissues can interconvert, let's take a look at how this process can work against us to make us not just too heavy but also unhealthy.

On a pro-inflammatory diet, our physiology starts making fat cells so fast you'd think it were some kind of nervous habit. When stressed, we head straight for the Häagen-Dazs. And in a sense, so do our physiologies, as transdifferentiation converts all kinds of cells into fat.

In patients with age-related dementia, grey matter gets replaced by cells containing excessive amounts of fat.[281] Osteoporotic bones have had bone-forming cells replaced by fat cells.[282] And fatty liver, a common cause of chronic indigestion and GERD symptoms (like heartburn), is caused by fat cell formation at the expense of normal, functioning liver cells. To put all this in terms of the larger regulatory picture, when muscle, bone, gland, and nerve cells are denied a full complement of vitamins, amino acids, minerals and so on, they seem to take that denial as a signal to dedifferentiate and start storing fat. With so many cells abandoning their posts in healthy tissues to join the growing ranks of fat cells, you can imagine how poorly these tissues function. This whole degenerative process can be expedited in the presence of cortisol from stress and lack of sleep, or from the many inflammatory factors that build up from a lack of exercise. An imbalanced diet, which releases still more inflammatory signals, makes things even worse.

Fat-making may seem like the body's default reaction, but really it's just the default reaction in periods of stress and nutrient deprivation. When the body gets all the real food, exercise, and rest that it needs, the default reaction is to convert unwanted fat cells into something better. Which physiologic directive your body follows is ultimately up to you.

Some nutrient deficiencies and stress levels are so severe, however, that it becomes increasingly difficult to ship nutrients throughout the body effectively. If sugar and fatty acids can't make the journey from wherever they were (usually your digestive system) into a proper fat-storage cell, then they end up lining your arteries, seeping into your tendons, and polluting your body. Now, instead of building fat, you just get sick. White blood cells will have to enter these polluted segments of artery, joint, or any other compromised tissue and try to clean up the mess. But white blood cells cause inflammation, which damages tissues (including arterial walls), makes your joints hurt, and clots your blood. This is why a diet that makes you fat also makes you feel bad, raises your blood pressure, and causes diabetes, heart disease, kidney problems, and so many other diseases. It's also why white blood cells filled with fat are found in so many degenerated organs.

Cancer is a consequence of unhealthy cell communication: The cell mutates because it receives abnormal chemical instructions. When these mutants divide rapidly and invade other tissues, they are called *metastases*. Many cancer cells produce hormones to maintain a state of constant growth, unrestrained by the body's instructions. Like cancer, fat produces pro-inflammatory factors that stimulate its own growth.[283] More fat sends a louder signal to the body to create still more fat. And fat cells invade other tissues, just as cancer does. Even thin people can, through poor diet, encourage fat to infiltrate healthy tissues. When fat invades, we develop cellulite, weakened bones, and brain and muscle atrophy. Finally, like cancer, obesity is associated with blood clots, fatigue, and premature death. Obesity behaves like a self-sustaining tumor, and anyone who is overweight can feel trapped in its vicious cycle. I see people whose losing battle against their weight has them as frightened as someone with cancer, willing to pay anything for a cure.

Fortunately, fat cells *can* be retrained.

And that's the word I want you to keep in mind, *retraining*. People are often amazed how amenable their pets are to training—once they learn to communicate with them effectively. The same goes for our cells. A key point of my message is that our cells react to the signals we send them through diet and activity, and they do their best to comply. Once you've cleared your body of inflammation, then exercise helps your body know what to do with the food it gets. It's like sending a wish list to your cells: *I'd like more muscle in the pectorals, less flab on my thighs, and—oh yes, I've been clumsy lately—I'd like*

Weakened Collagen Can Make Fat Look Lumpy

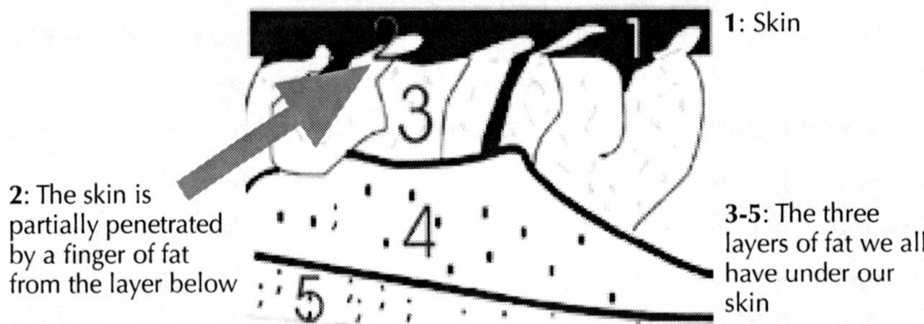

Figure 3. Why Some People Develop Cellulite. In this diagram of a cross section of skin and the fat below, collagen is shown in black, fat in white. Layer 1 (the skin) looks black because skin is collagen rich. Layers 2-5 are fatty and contain very little collagen, so they look white. In people with cellulite, fat in layer 3 produces pro-inflammatory chemicals, called *cytokines*. This weaken the collagen, literally melting it away to create thin spots in the skin and allowing the fat sitting below it to extrude (ooze) upward, filling the defects. The resulting fingers of fat cause the skin to dimple, giving cellulite its lumpy, cottage cheese appearance.

Source: Pilot study of dermal and subcutaneous fat structures by MRI in individuals who differ in gender. Skin Res. Technol. 2004 Vol 10, 161-168.

more proprioceptive neural tissue coordinating motion of my ankles and my lower spine. For most of us, the wish list includes a trimmer waistline, more energy, and a sexier physique. To accomplish that, we need an exercise program that will send that message, which means—since each sends a distinct set of signals—one that includes both aerobic *and* anaerobic activity.

Step 4: Exercise

Aerobic Exercise—Make Sure to *Feel* It

Ah…the 80s. Purple spandex and hot pink leg warmers. In Syracuse, New York, through the long grey winters, I'd drive through the slush to my local YMCA to avoid freezing my lungs running outside. I would sweat buckets into my rather unfashionable T-shirt-and-shorts ensemble, grasping the handles to keep from falling over the edge of my treadmill machine, shifting posture, and creating more commotion than the women in matching outfits over on the stationary bikes sedately reading a romance novel and listening to a walkman while their legs rotated in tiny circles beneath them.

Given the kinds of lousy foods I was eating in those days, my extreme exercise regimen might have been doing me more harm than good. Without adequate nutrition, all that full-throttle effort may very well have been breaking down my tissues. In terms of sending the message to build muscle, I was perhaps overdoing it, while the ladies on the bikes might as well have been window-shopping. Exercise, rest, and eating right all work together to give you the kind of body you want. But in order for exercise to contribute as much as it can, you have to know how to get the most out of your workout.

Don't let anyone tell you that—just because you're dressed to workout, you're in a gym and you're using a fancy new machine—you are doing aerobic (oxygen-requiring) exercise. Don't get me wrong. Even strolling along tra-la-la on an elliptical station beats sitting on the couch eating fruit roll-ups. But unless your workout makes your lungs work harder and makes you break a sweat, you aren't doing aerobic exercise; you're just breathing.

This level of workout demands your concentration. Yoga instructors call it *mindfulness*. Weight lifters who argue for the benefits of free weights over universal machines think they get faster results when they have to concentrate on things like balancing a heavy barbell above their chests. The more aware we are of the act of exercising, the more we engage our muscles. Concentration level influences how nerve and muscle cells respond, so whether for an intense run or just walking up the stairs, you'll see more results if you *focus* on every motion—the swinging of your arms, your calves lifting your spine, your hip rotation. If you're running, focus on really filling your lungs. If going up the stairs at work, focus on working the calves for one flight, then try to engage the butt muscles the next. Focus on the contra-body motion—different parts of your body rhythmically moving in opposing directions. Dancing, swimming, golf—each involves contra-body motion, which helps you to involve the whole body. Mindfulness of motion applies to all forms of exercise and is a prerequisite to improving performance.

A good walk, as with any exercise, works out more than your legs, and you get a better workout if you are conscious of your body's balanced involvement in contra-body action. Opposing motions across the fulcrum of your hips and spine allow you to take advantage of a physiologic "spring" built into your muscles, which cardiologists first recognized as the means by which heart failure patients survive. It's called the *Starling* effect. When a muscle is stretched before it contracts, it magnifies the force of the contraction automatically, without any additional input from the nerves. In a failing heart, the muscle needs the extra energy generated by the Starling effect to pump blood effectively. In a dance move, a happy walk, or a properly executed golf swing, extending your limbs to the edge of the swing allows your muscles to stretch and then rebound effortlessly. Paying attention to how your muscles react helps you to hone the technique of whatever it is you're trying to accomplish. That's thinking like an athlete, and it really does make any exercise more fun.

I let all my patients suffering from depression in on a little secret: Studies show that exercise is at least as effective as the best antidepressant medications.[284] Aerobic exercise releases *endorphins*—chemicals your body

Overweight and Pregnancy

If you're overweight, your body is almost certainly suffering under a constant state of low-level inflammation. This inflammatory chemical static is so powerfully disruptive that it can interfere with some of the most important signals in the biological world, those that the next generation depends on. In Chapter 5, we learned that the baby's placenta sends signals to the mother's body, demanding her tissue relinquish nutrients for the benefit of her fetus. But when mom's significantly overweight, the message can't get across. As a result, blood vessels supplying baby with nutrients become thin and shriveled, leading to "major placental growth restriction" when compared to normal weight moms.* So if you're planning on getting pregnant, it's essential to get yourself to a healthy weight first. This will not only facilitate a happy pregnancy but will help with fertility so that you can get pregnant in the first place.

* Effect of nutrient intake during pregnancy of fetal and placental growth and vascular development. Redmer DA. *Domestic Animal Endocrinology*. Volume 27, Issue 3, October 2004.

makes that activate the reward centers of your brain. Not only do these natural feel-good chemicals regulate and improve mood, they act directly on muscles to help them burn more energy and contract with more power.[285] Exercise also cleans the bloodstream of a chemical that makes us feel bad, something called tumor necrosis factor. TNF is a powerful, pro-inflammatory signal that increases sensitivity to pain (it also inhibits muscle growth, and makes blood clots form more easily).[286 287] So aerobic exercise doesn't just pump up your muscle, it pumps up your mood.

It can also pump up your brain—literally. These days, aging baby boomers who forget where they left their car keys jokingly call it early Alzheimer's. But if you've had personal experience with this progressive disease you know it's no laughing matter. In search of ways to combat this terrifying illness, scientists put 30 sedentary older adults (ages 60-79) to work. Over a six-month period, test subjects exercised for an hour a day, three days per week, doing aerobic muscle toning and stretching exercises. Amazingly, brain MRIs showed "[s]ignificant increases in brain volume, in both gray and white matter" in four areas of the brain, several of which are related to making new memories.[288] As I alluded to earlier, the life of a cell is far more unpredictable than we thought, and even nerve cells can grow and divide throughout our lives.[289] If you want your brain to work better, take it for a hike.

Anaerobic Exercise—Why Intensity Matters

The main thing that distinguishes aerobic and *an*aerobic exercise is the level of intensity. Aerobic exercise is easier to do while thinking about something else. Anaerobic exercise requires single-minded focus, a higher level of concentration. But the payoff is a whole new level of muscular coordination and capability. Anaerobic exercise generates a flood of body-sculpting signals so that you get stronger, faster, and more athletic.

When you work so hard that your oxygen demand exceeds the capacity of the body to deliver blood to the tissue (which is why it's called anaerobic, as in "without air"), you have entered that higher realm of exercise called the *anaerobic threshold*. It burns. That burn means you have seconds to minutes before your muscles begin to fail. The time limit has to do with the fact that the metabolism of sugar to energy occurs in two stages.

The first stage, called glycolysis, doesn't require oxygen and is therefore an anaerobic process. It produces the starting materials for the second stage (pyruvic acid), along with some energy for your cells, called adenosine triphosphate (ATP). The second stage uses oxygen to burn the products of the first reaction, and is therefore an aerobic process. The aerobic stage of sugar metabolism produces lots and lots of ATP.

If the muscles don't get enough oxygen to burn all that pyruvic acid, the acids start building up and you feel the burn, telling you your muscles are about to fail. And that's a useful signal. If you were being chased by a lion, for example, the burning signal would warn you that your muscles were on the verge of seizing up. Time to start looking for a tree!

Once the anaerobic activity is over, your metabolic management team furiously takes notes on the physiologic event that just took place, taking record of which muscles worked the hardest and will need to be tweaked for better performance in the future. From the crucible of intense activity emerges a stronger form of muscle that will last longer than it did before. On the savannah, this would make you a more elusive prey and a better hunter, enabling you to run a little faster and chase your quarry a little farther next time. Anaerobic exercise is *the* classic example of no pain, no gain. In the modern world, anaerobic exercise can help transport a dedicated athlete into the zone of superstardom. For the rest of us, however, it's a really great way to burn fat because it flips the body's muscle-generating switch to overdrive, and you start converting flab into firmness like nobody's business.

How much of this kind of intense exercise do you need to do any good? Less than you might think: *Try eight minutes a week!*

For years muscle-bound men and women have encouraged us to *feel the burn*. But nobody suggested that fairly sporadic activity would do the job. Doctors at the Exercise Metabolism Research Group in Ontario, Canada suspected that chronic fatigue induced by *daily* training could actually hamper athletic improvement. They investigated how a *minimum* of super-intense exercise affects muscle work capacity. The test subjects started with four intervals and gradually increased to seven over a two-week period of training performed on Monday, Wednesday and Friday. The intervals consisted of 30 seconds of all-out cycling with four-minute rest periods, totaling just 15 minutes over the two weeks. The subjects improved their exercise capacity by 100 percent. You read that right. Over a two-week period a *total* of 15 minutes of cycling as if their lives depended on it *doubled* their muscle power! Incredibly, the body is so ready and able to respond to signals, that the most urgent signal of all—*run for your life*—produces astonishing gains in performance.[290]

How? Our physiology is our patient and faithful servant. And it is logical—you could say intelligent—in the way it responds. When stimulated to build more muscle, the body does exactly what a smart city planner might do in an expanding metropolitan center: It increases enzyme activity in the muscle to handle the increased workload (the equivalent of hiring more policemen, firemen, and so on), it increases blood flow to handle more nutrient and oxygen traffic, and produces more mitochondria to generate plenty of energy. We call this synchronized set of responses *increased metabolism.*[291]

All this infrastructural development—making more of these complex tissues—can't be accomplished with exercise alone. You need more nutrients to manufacture new enzymes, build more cell organelles, reproduce more cells, pave more blood vessels, and then to maintain all this new equipment. Without a healthy diet, anaerobic exercise can't build these tissues, and can actually break your body down. Healthy diet, along with a balance of aerobic and anaerobic exercise, helps generate the perfect internal environment to clear away the fat-building signals and replace them with a new message: *Get fast. Get tough. Get strong.*

These benefits exist for persons of every age. As we get older, we gradually lose the growth factors that help maintain our fat where we want it and keep our muscles, bones, and joints strong. But during and immediately after exercise, growth factor and hormone levels spike, so you get an infusion of youth serum every time you work out.[292]

Three Habits of Successful Exercisers

One: *Mindfulness*. Use your body consciously. The best exercises involve the entire body. I don't care if you are thumb wrestling; think about your stance, your balance, your breathing, and you'll fake-twitch faster, grab harder, jive better, and bring the opposing thumb to its knees. Never forget that exercise should be fun. Don't allow yourself to do anything that causes a pinch or a dull ache. Listen to your body. If it's objecting, take time off or change what you're doing. Keep in mind that exercise builds more than just muscle, it builds practically all functional tissues; it increases their investment with nerve endings and blood vessels, builds bone, strengthens ligaments, and so much more. Many exercise physiologists firmly believe that conscious intention during and after exercise—visualizing what you are doing *and what you hope to accomplish*—is key to getting the most from a workout.

Two: *Time management*. Aerobic exercise takes time. The more time you give it, the more it gives you. (Up to a point. A reasonable cap is an average of 30-40 minutes per day.) Want to detox? Aerobic exercise cleanses your system of inflammatory debris. If you're new to exercise, start with ten minutes a day and increase by ten percent each week. And don't forget to get plenty of sleep. If your bed's uncomfortable, get another one. And nice pillows and sheets—it's all money well spent. It's mostly during sleep that our bodies heal and rebuild tissue, so sleep is crucial.

Three: *Push yourself.* Anaerobic exercise demands more concentration than aerobic exercise. If your doctor says you're healthy enough for intensive exercise, then you should get to the point where you feel a burn and then keep going for another minute or two. Do that ten times per week and you will see improvement. Make sure you can distinguish a healthy anaerobic burn from the pain of an overstressed muscle. Keep in mind, even an aerobic workout can include elements of anaerobic strain, which helps you build healthy tissues faster.

As we've seen, fat storage is a kind of default action the body performs during periods of nutritional imbalance. When too much fat invades healthy tissues, it weakens them and impairs function. If you want to be healthy, if you want to build bone and muscle and reduce your stores of malignant fat, you must send your cells the clearest possible message. If you fill your metabolic airways with static, the message won't arrive, keeping you from getting the results you want.

The bad news is, the battle between clarity and static isn't a fair fight. In a universe that tends toward disorder, there are all kinds of weird food products and distorted chemicals that can disrupt our physiologies, but only one class of foods—the natural kind—that can maintain internal order. Makes sense, right? Painting the Mona Lisa takes more energy and talent than shooting at it with a pistol. Dietary imbalances rapidly generate inflammation and static that can take weeks or months to clear. So when people tell me they only eat junk food "occasionally," I try to help them realize that they're setting up a competition in their body that they're bound to lose. If you are struggling with weight, or have any chronic medical issue, you can't afford to ship fresh ammunition across the front lines to the enemy.

That means no junk food, period.

Here's the good news: For every junk food you love, there's a healthier, and tastier, alternative. Seriously! If you like McDonalds French fries, you'll get even better flavors using traditional ingredients at home. You can make fries using peanut oil or animal fat (lard, tallow, duck fat, etc.), or make home fries seasoned with spices and baked in pan drippings. If you like sitting down with a sack of chips, you'll get similar, but far more intense, flavors from a few slices of quality, aged raw milk cheese—so satisfying you *can* have just one. While junk food flavorings make you hungrier, naturally flavor-rich foods contain appetite suppressants like cholesterol and saturated fat.

In this chapter, I've focused on the problem of weight. But the same signal disruption (from inflammation and trans fat) that leads to the generation of excess fat also leads to the *de*generation of bone, nerve, and organs. It even causes immune system dysfunction. In fact, because pro-inflammatory foods disrupt normal cell development, the same foods that make us fat also lead to problems we typically associate with aging, from heart disease to Alzheimer's to cancer. What this means is that the Four Pillars do more than make weight loss automatic. They'll keep you from developing all these diseases of aging. In other worlds, they'll help keep you young.

But while all the cells described in this chapter can be born anew at any stage of life, there's one type of tissue that depends—more than anything else—on being built right in the first place. I'm talking about connective tissue. *Feeling* old comes primarily from having connective tissues that are breaking down prematurely. If your connective tissue was built as well as possible, your joints will stand up to incredible abuse, both physical and nutritional. In the next chapter, you'll learn how to gauge your connective tissue health and what you can do (even if it wasn't built as well as it could be) to prevent your body from aging faster than it should.

Eleven

Forever Young
Collagen Health and Life Span

The day after Christmas, a woman ran into our office shouting, "My baby! My baby!" and disappeared back out into the parking lot. The nurse on duty raced out front to find a panicked mother struggling with a car seat where a baby lay listless, strawberry red and covered in blotchy hives, his lips purple and swollen. The infant was having a severe inflammatory reaction and was struggling just to breathe.

Baby Kyle, who was never breastfed, was in the throes of an anaphylactic reaction, triggered by a few spoonfuls of low-fat, high sugar blueberry yoghurt. Anaphylaxis is an allergic reaction involving inflammation of the blood vessels throughout the body, and it can kill. In the last chapter, we saw how inflammation interferes with cell communication and leads to weight gain. Anaphylaxis is a classic case of inflammation gone completely out of control. Fortunately, the pediatrician administered powerful anti-inflammatory medications, which saved little Kyle's life.

Pro-Inflammatory Fats and Sugar Age Us Prematurely

Food allergies, some serious like this, are on the rise. In fact, the number of children with food allergies has risen 100 percent in the past five years.[293] This and other disturbing medical trends are mysteries to medicine and frustrating to parents. But now that you know that sugar and vegetable oil (the

Feeding Your Skin With Beauty Cream

The highest quality skin products contain the collagen-building nutrients your skin needs to restore itself. Even skeptical doctors admit that regular use of these expensive products can have impressive results. However, skin care expert Dr. Dennis Gross, MD, warns that it's not an overnight solution. "It takes time, molecule by molecule, to build collagen fibers." Dermatologists advise patience, and regular application to get anti-wrinkle creams in contact with skin as much as possible. Why not also feed your skin from the inside?

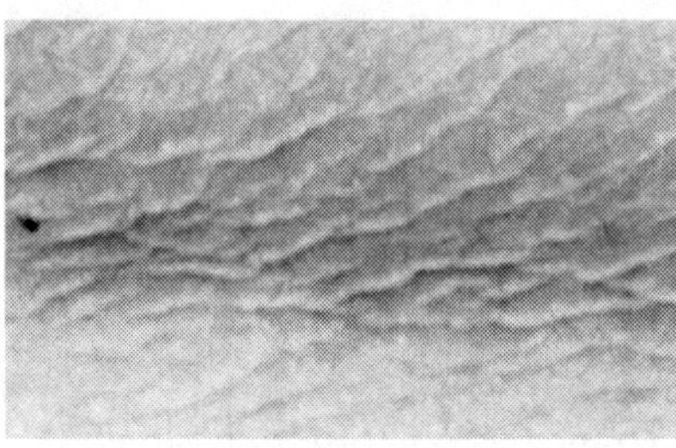

Figure 1. Fine Wrinkling on a 84-year-old Woman's Arm. The right side shows her skin after just three months of applying a vitamin A cream.

Feed Your Skin Soup

If rubbing a cream containing two or three collagen-building nutrients can help your skin, imagine how effectively you could nourish and rebuild your dermal collagen if you ate a meal containing *dozens* of growth factors. The nutrients in bone stocks switch the genes for collagen manufacture to "on." This effect is magnified by vitamins A, D, E, and C, and a few common minerals. Whether in a skin cream or your soup bowl, the same natural ingredients help you look young. But when you ingest them, you infuse all the layers of your skin, and all the other tissues of your body, with rejuvenating nutrients.

Image Source: Improvement of Naturally Aged Skin with Vitamin A. Kafi R. Arch Dermatol 2007 Vol 143, May

main ingredients in infant formulas) combined with nutrient-deficient foods make up the perfect pro-inflammatory diet, you already know what's wrong with Kyle and what should be done to make him healthy.

But what if Kyle kept eating the same kinds of foods? This chapter will discuss what kind of health children with food allergies, or anyone raised on pro-inflammatory fats and sugars, can look forward to as he grows older. That discussion will focus on the effects of poor diet upon collagen-rich connective tissue, since healthy collagen is key to healthy aging. If your parents aged well or lived a long time, you can be sure they had good, strong collagen.

Unfortunately, however, you can't count on inheriting collagen of the same quality. The quality of a person's collagen is not written in genetic stone. (As you now know, there's no such thing as "genetic stone" since your genes are always changing.) Like other tissue types, collagen is made from raw materials you must eat. Unlike other tissues, however, collagen is uniquely sensitive to metabolic imbalances. When your body is making collagen, it's performing a physiologic high-wire act, a feat of extraordinary timing and mechanical precision. This level of complexity makes collagen more dependent on good nutrition and more vulnerable to the effects of pro-inflammatory foods than other tissue types.

When we talk about people who have aged well, one of the first things we think about is healthy skin. But if you've read any beauty magazines in the past decade, you know that skin health depends on collagen health. Mi-

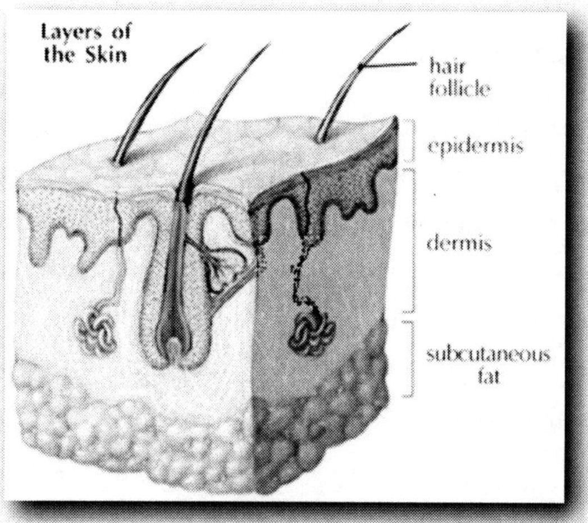

Figure 2. Anatomy of Skin: Epidermis, Dermis, and Subcutaneous Fat. The outer layer, called the epidermis, is a husk of dead cells that are filled with waterproofing material and pigment. The middle layer, called the dermis, is the support system of your skin, containing blood vessels, nerves, sweat and oil glands, and the muscles controlling hair follicles, all held in place by strong and elastic fibers made of collagen. The innermost layer is called the subcutaneous fat. It's where the bulk of our body fat is stored.

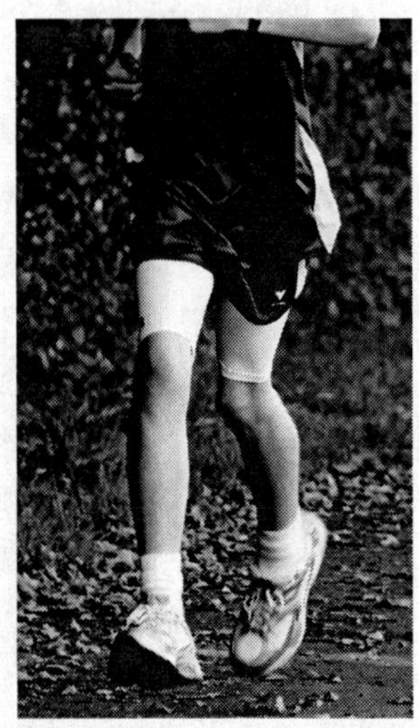

Figure 3. A Classic Sign of Weak Collagen. This child has a mild case of *intoeing*, which is associated with abnormal collagen growth and lax ligaments. Were he to play soccer or ski, this child would be at higher than normal risk for joint injuries (like ligament tears). Today, more children than ever need joint reconstruction after sports injuries. Unlike my medical colleagues, who believe the problem is increased physical activity, I believe the root of the problem is decreased collagen strength. To protect their joints, children must expose their tissues to the stimulus of exercise and give their bodies the collagen-building foods needed for growth and repair. (See Chapters 7 and 10.)

chelle Pfeiffer is one of the most beautiful actresses working today, but whether she retains that beauty as the years wear on depends not so much on the superficial layers of her skin but on what lies beneath.

Collagens: Molecules That Make Us Strong

Collagens are a family of extra-cellular proteins that give skin its ability to move, stretch, and rebound into shape. Thin wisps of tough, elastic collagen molecules run between adjacent cells in the outermost layer of skin, called the *epidermis*. And larger bundles of collagen form strips that weave together in a continuous layer beneath the epidermis, in a part of the skin called the *dermis*.

Collagens aren't just in skin; they're everywhere, imparting strength to all your tissues. Just as strands of collagen running between skin cells hold our outermost layer of skin together, collagens unite adjacent cells in all your glands and organs, from your brain to your bones to your liver and lungs. Larger bundles of collagen form strips and sheets in the ligaments and tendons surrounding your joints to hold your skeleton together. Collagen is the most prevalent kind of protein in your body; about 15 percent of your dry weight is pure collagen. Without it, we wouldn't just fall apart at the joints;

we would literally disintegrate into small piles of individual cells. While it may seem like an obvious connection, doctors are only now beginning to appreciate the relationship between collagen strength and sports and job performance. Research now reveals that people with weak collagen experience more injuries throughout their lives.[294,295,296]

The reason collagen health is so dependent on a healthy diet has to do with the complexity of the individual collagen molecules. You can get some idea of how hard collagen is to manufacture from the wound healing process. If you've ever cut yourself so deep that you needed stitches, you may have noticed how long the scar takes to heal—sometimes a full year. When new collagen is formed in a wound, it's composed of shorter, less organized strands than the original. By six weeks, the collagen fibers are far more organized and longer, but only back to about 75% of the original strength. As the supporting collagen becomes gradually more organized, the scar on the surface fades. In about a year, the skin strength is just about what was before the injury, though a small scar may remain if the collagen fibers below could never quite iron out smooth.

All collagens are made from chains of amino acids coiled around each other in sets of three to form a triple helix. The longer they are, the more strength they give to the tissue they're in. But the longest, strongest collagens are also the hardest to make. All collagens carry special molecules called *glycosaminoglycans* (which we first read about in Chapter 7, in the section on bone stock) attached like bangles on a necklace to the triple helix backbone. Each class of collagen varies in length and amount of attached glycosaminoglycan bangles, allowing for all sorts of variation in strength, flexibility, water retention and lubrication. Once manufactured, collagen molecules get anchored to the exterior of the cell and unfurl throughout the extra-cellular matrix where molecules from adjacent cells can intertwine. The structural biology of collagen is incredibly complex, a masterpiece of extracellular engineering. If you are one of the lucky people to be endowed with good quality collagen, not only will your skin resist wrinkling, you will have a better chance of avoiding joint and circulatory problems down the road.

Tiger Sidelined by Cross-Linked, Degenerated Cartilage

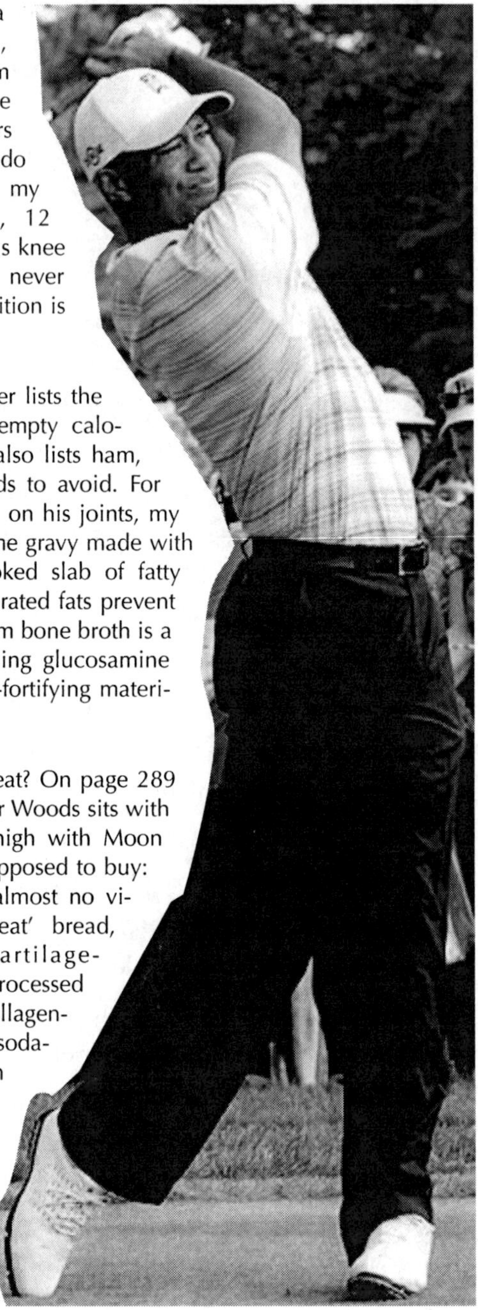

After making sports history with a dramatic win at the 2008 US open, Tiger's knee gave out, forcing him into temporary retirement. "I've been trying to adjust over the years to alleviate some of the stress I do put on my left leg. But basically, my left knee's been sore for 10, 12 years..." Tiger originally injured his knee skateboarding as a child but it never fully healed, and I think poor nutrition is partly to blame.

In his book, *How I Play Golf*, Tiger lists the ten foods his nutritionists call "empty calories." One of those is gravy. He also lists ham, roast beef, and prime rib as foods to avoid. For someone who depends so heavily on his joints, my prescription would be to pour some gravy made with bone broth over a properly cooked slab of fatty meat. By now you know that saturated fats prevent inflammation, and gravy made from bone broth is a natural joint supplement, containing glucosamine as well as a battery of other joint-fortifying materials.

What does this world champion eat? On page 289 of *How I Play Golf*, a cartoon Tiger Woods sits with knife and fork at a table piled high with Moon Foods, the same junk we're all supposed to buy: canned vegetables, which have almost no vitamins, fluffy store-bought 'wheat' bread, which is converted into cartilage-crosslinking sugar molecules, processed skim milk which is full of collagen-damaging glycated proteins, and soda-pop style "fruit juice," loaded with more sugar. He also throws away the yolks, the most nutritious part of the eggs. Please, Tiger, for healthy, long-lasting joints, give your joints what they need: the Four Pillars.

If any one of the thousands of steps involved in making collagen goes haywire—which is likely to happen if your diet was poor during critical growth periods (low in nutrient-rich foods from the Four Pillars and high in sugar and vegetable oils)—the integrity of the finished product is compromised and may break down prematurely. You might imagine that, with lesser quality collagen holding us together, our tissues would start pulling apart and separating after a certain number of years. That's exactly what causes wrinkling, arthritis, and even circulatory problems. Unless baby Kyle's mother starts treating vegetable oil and sugar like the poisons they are, these are the kinds of medical problems that will plague him as he grows older.

No matter the strength of your collagen today, how good you feel tomorrow depends a lot on your diet. People who eat pro-inflammatory foods experience more joint damage on a daily basis because sugar acts like an abrasive in the joints.[297] At night, the small frays and tiny breaks in the collagen that formed during the day must be repaired. But inflammation interferes with healing. Instead of waking up feeling recovered, people on bad diets wake up with stiff joints. Their scars and stretch marks will be more obvious, too, because inflammation disorganizes the collagen fibers so that, as tissue heals, it forms irregular lumpy mounds or deep pits, with more disfiguring results.

One of the best ways to help collagen heal is, not surprisingly, to eat some. Eating meat on the bone or using bone broths in soups, stews, and sauces floods your bloodstream with glycosaminoglycans, which head directly to the parts of the body that need collagen most.[298] These extraordinary molecules attract enormous amounts of water, up to 1000 times their own weight, which coats your joint tissues in tiny, electrically charged clouds, transforming ordinary water molecules into a protective layer of super-lubricating fluid.[299] Glycosaminoglycans will naturally adhere to collagen anywhere in your body, moistening dry skin, helping your tendons and ligaments stay supple, and generally making you look and feel younger.[300]

Eating homemade bone stock in childhood has fantastic joint-strengthening and collagen-fortifying effects that can last a lifetime. The benefits are so dramatic that it's astounding to me more people haven't noticed the connection. My patients who ate traditional cuisine with meaty stocks and rich bone broths on a regular basis tend to enjoy all the hallmarks of well-built bones and connective tissue. They have broad hands with wide knuckles and relatively large feet that are proportionately wide from toe to heel. Their skin is smoother, with tighter pores and smaller hair follicle openings, reflecting greater tensile strength. Because their bodies are so well-built, these are the people who can enjoy their golden years to the fullest, or work past retirement if they so choose.

A lot of people think cellulite comes from being too fat. But extra fat where you don't want it is only part of the problem. Lumpy, irregular cellulite forms in fat deposits that lack adequate connective tissue struts to support a smooth shape.[301] When I see photos of celebrities with terrible cellulite on their thighs, I imagine how their nutritionists are probably telling them to

Cellulite Fat Lacks Collagen

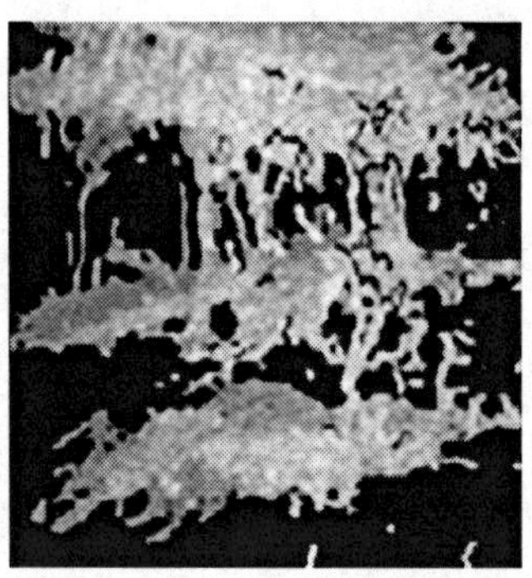

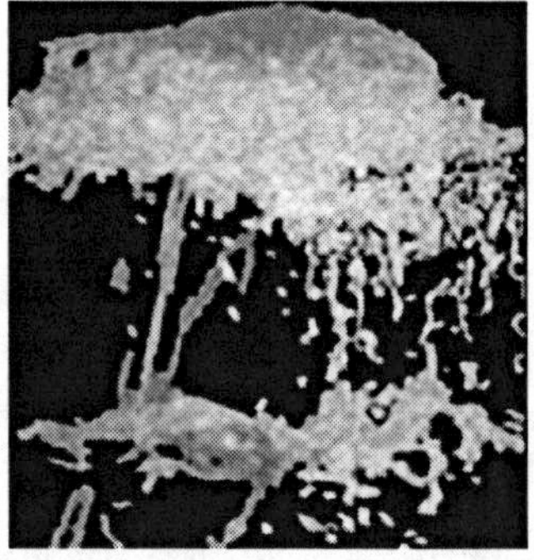

Figure 4. Advanced Cellulite. These are MRI reconstructions of the collagen supporting the fat layer in two different women's thighs. On the left, a woman without cellulite and on the right, a woman with cellulite. The MRI shows only the collagen within the fat, not the fat itself. The woman with cellulite has only two layers of collagen support, while the woman with no cellulite has three.

Image Source: *Skin Research Technology* **8**, 118-124 (2002), by Bernard Querleux avoid animal products, and how frustrated they'll be as their cellulite hangs on. To get rid of cellulite, combine exercise with a diet full of healthy, natural fats (including animal fat) and collagen-rich stocks. This will send the message that you want your body to replace the saggy fat pockets with smooth, toned curves.

Now that you know why collagen health is important not just to skin, but to every organ in your body, let's learn how inflammation affects your collagen day to day and over the years.

The Good and Bad Sides of Inflammation

Inflammation, as the name suggests, creates a burning sensation—but only when it reaches our nerves. Skin is full of nerves, so inflammation in the skin causes irritating sensations, including burning, stinging, and itching. Inflammation in the joints may cause an aching feeling. In the head, a headache; in the gut, nausea or cramping; in the heart, a crushing chest pain; and in the lungs, it can make us wheeze and cough.

Like pain, which alerts us to the fact that something is wrong with us, inflammation does have a good side. It's supposed to signal the body's repair systems that a section of tissue needs special care. A bee sting is a classic example of an inflammatory event caused by toxins injected under the skin, which swells up as surrounding blood vessels leak in an attempt to dilute and neutralize the toxin. An ankle swells a little immediately after a sprain. But the real swelling begins hours later, when inflammation signals capillaries to begin leaking serum, stem cells, growth factors, and all the other materials needed to lay the groundwork for the creation of replacement tissue. One of the most dramatic examples of beneficial inflammation occurs during bacterial infection and abscess formation. Inflammation triggered by bacteria invading our tissues releases powerful enzymes that chew through collagen to help the body drain the abscess and expel the invaders. The resulting scar is the small price we pay for avoiding deadly sepsis.

In the setting of dietary imbalance, however, inflammation can go from the physiologic equivalent of a mild-mannered Dr. Bruce Banner into a destructive and uncontrollable Hulk. You may have such a dietary imbalance and not have any symptoms, or only vague aches and a feeling of tiredness, but on a pro-inflammatory diet you are a true "ticking time bomb." When inflammatory responses are triggered with little or no provocation, or are overly vigorous, swelling tissues and destructive enzymes may become life threatening. That's exactly what happened to the strawberry-red baby in the introduction to this chapter. Let's take a closer look.

Red Rashes—Red Alarms Signaling an Imbalanced Diet

If you slap someone's cheek, it turns red. Ever wonder why? The injury triggers a healthy inflammatory response, which dilates the blood vessels of the skin. This allows more oxygen, white blood cells, and nutrients to give the injured tissue a little boost to regain normal function.

But what about red rashes that just appear for no apparent reason? I see patients with rashes every day in clinic. And I take every one of them seriously because they're a sign your body—and your diet—are out of balance, maybe severely. In the most severe cases of imbalance, anaphylactic reactions like baby Kyle's are a real possibility. Even slight immune system imbalance leaves you vulnerable to all manner of recurring problems, feeling fine one minute and horrible the next.

All kinds of allergic reactions can occur whenever someone's immune system has been so overwhelmed by conflicting signals from excessive, ongoing inflammation that its chemical programming gets confused. The confused immune system interprets normal body proteins as foreign and launches an attack. The affected tissues then ooze chemicals that increase blood flow and cause serum to leak into their surroundings. On the skin, you may see a number of red, raised so-called *wheal and flare* reactions that look a little like mosquito bites. The affected blood vessels can be anywhere: sinuses, lungs, kidneys, joints, etc. Depending on the location and the severity of the immune response, a person's symptoms may be mildly annoying—a runny nose or watery eyes—or they may be life threatening. Immune system confusion will vary day by day depending on stress, infection, sleep, and diet, making allergic reactions hard to predict. To get off the roller coaster, be confident that a good diet can straighten out even the most confused immune systems.

One of the most common rashes I see is eczema. People with eczema can develop itchy, blotchy red rashes all over their body. As with all allergic disorders, the symptoms of eczema can resolve but then flare up again and again throughout a person's entire life. People with eczema—just like people with food allergies—may also experience immune system imbalance elsewhere in the body, causing allergic rhinitis, sinusitis, and asthma. Food allergies, chronic runny noses, asthma—the underlying cause is the same, immune system imbalance caused by pro-inflammatory foods. And you already know what the cure is (see Chapter 7).

When Kyle's pediatrician referred him for allergy testing, his mother learned that her ten-month-old had already developed allergies to proteins in milk, shellfish, green beans, and eggs—some of which he'd never even eaten. As Kyle grows and his airway enlarges and better tolerates small degrees of swelling, he may overcome the breathing crises. But if his mother keeps feeding him the standard Food-Pyramid-compliant diet, he will develop more inflammatory problems. One of the most common and most disfiguring is acne.

How Inflammation Causes Scarring Acne

Earlier in the book, I explained how oxidation damages fats, and how those damaged fats lead to inflammation, making it nearly impossible to lose weight. Oxidized fats in our skin lead to the pustular inflammation that teenagers, and many adults, dread.

Right now, you're covered in bacteria—billions of them. Don't bother running off to the shower; you'll never get rid of them all. These beneficial skin bacteria protect us from infection. They make their living off the shed husks of dead skin cells, which are so loaded with protein and fat that they offer a reliable food source for all kinds of microbes.

If bacteria were to penetrate the dead outermost layer of skin, patrolling

A Scar Is Born

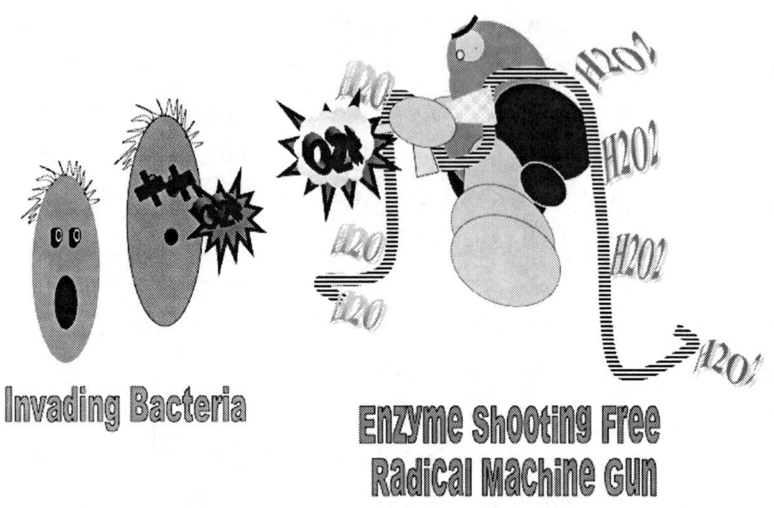

Figure 5. Free Radicals Help Kill Bacteria but Also Damage Collagen. Here we see an enzyme that generates free radicals to destroy bacteria. Without these enzymes, invasive bacteria would take over our bodies and kill us. Unfortunately, an enzyme's aim is not so accurate and many innocent body bystanders also get hurt—the cost of doing business.

white blood cells would go berserk. To them, the foreign proteins and oxidized fats adorning cell membranes of invasive bacteria are signs of trouble and, like beat cops spotting a couple of hoodlums carrying weapons into a playground, they sound the alarm. Like a well-trained swat team, swarming white blood cells bust down doors and break through walls to get to their target, shooting free radicals and releasing those collagen-chewing enzymes (called *collagenases*). If it was all a false alarm caused by diet-induced accidental inflammation and in reality no real infection—well, too bad. White blood cells aren't disposed to quibbling over such nuances, so you'll just have to deal with the scars. If you've ever had an abscess, you know that the first thing the doctor wants to do is drain it. That's all the body is trying to do by unleashing its collagenases.

Acne is a problem of oil oxidation. When we eat easily oxidizable, unnatural oils, they wind up everywhere—our arteries, our nervous system, and the skin on our face. White blood cells mistake oxidized oil for the fatty acids that coat the surface of invasive bacteria, and squads of white blood cells rush to the scene. And as you know, they show up swinging and strike at everything within reach. The acne lesion swells and reddens. Once the battle is over, the site is commemorated with a permanent pit. This is called *cystic-nodular acne*, an example of an inflammatory false alarm generated not by infection but by oxidized oils. So if you or your teen is fighting acne, step one is getting off of vegetable oil. And while you're at it, get off sugar too. Sugar suppresses the immune system and feeds the bacteria living in acne pustules.

When I see a person with acne, it suggests they've been eating pro-inflammatory foods full of sugar and vegetable oil. Pro-inflammatory foods send powerfully disruptive signals that will override signals for less urgent metabolic needs (like muscle development, as we saw in the last chapter). So people with bad acne are also prone to hormone imbalances, reproductive challenges, and a variety of other problems.

Today acne is the most common skin disease, with nearly 90 percent of adolescents affected.[302] But there's little evidence that acne occurred at anything near these rates in the distant past, and many dermatologists believe it is a modern disease. Not only were the fats ancient people consumed healthier than what we eat today, they may have enjoyed protection from acne and other skin infections because of a secret ingredient in their makeup.

Beauty Secrets of the Ancient Egyptians

Archaeologists have found the earliest evidence of cosmetics being used in Egypt dating back to 4,000 years BC. The Egyptians made their makeup using fat blended with special saps and either red ochre or ashes. Around the world today, indigenous people still go to great lengths to find the right ingredients to make their own makeup. For instance, the Himba, a nomadic tribe of goat herders in Northern Africa, mix goat-butter with ochre and finely crushed herbs, and the paste gives their skin a beautifully smooth red-brown hue. In Hawaii, people used coconut butter that had been left in the sun for a few weeks to give themselves a shiny glow for (frequent) festival occasions. This common practice of applying carefully blended fats to our skin has several purposes.

For one, fat holds moisture in our skin, which helps it to stay smooth and soft. Today, high-quality skin care products still contain cocoa butter, avocado, olive oil, and even egg yolk. As good as modern cosmetics may be, they lack the secret ingredient of their aboriginal counterparts: probiotics. The blends of goat butter, cocoa butter, and probably even the ash and fat the Egyptians used, all were loaded with beneficial bacteria, thanks to the fact that their raw materials and containers were colonized with microbes. Applying creams with beneficial bacteria has the same benefits to your skin that eating probiotic-rich foods like yoghurt has to your intestinal tract: healthy numbers of beneficial critters outnumber any potentially invasive bacteria. This would have helped people in the past—who generally had little or no clean water to wash with—from getting infected after cutting their skin.[303]

Next time you're having lunch with one of your girlfriends and she's pouring on the low-fat dressing, ask her if she'd use the same ingredients to condition her hair or moisturize her skin. Probably not. Quality beauty products are made with natural saturated fats. Vegetable oil is less suitable because it oxidizes too easily, gets sticky, and irritates our skin. The cosmetic manufacturers would probably love to use these cheap oils instead of more expensive natural fats, but they would never get away with it. Putting this stuff in make-up would lead to obvious allergic skin rashes and acne. Of course, food manufacturers *can* get away with putting vegetable oil in everything—while telling us that it's good for our heart! Lucky for them, we can't see the inflammatory damage it does to our arteries. And because we don't have nerve endings in our arterial lumens, we can't even feel it. But we can think in the more naturalistic common sense terms of our ancestors and say, *If I can't put it on my skin, I won't put it in my mouth.*

The Sun *Can* Damage Skin, but It Doesn't Have To

So far, we've seen that vegetable oils and sugar can create imbalances in the immune system and cause acne, and both diseases can damage our collagen. But one of the most well known collagen-destroying factors is the sun.

Given the near-obsessive use of sunscreen in all but the dimmest of light, you'd think that UV radiation passed right through our bodies, like X-rays. In reality, UV has little penetrating power, and most UV (95 percent or more) is blocked by the rapidly regenerating epidermis. The collagen beneath the epidermis absorbs much of the rest.[304] Depending on your diet, that five percent may lead to inflamed, sunburnt skin—or it may not. (Of course, if you get way too much sun, you'll get redness and inflammation even on the best diet.) Inflammation leads to the release of those collagen-chewing enzymes and can greatly exacerbate the damage done by UV light, leading to wrinkling down the road. A diet full of nutrients will keep those enzymes on a short leash and keep your skin looking young.

So should we avoid the sun as much as possible? If your diet is full of pro-inflammatory fats and sugar, then the answer is a guarded yes. But if your diet is healthy, then your collagen won't be seriously injured unless you get so much sun your skin actually burns. I'd like you to get sunlight regularly. But I'd also like you to give your skin what it needs to protect itself while you do.

Like plants, we use sunlight to grow. We used to get most of our vitamin D—the sunshine vitamin—directly from sunlight. When UV smashes into the epidermis, it strikes cholesterol molecules, transforming them into a precursor of vitamin D which gets fully activated in the liver and the kidney. You need D to metabolize calcium, so if a child doesn't get enough, it can weaken their bones and stunt their growth. We also used to eat a lot more liver than we do today, which happens to be the best dietary source of vitamin D. As you know from previous chapters, few of us get enough D these days. Even fortified milk rarely contains the amount of vitamin D it's supposed to, and only *cholecalciferol* supplements work like the real thing (*ergocalciferol* can even be toxic).[305][306] No matter where human beings live on the

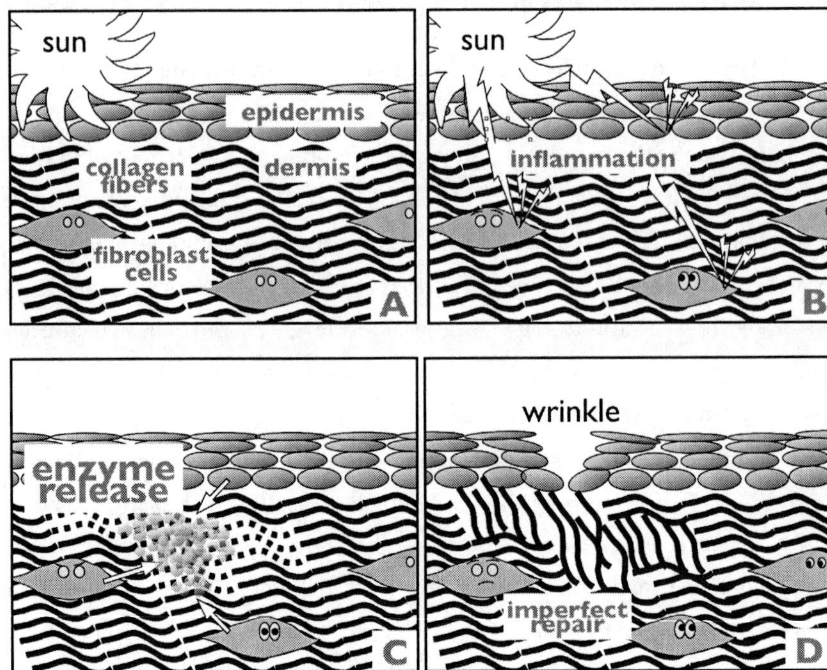

Figure 6. How Sun Causes Wrinkling. On a pro-inflammatory diet, sun exposure (panel A) causes excess inflammation (panel B), which induces fibroblast cells to release enzymes that chew apart your collagen (panel C), leading to the imperfect repair (panel D) that distorts the smoothness of your collagen fibers and enables a wrinkle to form. The more cycles of collagen destruction your skin goes through, the more you wrinkle. Both inflammation and UV radiation damage your DNA, potentially leading to skin cancer.

Warning: To prevent aging, you have to block UVB *and* UVA, and no known sunscreen can yet block UVA. Fortunately melanin, which makes our skin dark, can. Sun*blocks* (opaque creams like zinc oxide) also block both UVA and UVB.

By the way, the SPF factor refers only to UVB blocking ability. The FDA doesn't have any standards for UVA blocking creams, so labels claiming to block UVA are meaningless.

planet, they've got to get their sunshine vitamin one way or another, whether directly from the sun or indirectly—as they do in Norway and Alaska—by consuming liver oils from fish and other animals that did get sunlight.

Battle of the Diets

Compare how these two sixty-year olds have aged. The man on the right has spent most of his life out in the sun eating a traditional Himba diet composed of 50-80 percent animal fat. His smooth, tight skin represents what everyone's skin could look like at this age had we all been raised on balanced diets. The kind-looking man on the left is Dr. Dean Ornish, a non-smoking American physician, and a well-intentioned proponent of a low-fat, industrialized interpretation of a Mediterranean diet. Unfortunately, his collagen is sagging and deteriorated due to lack of fat-soluble vitamins and unintentional consumption of pro-inflammatory fats (trans and MegaTrans, see Chapter 8.)

Dr. Ornish is not overweight, yet we see fat deposits under his chin because of his pro-inflammatory diet. Inflammation also elevate insulin levels. Insulin is a powerful signal for storing both sugar and fat, and doing so in a hurry. The kind of fat receptors under our neck (and on our bellies) are called *alpha receptors*, which are the body's first responders to excess energy. So even on a low-fat diet, with alpha receptors turned on, your body is greedy for energy, and any sugar you eat is converted to fat and stored under your chin, on your belly, and around your internal organs.

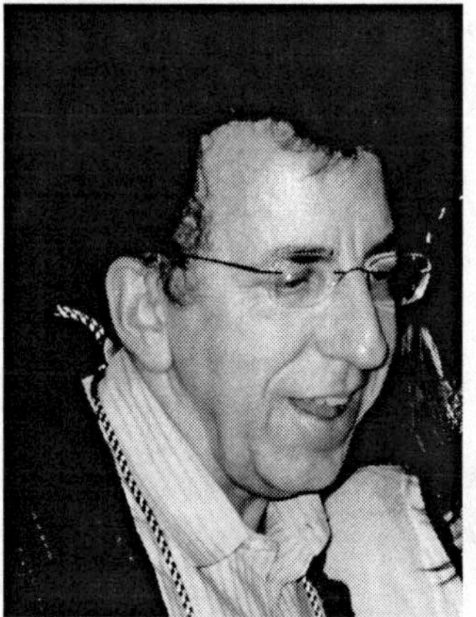

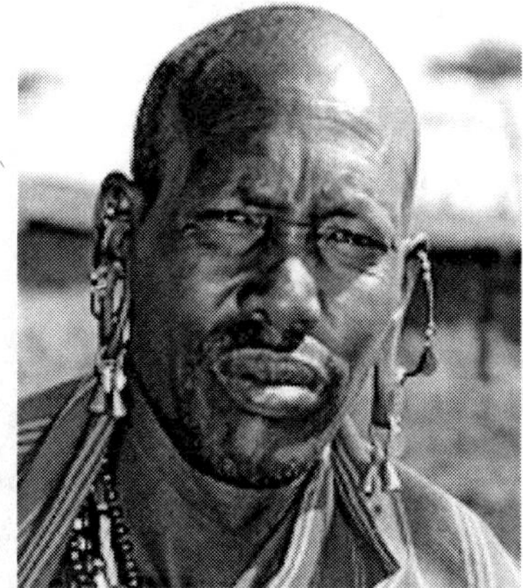

Figure 7. Low-Fat (left) Versus High-Fat Diets (right). Who Looks Tougher? Because sagging skin and bloated neck wattles belie a weakness within the connective tissues supporting our bones and joints as well as our skin, we can judge a person's potential strength by how well their skin holds up. Trans fat plus high carbs are largely responsible for the decline and fall of the American physique.

In the summer, a naked Caucasian (at around 35 degrees latitude at midday) can make enough D to last at least a week.[307] After that amount of radiation, ideally, we'd shut off the supply of UV because too much destroys collagen and vital nutrients, *including* vitamin D. Fortunately, your skin has a way of regulating the dose of UV you get. A skin pigment called *melanin* accomplishes this for us. Our genetics so perfectly modulate the amount of pigment in our skin that the skin tone of indigenous people can be used to predict their latitude of origin to within a few degrees.[308]

How does your skin accomplish the day-to-day regulation of melanin, say, when you go to the beach? By responding to an increase in the amount of radiation it gets. When UV light penetrates the thin outermost layer of dead cells, it enters special cells called *melanocytes*. Melanocytes contain a signaling chemical that acts like a tiny mechanical switch. When UV hits the chemical, it flips the switch to on: The chemical undergoes a shape change (because an electron is stripped away by the UV rays), which allows it to fit into an enzyme that turns on the melanocyte's melanin-production proteins, jump-starting your tanning systems. Within a matter of minutes to hours, depending on your genetics, your skin starts looking tan.

Melanocytes live in the outermost layer of skin where they can best protect the layer of collagen beneath. Unlike sunscreens, which can't stop

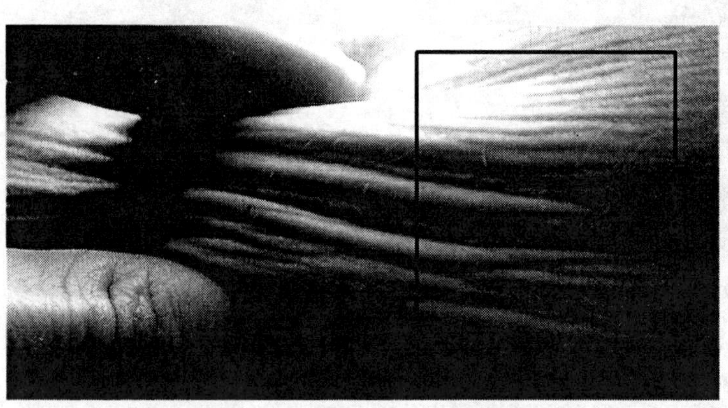

Figure 8. Test For Premature Wrinkling. This is my arm at age 40. My collagen was not formed properly, due to epigenetic damage on my father's side (he also aged prematurely), lack of cartilage/bone broth in childhood, and dietary toxins (my sugar habit, plus margarine). You can perform this test by starting with fingers two inches apart and pinching gently to bring your fingers one inch apart. Continuous wrinkling indicates inadequate elastin. If I don't watch my diet now, I'll age rapidly.

harmful, deeply penetrating UVA, melanin effectively blocks the entire UV spectrum. Though sunscreens don't block UVA and therefore don't directly protect collagen, they do prevent burning, which reduces inflammation. (See Figure 6).

Many of us Irish folk have sluggish melanocytes that can't pump out the color fast enough, and so we tend to burn. Then, after a day or so, the redness starts to tan. How do we get tan *after* sun? Too much sun inflames the skin. The inflammation releases free radicals. And the free radicals trigger the melanocyte-signaling chemical, which gets the tanning engine running. This delay feature may be by design; in higher latitudes, a hyper-reactive tendency to tan wouldn't allow people to make enough vitamin D. Even on a good diet, that whopping dose of UVA on your first day of hanging out in the sun can damage your collagen down to the deep dermal layers and age your skin prematurely, but on a bad diet, the damage will be worse.

So get your summer sun, but pace yourself—especially if you're light skinned. Ideally, before your Hawaiian vacation, get a base tan under controlled conditions in a tanning salon first. That melanin can protect your deeper tissues from UVA, while the sunscreen prevents UVB-induced inflammation. I know you'll be tempted, but please, when you're getting sun, stay away from pro-inflammatory vegetable oils and sugar even if you're on vacation. Not only will you be protecting your skin, but that move will help steer you towards your vacation destination's best traditional cuisine.

Defying Time and Gravity

When we see a 75-year-old who looks half her age, we might presume she's spent her whole life ducking into the shadows to avoid the sun. That, and maybe Botox. But when you hear that she loves the outdoors, hikes regularly, and spends three days a week out on the golf course, you think, *What gives? Why does her skin look so smooth?* The secret isn't avoiding the sun. It's avoiding inflammation.

If this woman, let's call her Mary, is so adept at avoiding inflammation, chances are good that the rest of her body is holding up just as well. She avoids inflammation by staying away from artificial fats and sugar—giving into none of those buffet-table temptations and steering clear of vegetable oil dressings and the sugary juices that could damage her nerves—so she's as sharp and feisty as ever. She remembers what happened sixty years ago and what happened sixty days ago. Mary and her husband have recently taken up ballroom dancing. Sometimes, when they get home after class, they waltz themselves straight into the bedroom to keep the music going. And they can, thanks to healthy arteries and the robust blood flow that comes with it.

Mary loves making stock, sauerkraut, her own fresh bread, and all the foods from the Four Pillars that her mother taught her to make and that keep inflammation away. When her friends come over for brunch, they complement Mary on her amazingly smooth skin—especially lately, as they've been noticing more blotches on theirs. On imbalanced diets, something as minor as a pimple, a rap on the shin, or even friction around the neck from clothing and jewelry, can produce enough inflammation to trigger the tanning machine by mistake, causing a dark spot. Their skin seems to have aged faster than Mary's. And it has: inflammation accelerates cell division, setting the aging process to fast forward, making skin thinner, weaker, and vulnerable to bruising. Mary's Four Pillars diet has slowed it all down.

Practically every nutrient studied plays a role in protecting collagen by acting as antioxidants and/or growth factors. Vitamin A, C, glutathione, glucosamine, and omega-3 fatty acids have each been shown to cut collagen damage from UV radiation by up to 80 percent.[309,310,311,312] Imagine the effects of getting enough of *all* of them combined, as Mary does. Cortisone has been studied too, and found to have similar anti-wrinkle effects. Cortisone is a hormone made from cholesterol by the adrenal glands, which, as with all organs, depend on their owner's good diet, exercise, sleep, and avoidance of chronic stress. By eating poorly and suppressing adrenal function, we reduce our body's natural cortisone production and prematurely age all our collagenous tissues—most conspicuously, our skin. By eating real food, full of genuine vitamins (not synthetic counterfeits), Mary has kept her collagen in superb condition.

Brains Like It Smooth

What happens inside our brain that makes us think young skin is more attractive? Like children, our brains can be easily frustrated. They can't stand confusion, even if it only exists at the subconscious level. When you look at someone, your eyes travel from feature to feature in jerky bursts of motion called *saccades*, darting between features as if magnetized by contrast. Young skin is smooth, with no distracting wrinkles. This enables us to focus on the person's expressions, facilitating safe and pleasant communication.

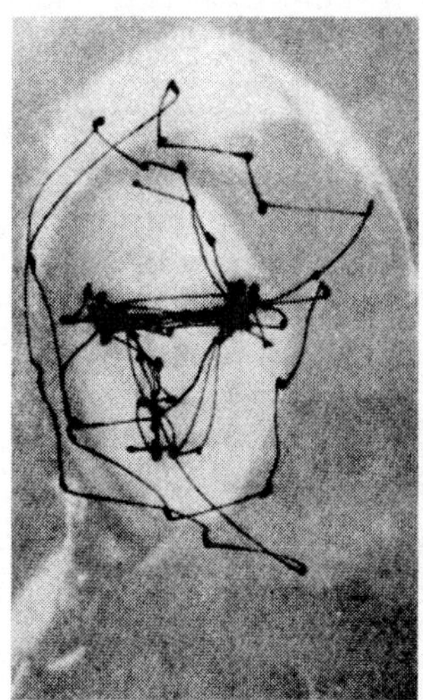

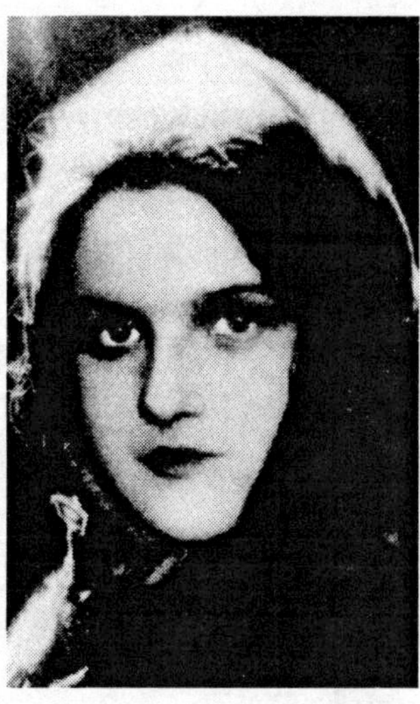

Figure 9. How We See Faces. The picture on the left shows the trace of a person's gaze while examining the portrait on the right. These two pictures are taken from the work done by Russian psycho-physicist Dr. Alfred Yarbus in the 1950s. Yarbus demonstrated that human beings do not scan a scene randomly. Our eyes move deliberately between points of interest, which tend to be areas of contrast, particularly around the eyes and mouth. The quick darting from feature to feature strongly suggests that, rather than assessing features individually, we measure their relationships to one another and to the face as a whole. When those relationships conform closely to the Marquardt mask, we want to keep looking! (See Chapter 3.)

Mary does strength training, but toned muscles alone can't prevent "the sag" that we all dread, which develops as gravity relentlessly tugs our tissues downward. Mary has a built-in anti-gravity device, a latticework of sturdy collagen woven throughout her body fat. Having enough healthy collagen in the *subcutaneous* fat (just under your skin, where most body fat is stored) doesn't just prevent cellulite and keep your curves looking taut, as we saw earlier. It also prevents the development of the chin wattle, the droopy butt, the floppy underarm, and even those creases on the sides of the nose and mouth. Mary's mother didn't have these things, and neither does Mary. The reason is healthy subcutaneous fat.

The Ultimate Connective Tissue Support: Elastin

More than anything else, the ability of your collagen to stand up to gravity depends on a very special member of the collagen family, called *elastin*. Skin, arteries, lungs, and ligaments have the most elastin, which gives these tissues their rubbery consistency and ability to rebound after stretching. Women like Mary have a healthy amount of elastin throughout their bodies, as does anyone who ages well or looks younger than they are. If any single molecule could be said to represent the fountain of youth, this would be it.

Mary's supple and resilient elastin molecules were built to last. With a half-life of 75 years, they're meant to last a lifetime. UC Davis anatomy professor Charles G. Plopper tells us "the half-life of elastin matches the life span of the species,"[313] suggesting elastin plays a central role in determining life expectancy. (Half-life means that half of something will be gone in the given time interval.)

Elastin's strength is also its drawback. Since it's supposed to be made to last, your body doesn't make much more after puberty. As far as we know, it's only possible to make elastin during periods of rapid growth. Elastin depends on a unique chemical bond, called the *desmosine* bond, that's extremely difficult to manufacture. It can be made only while your body is swimming in the hormones and growth factors that orchestrate its manufacture—during embryologic life, early childhood growth spurts, and adolescence. Although Mary's mother didn't know any of these physiologic details, she knew that the intricate and delicate growth processes going on inside Mary's little body were dependent upon the best nutritional environment she could provide. This applies especially to elastin, since elastin's complexity makes the process of manufacturing this vital tissue particularly easy to disrupt. Says Dr. Plopper, "It is now apparent that a range of intra-uterine and early postnatal factors, such as hypoxia, nutritional restriction and FGR [not having enough room in the uterus] can affect elastin deposition."

Mary's upbringing was a lot different than Kyle's, the sickly baby we met at the opening of the chapter. Thanks to the fact that Mary's mother, and her mother's mother, did everything right—from planning conception to fortifying their bodies to breastfeeding and cooking from scratch—Mary's life has been blessed with superior health, good looks, and happy fortune. The same mixture of hormones and nutrients that ensured Mary's strong elastin also ensured balanced skeletal growth. Her wide jaw and strong cheekbones allowed for straight teeth and a beautiful smile. And because optimal facial development leaves enough room for the eyes to develop normally, Mary never needed glasses. Even now, much to her eye doctor's amazement, good quality collagen in the lenses of her eyes has delayed the onset of presbyopia (the age-related lens stiffness that necessitates reading glasses). Though she's always enjoyed the sun, Mary's anti-inflammatory diet has kept her free of cataracts, macular degeneration, and other degenerative diseases that make us feel old.

The Ancestor's Tale

Mary is the hero of this book. As is her mother, and her mother, and hers—all the way back to her most distant ancestors who followed dietary practices that ensured the benefits of beauty and health. Mary is the manifestation of that dream. And because she appreciates her ancestors' gifts, she has fulfilled her duty to protect them and has passed the genetic vessel unbroken to her son and daughter.

The vessel is her family's epigenetic code. And Mary's granddaughter now benefits from it. If she's careful, and willing to take seriously her charge as curator of her family's genetic heritage, then her ancestors' dream will live on in the healthy, beautiful body of Mary's great-granddaughter.

The sacred vessel of epigenetic integrity does not belong to us. We receive it, benefit from it, and then pass it on. During our lives on Earth we must also protect it. And by eating food from the Four Pillars and celebrating the living art of ancient, traditional cuisine, we can do exactly that, engineering our bodies, and those of our children, into the forms that best represent balanced, uninterrupted, natural growth.

The requisites of perfect health are not hidden. We know what keeps us well, and we know what makes us sick. When we allow real food to connect our bodies to nature, nature speaks through that sustenance directly to our DNA, to the living, intelligent engines that drive our physiologies. Health is beautiful. Food informs physiology. Source matters. Your family's physiologic destiny is largely under your control. These are the central tenets of Deep Nutrition. If you adhere to the principles outlined in this book, you'll soon feel healthier than you do today. With every meal, you will support vital symmetry within your children's growing bodies and rig the genetic lottery to the benefit of those yet to be born. And in doing so, your legacy will sprout from the earth hundreds of years from now, in the form of a beautiful child. That child's beauty and health is your beauty and health, an unending renewal that promises to keep you forever young.

Epilogue
Health Without Healthcare

In *Selling Sickness,* authors Ray Moynihan and Alan Cassels explain "there's a lot of money to be made telling healthy people they're sick." The prologue to their book, published in 2005, paraphrases a candid interview of Merck's now retired chief executive Henry Gadsen, originally published in *Fortune* more than 30 years ago. "Suggesting he'd rather Merck be more like chewing gum maker Wrigley's, Gadsen said it had long been his dream to make drugs for healthy people. Because then, Merck would be able to 'sell to everyone.'" The case that the healthcare industry does not exist for the betterment of our health has also been well-argued by a number of experts from respected institutions including Harvard[314] and *The New England Journal of Medicine,*[315] and so for the most part I've resisted making grand indictments of the healthcare industry and attacking its failure to keep us well. But it's not just industry that's to blame. This kind of corporate thinking trickles down from the boardroom into your local clinic, contaminating individual doctors—like yours.

While I was building my practice, my boss explained to me that to be "successful" I would need more chronic patients in my panel. He explained that putting people on blood pressure and other medications, which would need periodic monitoring, was key to building a practice. I understood that from his perspective keeping my patients healthy—and medication free—was bad for business. This entrepreneurial mentality is endemic in today's healthcare model.

But these days it's gone beyond populating one's own practice with as many unhealthy people as possible and doing little to improve their health. As I discovered in 2007, now the name of the game is to push as many drugs as you can by whatever means you can get away with. When I interviewed with the chief of family medicine at a large medical corporation on the West Coast he explained that, since he was part of a team of people who arranged for pharmaceutical companies to issue cash grants, he was in a position to offer me a particularly enticing salary.

"What are the grants for?" I asked.

"We have a quality improvement program that tracks physician prescribing patterns. We call it 'quality' but it's really about money."

And that's all it's about. It works like this. In his organization, any patient with LDL cholesterol over 100 is put on a cholesterol lowering medication. Any person with a blood pressure higher than 140/90 is put on a blood pressure medication. Any person with "low bone-density" is put on a bone-remodeling inhibitor. And so on. The doctors who prescribe the most get big bonuses. Those who prescribe the least get fired. With a hint of incredulousness in his voice he explained, "So far, every time we've asked for funding for our program, the drug companies give it to us." If this is where healthcare is headed, then these hybrid physician/executives will instinctively turn their gaze to our children and invent more creative methods to bulldoze an entire generation into the bottomless pit of chronic disease.

Merck CEO Henry Gadsen's 30-year-old dream was to make healthy people buy drugs they didn't really need. But he was dreaming small. What I see happening now is more sinister, more profitable, and promises to have longer-lasting repercussions than merely creating diagnoses that lead to unnecessary prescriptions. What I see is a massive campaign of nutrition-related disinformation that has reordered our relationship with food and reprogrammed our physiologies. Industry has moved past selling sickness and learned how to create it. Whether by intent or simply fortuitous coincidence, today's definition of a healthy diet enables corporations to sell us cheap, easily stored foods that will put more money in their pockets and more people in the hospital. By denying our bodies the foods of our ancestors and severing ourselves from our culinary traditions, we are changing our genes for the worse. Just as corporations have rewritten the genetic codes of fruits and vegetables to better suit their needs, they are now in effect doing the same thing to us.

But there's one thing they've overlooked. Fruits and vegetables can't fight back. We can.

Appendices

Cod Liver Oil

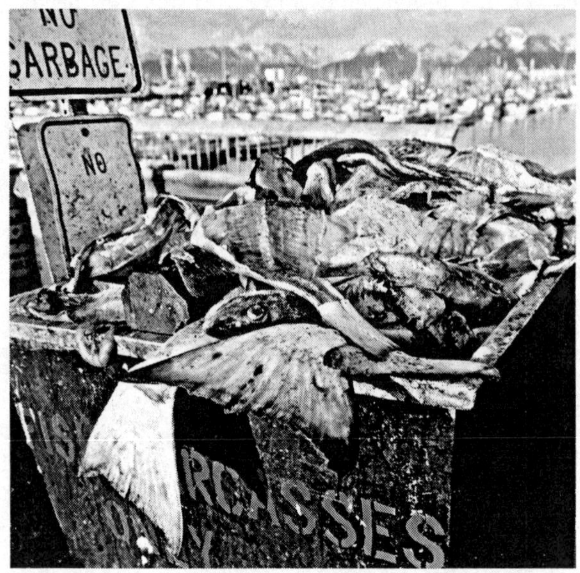

Deep Nutrition offers a new mode of thinking about health, one that involves an appreciation for the way food tethers us to the natural world and communicates to our bodies the health and beauty of the environment from which that food was collected. This relationship to the environment is both life sustaining and, in modern times, dangerous in that our foods represent *all* aspects of their sources, both good and bad.

Fish liver oils exemplify this complicated relationship perfectly. Cod liver oil, for instance, contains high levels of vitamins A and D, as well as essential fatty acids —all of which may be difficult to acquire without supplementation. They also may contain high levels of mercury and PCBs (the removal of which can destroy nutrients). Everything in the fish liver oil says something about the fish's environment and, therefore, its relative value to your health. Consumers should judge the quality of fish oil supplements as they would any other food, taking into consideration source, production, freshness, sustainability, and taste.

Tests to Measure Your Health

For the past few decades, researchers have noticed a strong association between type 2 diabetes and cardiovascular disease. So strong is this correlation that, according to one recent article, "the risk of major cardiovascular events in Type 2 diabetic patients without history of coronary heart disease (CHD) is equivalent to that observed in non-diabetic subjects with CHD."[316] Some researchers have hypothesized that this strong correlation implies a single underlying cause for both diseases. This has come to be known as the *common soil hypothesis.*

The correlations don't stop there, however. Both CHD and type 2 diabetes are also strongly associated with a long list of other diseases, including obesity, asthma, arthritis, osteoporosis, cancer, gout, sleep apnea, learning disorders, mood disorders, autoimmune diseases, and fertility problems. Given this web of correlation, it follows that the discovery of a "common soil" cause would help to explain the appearance of all these modern diseases now plaguing a huge segment of the population.

It is encouraging that some researchers in recent years have come to recognize the role of inflammation and oxidation in the development of diabetes and heart disease. But progress has been painfully slow. Researchers continue to jockey about the more fundamental physiologic reality: The underlying cause of modern disease is a low-nutrient diet high in distorted, manmade fats and sugar (along with a sedentary lifestyle). The competing influences of scientific fidelity and financial gain pull research in opposite directions, like gravity and centrifugal forces upon an a satellite orbiting the obvious.

The simple fact is that all "modern" diseases are caused by the same three dietary factors, and their pathogenic courses largely overlap. In this sense, they could be considered aspects of a single devastating disease (caused by what we might call "deep malnutrition").

The first of the following two tables maps out the progression of this disease—in its three most common manifestations—from onset to full-blown, acute illness. The second table lists useful indicators (from simple, inexpensive tests) associated with each stage of the disease's progression.

Use these tests to estimate your current health status and to gauge your progress as you apply the principles of Deep Nutrition to your life.

The four stages of health degradation due to glycation (high sugar), lipid oxidation (vegetable oils), and malnutrition and their associated physiologic effects			
	Arterial health	Glucose metabolism	Immune system and hormonal health
stage 1	•lipid cycle disruption (see page 187) •fatty streaks develop inside arteries due to lipoprotein damage and the resulting deposition inside arteries •Intimal thickening develops in damaged areas due to lower oxygen tension	•cross-linked cell membranes •upregulated RAGE receptors •glucose transporters slow to respond to insulin due to stiffened cell membranes •exaggerated insulin response after meals	•hyper reactive inflammatory responses due to chronic upregulation of pro-inflammatory cytokines and other mediators
stage 2	•diffuse intimal thickening develops •in the kidney, this reduces oxygen delivery to juxtaglomerular cells resulting in elevated diastolic blood pressure and exaggerated response to stress, or "white coat hypertension"	•insulin levels become chronically elevated due to increased burden of cells with stiff and abnormally functioning membranes	•increasingly over-reactive inflammatory responses disrupt hormonal and growth signals •cross-linked cell membranes further disrupt hormonal signalling
stage 3	•hypertension develops due to chronic renin-angiotensin stimulation •increased lipoprotein deposition in arterial lumen leads to atherosclerosis	•prediabetes develops •reduced oxygen and nutrient delivery to heart muscle leads to collagen deposits in the myocardium, stiffening the muscle and leading to diastolic heart failure	•disrupted repair cycles due to lack of sleep and chronic inflammation leads to connective tissue swelling •hormone receptor down-regulation
stage 4	•continued shear stresses and fat buildup in the artery lead to "vulnerable plaques" which can rupture, leading to heart attacks (see pages 196-7)	•chronically elevated glucoses accelerate the process of membrane damage and collagen cross-linking, leading to full-blown diabetes	•hormonal disruption leads to osteoporosis, circadian rhythm disruption •immune disruption impairs immune surveillance

Typical test results and symptoms associated with the four stages of health degradation due to glycation (high sugar), lipid oxidation (vegetable oils), and malnutrition			
	Arterial health	Glucose metabolism	Immune system and hormonal health
stage 1	•high *post-meal* triglycerides	•feeling a "sugar low" or tiredness resolved by eating sweets	•allergies and asthma •hives/itchy rashes •slow resolution of colds and other infection •frequent headaches
stage 2	•suppressed HDL •chronically elevated LDL and/or triglycerides •carotid ultrasound test shows abnormal intima-media ratio •blood pressure over 130/80 when stressed or sick	•glucose tolerance testing shows glucose intolerance •blood test shows elevated insulin levels •weight gain	•irregular and/or painful periods •weight gain •skin changes: acne, dark blotches, dryness •short and/or narrow-boned stature •crooked teeth •narrowed airways
stage 3	•blood pressure over 140/90 •endothelial dysfunction develops, causing ED and exercise intolerance	•fasting sugar level over 90 •HgbA1c (reflects average blood glucose) over 5.5 •exercise intolerance due to diastolic dysfunction •echocardiogram shows diastolic dysfunction •nocturnal foot pain and heel callous thickening	•joints stiff on wakening (due to connective tissue damage) •low estrogen and testosterone levels •infertility and early menopause •low bone density (due to reduced hormone receptivity)
stage 4	•blockages on angiograms, vulnerable plaques on intra-arterial ultrasonography	•fasting sugar level over 125 •HgbA1c over 6.5 •urinalysis shows *microalbuminuria* (protein in urine) •retinal exam shows abnormal blood vessels	•chronic fatigue •osteoporotic bone fractures •cancer •autoimmune disease (lupus, multiple sclerosis, myasthenia gravis, thyroiditis, etc.)

Steps for Including The Four Pillars in Your Diet

Starting with the Easiest First

1. Drink more milk.
   Best choice: raw, organic, whole.
   Next best: whole, organic.
   If lactose intolerant, choose yoghurt. Do not buy low-fat or fat-free dairy.
2. Buy sugar-free peanut and nut butters, the kind with the oil on top (all that oil is typically absorbed by sugar molecules in brand-name peanut butters). Avoid those that use palm oil, they tend not to taste very good.
3. Buy sprouted grain bread instead of whole wheat or white. Popular brands are Ezekiel and Alvarado street Bakery. These are usually sold in the refrigerated or freezer section because they are preservative free and you need to store them in your fridge. Many are wheat-free as well.
4. Instead of boxed cereals or instant oatmeal, eat toast with butter, sugar free peanut butter, or poached eggs for breakfast instead.
5. Use fresh, seasonal vegetables instead of frozen whenever possible. Season with salt and add generous amounts of butter and your kids will love them. Steam vegetables (like broccoli, asparagus, carrots, and cauliflower) instead of boiling, which leaches vitamins and minerals.
6. Buy Bubbies or other brand lacto-fermented pickles and sauerkraut and use as condiments/side dishes instead of chips or cookies at lunch. Save the juice when the jar is empty for salad dressing and to use as a starter for making your own sauerkraut.
7. Never use margarine or low-fat, low-cholesterol "spreads." Buy organic butter from pastured animals. Popular brands are Organic Valley and Horizon.
8. Choose healthy oils, see table listing of Good Fats and Bad on page 173.
9. Make your own salad dressing.
   Even easier, pour olive oil then balsamic vinegar over your salad (pouring the oil before the vinegar helps it stick better). Use a ratio of approximately 2:1 oil to vinegar. For extra flavor fast, add 1 Tbsp of the juice in the Bubbies pickle or sauerkraut jars.
10. Boil a dozen eggs and eat with salt for a quick lunch.
11. Eat large salads three to five times a week. Don't bother with iceberg lettuce. For variety, experiment with other greens, including radish leaves, arugula, beet greens or whatever looks particularly fresh. Add celery, carrots, sprouts, capers, pine nuts, sunflower seeds.

12. Use fresh herbs often. Add basil to salads with tomatoes; add parsley to hamburger; add garlic to butter for vegetables; rosemary to chicken; mint to beef stews or fatty roasts; ginger to stir fries.
13. Instead of canned tuna, buy salmon or mackerel *with bones in*. Mix with olive-oil based mayonnaise or small amounts of regular mayo and mustard to use for lunch as a replacement for nitrate-laden sandwich meats.
14. Eat liver once a week.
15. Eat soups made with bone stock once or twice a week.
16. Use bone stock rather than water as the base for making rice, mashed potatoes, noodle dishes, etc.
17. For variety, substitute beets or turnips for baked potatoes.
18. For light desserts that give a sweet finish to your meal, drink Kombucha or wine.
19. Use bone-in chicken, turkey, and red meats whenever possible.
20. When eating boneless cuts or beef, like fillet, serve with bone-stock gravy (also known as demi-glace).
21. Buy fatty cuts of meat, like New York strip, and sear the fat on the grill before cooking to enhance flavor.

What You Need to Cut from Your Diet:

1. Vegetable oil
2. Added sugar and honey (to tea, coffee, etc.)
3. Soda
4. Juice, except fresh squeezed. (Why not just eat the fruit? It's got more fiber and more antioxidants!)
5. Energy bars and "health" bars
6. Boxed cereals
7. Fried fast foods
8. Powdered "proteins," and powdered milk
9. Salad dressings made with any kind of vegetable oil, including canola
10. Low-fat products, including milk, cheese, salad dressings, cookies and other baked goods
11. Snacks and desserts—if you want to lose weight

Our Four Pillar Menu

Breakfast

Cream-top yoghurt flavored with any combination of:
jelly, vanilla extract, chopped fresh fruit, dried fruit, nuts

Raw whole milk (1 cup) with cream (2-3 Tbsp) added to 1/4-1/2 cup toddy (cold-brewed coffee)

Breakfast porridge:
Can be made with steel cut oats, barley, brown rice and more, including wheat berries and quinoa, both of which can be germinated first
Non-germinated cereals/etc. can be live-culture processed overnight by soaking in warm water with whey, miso, yoghurt, sourdough starter or other activating agent
Flavor with cream or butter, and experiment with spices, especially cinnamon and nutmeg, as well as herbs (mint) and citrus zest, or nut and dried fruit combinations (walnuts and cranberries, raisins)
If making without overnight soaking, use stock as the flavor base instead of water

Sprouted-grain bread, toasted and spread with butter, butter and fish eggs, peanut butter, or your favorite sugar-free nut-spread

Poached eggs on sprouted-grain toast

Crepes with vanilla-extract-flavored whipped cream and chopped fresh fruit

Avocado halves with coconut cream and a pinch of salt

Lunch: Healthy "Fast Food"

Hard boiled eggs with salt

Sardines with sauerkraut in a bowl

Sardines on sprouted-grain toast with mustard and sauerkraut

Liverwurst with mustard on crackers or sprouted grain toast

Peanut butter with wheat germ on you name it: sprouted grain bread / apples / celery

Smoked oysters on crackers

Fresh and sprouted tahinis and "spreads" (chickpea and / or sesame seed based; often sold by raw / vegan organic food manufacturers) on sprouted grain tortilla topped with fresh salsa

Milkshake or eggnog with banana and hazelnut extract (eggs must be washed and from a safe source)

Melted cheese on sprouted grain corn tortilla, topped with fresh salsa

Cucumber and tomato squares sprinkled with pine nuts, olive oil, balsamic vinegar, and a splash of (preferably lacto-fermented) pickle or sauerkraut juice (for salt)

Assemblage: raw nuts, peeled carrots, boiled eggs, slices of raw milk hard cheeses

Beverages

Kombucha
A live-culture fruity, bubbly brew with a trace of alcohol content

Brewed teas

Tomato juice

Unsweetened fruit juice, especially if home-grown fruit is available

Toddy coffee topped with whipped cream sweetened with vanilla extract and sprinkled with 1 tsp chopped up chocolate bar

Dinner With Luke and Cate

Nitrate-free chunk-style sausage on spouted-grain tortilla topped with cheddar cheese and fresh salsa

Liver (see recipe, following page) with fresh salad

Beef heart strips, grilled rare and topped with bone marrow medallions and demi-glace sauce, side of broccoli and garlic butter sauce

Home-made pasta and tomato-sausage sauce, side of fresh salad

Roast whole chicken with rosemary and giblets, sliced potatoes, and string beans

Chicken soup made with chicken stock, legs/thighs/and wings with home-made dumplings, side of fresh salad

Oxtail soup, side of fresh salad

Home-made pizza dough topped with pasta sauce, organic mozzarella, and whatever topping we have on hand: mushrooms, pepper, pine nuts, chicken, onions, cheddar and other cheeses, etc.

Zucchini, tomato, and onion trio fried in garlic butter and topped with vinegar-beef stock reduction sauce and finely chunked feta cheese

Filipino-style salmon head soup

Scrambled eggs with cheese, naturally cured bacon, and buttered toast

Steak with mushrooms flavored with bacon fat and drizzled in onion demi-glace sauce, asparagus with fresh Italian dressing

Grilled New York strip or porterhouse steak with wild rice and garbanzo beans cooked in chicken broth, with curly purple kale

Desserts

Kombucha or unpasteurized beer

2 oz dessert wine

Home-made cookies and milk

Dark chocolate, 1/2 oz max

Selected Recipes

Homemade Chicken Broth/Stock

The most common cooking question I get is, *How do I make bone stock?* Here is an easy chicken stock recipe from my friend Larry Ells, executive chef at the Grand Hyatt Kauai in beautiful Poipu. We've added white wine to his recipe for flavor and because the acid extracts more bone minerals into the broth.

Ingredients

Chicken bones, either fresh, or freshly frozen, 5 lbs. If you can find a butcher who sells them, include up to 50 percent chicken feet, thoroughly washed and toenails clipped off, for extra collagen
Carrots, washed and cut into slices or cubes, 2 medium
Celery, washed and cut into slices or cubes, 3 stalks
Leek (optional but very good) well washed and cut, 1 each
Onion, peeled and diced, 1 large
White wine 4-6 oz
Bay leaf, 2 each
Kosher salt, pinch
Black peppercorns , 6 to 8
Italian parsley, fresh and rinsed, whole, small bunch

How to Make it:

Cover the chicken bones and feet with cold water. Bring to a simmer and drain, and then rinse well. Return the bones and feet to the pot, again cover with cold water and add all other ingredients. Bring pot back to a low simmer, and simmer uncovered for about 4 hours. As the stock cooks, some grey foam will collect on top. Skim the foam with spoon and discard it.

When the stock is done, allow to cool for about 10 minutes and then very carefully strain stock into a metal or glass container, cool, loosely covered, at room temperature for about 30 minutes and then chill thoroughly. Use immediately or store in 3/4 full tupperware containers and freeze.

Use for making mashed potatoes, gravies and sauces, or quick soups for the family, with the addition of fresh vegetables and meats.

This recipe yields about 3 gallons of very good stock. The shelf life if refrigerated is 3 days. If frozen, 3 months. One large, fresh stewing hen may be substituted for the chicken bones and feet. Blanch, and rinse as you would with the bones and feet. Remove the meat from the hen as soon as it is cool enough to handle, and chill thoroughly as well. The meat has a shelf life of 3 days. If frozen, one month.

Sandy's Miracle-Liver Recipe:

We include this one organ meat recipe to show that you can get such tidbits to taste good and it doesn't take a culinary arts degree. This Filipino adobo-style (marinated in soy sauce) dish is Sandy's own creation. Her children love it and so do we!

Ingredients

1 cow's liver, cleaned (about one pound)
4-6 cloves garlic
1/8 cup soy sauce (naturally brewed, not hydrolyzed)
2-4 Tbsp Olive or peanut oil
Pepper

Prep and cooking time: 20 minutes
Serves 3 to 4

How to Make it:

Using a sharp chef's knife, dice the garlic and set aside. Slice the liver into one inch cubes. Pour oil into a large, flat-bottomed frying pan, coating the bottom, turn heat to medium, toss in the garlic and heat until it starts to sizzle. Saute garlic a few seconds, stirring. Add liver and cook briefly on each side until evenly brown and the blood starts oozing out, about two to three minutes. It should smell savory and good by this point.

Working quickly, grind very generous amounts of black pepper over the meat, about 1/4 to 1/2 tsp, then add the soy sauce into the pan, not pouring over the liver (to avoid washing off the pepper) and place lid over the top. Turn off heat, leave on hot stovetop and let sit for five to ten minutes until the blood turns pale brown. Serve au jus (that's what we do), over rice, or over noodles and with a sprinkle of parmesan cheese. Oddly enough, this liver will also taste good the next day!

Have a Favorite Four-Pillar Recipe? Share it Online at:

DrCate.com

Shopping, Reading, and Resources

Shopping Rules for Finding Quality Food:

1. Natural: If something couldn't have existed 200 years ago, skip it
2. Variable: If all units (chickens, cheese, tomatoes, etc.) are identical size and shape, that's a bad sign
3. Flavorful: If a given item lacks intensity of taste (without added MSG, hydrolyzed proteins, or sugar), don't buy it again
4. Seasonal: Avoid foods that are frozen and canned
5. Local: Packages should identify source

Reading:

A Revolution in Eating: How the Quest for Food Shaped America, Columbia University Press, 2005

Evolution in Four Dimensions: Genetic, Epigenetic, Behavioral, and Symbolic Variation in the History of Life, The MIT Press, 2006

Excitotoxins: The Taste That Kills, Health Press, 1996

Handbook of Food Additives, The Chemical Rubber Co, 1968

Health and the Rise of Civilization, Yale University Press, 1989

In Defense of Food: An Eater's Manifesto, Penguin Press, 2008

Mirror, Mirror...The Importance of Looks in Everyday Life, State University of New York Press, 1986

Mrs. Hill's New Cook Book: A Practical System for Private Families, In Town and Country. With Directions for Carving and Arranging the Table for Dinners, Parties, etc., Together with Many Medical and Miscellaneous Receipts extremely useful in Families, Applewood Books (Facsimile Edition of the 1867 original)

Natural Causes: Death, Lies and Politics in America's Vitamin and Herbal Supplement Industry, Broadway, 2006

Nutrition and Physical Degeneration, Price-Pottenger Nutrition Foundation, 2008

On the Take: How Medicine's Complicity with Big Business can Endanger Your Health, Oxford University Press, 2004

Overdosed America: The Broken Promise of American Medicine, HarperCollins, 2004

Preserving Food without Freezing or Canning: Traditional Techniques Using Salt, Oil, Sugar, Alcohol, Vinegar, Drying, Cold Storage, and Lactic Fermentation, Chelsea Green Publishing Co, 1999

Seeds of Deception: Exposing Industry and Government Lies about the Safety of the Genetically Engineered Foods You're Eating, Yes! Books, 2003

Selling Sickness: How the World's Biggest Pharmaceutical Companies are Turning us All into Patients, Nation Books, 2005

Survival of the Prettiest: The Science of Beauty, Anchor, 2000

The Cambridge World History of Food, Cambridge University Press, 2000

The Cholesterol Myths: Exposing the Fallacy that Saturated Fat and Cholesterol Cause Heart Disease, NewTrends, 2000

The River Cottage Meat Book, Ten Speed Press, 2007

Wild Fermentation: The Flavor, Nutrition, and Craft of Live Culture Foods, Chelsea Green Publishing Co, 2003

Resources:

EatWild.com: Excellent information on where to buy pasture-raised meats and eggs. Organized by state.

RealMilk.com: Volunteer chapter leaders from the Weston A. Price foundation post sources of fresh dairy on this web site.

SlowFoodUSA.org: Supports consumption of good, clean, and fair food. Members join local convivia.

LocalHarvest.org: Interactive map for finding farmers markets, CSAs (Community Supported Agriculture), and events, including workshops for learning artesanal food production techniques.

About The Authors

Luke Shanahan, MFA studied creative writing at the University of Iowa workshop and earned his MFA from the University of Arizona where he won several awards for fiction. He has taught college English, has freelanced for a number of newspapers and magazines including The Pacific Journal, the Garden Island Newspaper, and runs creative writing and screenplay workshops on Kauai. He is building a nonprofit organization FRESH that will bring families together around food and reconnects people to their culinary roots.

Dr. Cate Shanahan studied epigenetics and biochemistry at Cornell University's Molecular Biology program, attended Robert Wood Johnson Medical school, and completed specialty training in Family Medicine at the University of Arizona. In 2001 the authors moved to Hawaii, where Dr. Shanahan noticed that older patients who were raised on an entirely different, more natural diet tended to be the healthiest in their family, and that they also look different, with angulated facial features, better-aligned joints, and sturdier bones. Applying her knowledge of biochemistry and molecular biology to the study of food and human growth, she recognized that cheap fats and refined carbohydrates interfere with normal cell signals, and that traditional diets can help restore function. She traveled across the country to share this information with fellow physicians in formal lectures and meetings.

Other Publications:

Aging Skin: What Lies Beneath? The Pacific Journal, Fall, 2008

Friendly Bacteria: Can they Stop the Superbugs? The Pacific Journal, Fall, 2009

Lecture Titles:

Rich Cell, Poor Cell: How Peasant Food Can Save Your Life

The Third Parent: Why Your DNA Depends on a Healthy Earth

Index

Numbers in *italics* indicate subject is discussed in the figure or boxed text on the given page

A

Abramson, John, MD, 200
acne, 62, 271-4
adipose (see fat tissue)
adrenal gland, 212, 280
  vitamin C in, 6
adrenaline, 139, 210, 212
  sugar and, 217
advanced glycation end products (AGEs), 151, 204-6, 242, 246
Aesculapius, 14
affluence
  access to nutrients and, 89, 100, 117, 125
  of hunter-gatherers, 107
Africa, 119, 121, 123, 154, 162, 273
aging, inflammation and, 260, 280
aging, prevention of: 262-3
  brain, 255
  bones, 163
  joints, 204
agribusiness, 157, 176
agriculture, 107
alcohol, 207-8, 218, 228-9
  effects on growth, see *fetal alcohol syndrome*
allergen, 143, 149, 161
allergies, 38, 148-9, 162-3, 218, 261-2, 270-1, 274
  see also: children, food allergies and
Alzheimer's *see also:* brain
  exercise and, 255
  sugar and memory, 221-2
  stem cells and, 243
American Heart Association, 168, 180
American Medical Association, 13
amino acids, 129-31, 135, 146, 158-9, 161, 246
  collagen and, 265
  cooking and, 127
  deficiency and weight gain, 250
anaphylaxis, 261, 270
ancestral wisdom/science, 58-9, 105-6
  child health and, 4-5
  culinary arts, and, 19-21, 121-65
  ordered universe, perception of, 45
  production of health, 12-3
  skin health and, 273-4
  web of life, concept of, 6
anemia, sickle cell 71
animal products, 20, 123, 130, 140, 165, 268
  cooking, effect on nutrients, 153
  concept of whole foods applied to, 131
  effects of consumption on growth, 106, 134
  humane production, 72
  organic, added benefits of, 133
animal protein, 130
animals, earliest domestication of, 155
angiogram, 199, 213-4
animal fat, 13, 131, 138, 169, 173, 175-6, 269
  anti aging/ anti-inflammatory effect of, 275
  declining consumption of, 170
  vitamin content of, 176
  weight loss and, 249
antioxidants 15, 118, 152
  fermentation and, 146
  flavor of, 132
  presence in most whole, fresh foods, 152, 164
  loss during cooking, storage, etc., 152, 180
  supplements, 151
antibiotics, 11, 143, 164
antidepressants, 254
anxiety, 211-2, 218
apple shape, *see* female body type
apoptosis, 235, 246-8
arteries, healthy *182*
arthritis, 135-6, 141
  causative factors, 204, 246 , 267
  maternal smoking and, 29-30
  prevention by diet, 154
asthma, 37, 79, 97
  causative factors, 29, 30, 161, 271
  prevention by diet, 139
atherosclerosis, 161, 195-99, 204

Atkin's diet, 239, 241
attention deficit disorder, 74, 97

B

baby formula, 67, 146, 220, 262
bacteria, 144-7, 153, 156, 158-9, 271, 273
  pathogenic, 156, 160, 162, 269, 273
  see also: microbes, probiotics
Bassler, Bonnie, PhD, 147
beans, sprouting 150
beauty, 99, 263, 283
  birth order/timing and, 80-6
  Egyptians/Ancient cultures and, 4,5, 36, 274-5
  geometry, and 39-50, 109
  instinct for, 35, 50-5,63
  nutrition and, 64-80, 175
  significance of, 35, 36-57,61-4, 109
beef 113,115,132, 138
Berry, Halle, 1, 22-3, 35, 45
beta-carotene, 140
bile 159, 191, 249
bioconcentration of nutrients/toxins, *66,* 133-4, 152
biomathematics, 45-50
birth canal, 5
birth defects, 37-9, 91
  cause of, 79, 199-200, 207-8
  prevention of, 88, 91
blindness, cause of, 207
blood clot, *196-7,* 198, 205, 252, 255
blood lipids *see lipoprotein, cholesterol*
blood pressure 3, 9, 77, 79, 187, 251
blood sugar, 194-5, 203, 209-10, *228*
  cholesterol levels and, 192-5, 215,6
  headaches and,216-8
bone broth and stock, 134-8, 267-8, *266*
bone health, nutrition and, 26, 77, 97, 136, 154, 163, 258, 267-8, 275
  see also Joint health, osteoporosis
borage, 235
Bourdain, Anthony, 19-20, 128
brain
  development
    foods that promote, 13, 68, 141, 153, 162
    sleep apnea and, 38
  changes with childbearing, 77
  function
    during menopause, 211
    sugar and, 212, 217
  size, changes in, 106
  see also cognition, intelligence
bread, 143, 229-30
  ancient, 149
  sprouted, 148-151, 164
    fewer calories in, 230
  unleavened, 145
breast milk, 66-7, 160
Bush, GHW's inaugural dinner, 166
butter, 168-78, 273-4
  melting point, *170*
  weight loss and, 239, 241

C

calcium 198, 275
  dietary sources, 130, 136, 140, 158-60
  nerve damage and deficiency, 131
  requirements 65, 71
calories, 189, 233, 235
  exercise and, 203, 245
  refined foods versus whole, 164, 230
  weight gain and, 234, 241-3, 245, 248-9
cancer 2-4, 8, 134, 238, 250-3
  ancient cultures' resistance to, 59, 122
  birth order and, 79
  genetics and, 28, 79
  ideal geometry and, 37-8
  inflammation and, 236, 260
  mutation and,
  prevention, 146, 235-6
  sugar and, 204-5
canola oil, 180-1, 183
carbohydrates, 201-233
  consumption: Dr. Shanahan's recommendation, 210, FDA's, 233
  conversion to sugar, 226-30
  roll in chronic disease, 175
  scientific reductionism and, 112, 114
  taste of, 132
carrots 153, 224
cataracts, prevention, 283
celiac disease, *see:* wheat intolerance
cell membrane, 182, 187, 198, 203, 223

cellulite, 252, ***252***, 268, *268*, 281
children 4-5, 8, 63
ancient cultures and, 68-70, 115
brain development, 199-200, 219-23
diseases of, increasing, 97-8
effects of cholesterol-avoidance upon, 13-4, 199-200
epigenetics and, 27-30
food allergies, and 260-1
food aversions, and 118, 209
growth of, 37-8, 61-2, 76-102, 282
disturbance by bad diet, 175, 199-200, 202-3, 207, 267
height, relation to diet, 136, 145, 157, 267
joint health, relation to diet 135-6, 163, 267
Latina paradox and, 125
nutrient levels, USA, 71
planning for, 17, 68-9, 76-102, 163, 283-4
chocolate, 143, 162, 224
cholecalciferol, *see* vitamin D
cholesterol, 194, 198
appetite suppression, 176
brain growth and, *116*
controversy 12-15, 166-7, 199-200
drugs to reduce, 192
normalization by diet, 215-6
testing, 187-9
theory of heart disease 167-70
fallout from theory, 21, 171, 203
vitamin D, made from 275
see also: HDL, LDL, lipoproteins
chondroitin, 129
Clooney, George, 1, 35
clot, arterial *196-7*, 198-9, 205, 237, 251-2, 255
cod liver oil, 89, 288
coffee, 143
cognition, 47-50
cognitive development, sugar and 221
colds, 15, 71
collagen 13, 134-5, 163, 244, 267-90
damage to, by sugar, 204
damage to, by vegetable oil, 198
damage to, by UV, 274-9, *276*
foods that strengthen, 14, 134-6, *266*, 267-8, *277*
overall health and, 264-6
collagenase, 269, 272
cooking 121-65
traditions, value of, 21, 121-2
vegetables and nutrient availability, 152-3
see also ingredients ie fish, eggs, etc.
corn oil, *173*, 179
corn syrup (high fructose), 220, 226-7, *226*, 231, 242
cortisol/cortisone, 246, 251
beneficial effects of, 280
cow's milk, *see* milk *also* dairy
culture, bacterial (communication), 147
see also bacteria, probiotics
culture, human
beauty and, 50-1
food, significance to, indigenous 5-7, 66-69
to American, 105
culture, medical, 93

D

Dairy products 17,
bone health and, 26
human dependence on, *120*, 123, 154-5
pasteurization, historical need for, 156
pasteurization, effect of, 158-62, *160*
quality of, *66*, 95, (organic) 161-2
Deep Nutrition, 18-21
deer, fat content and hunting season, 131
dentition, as proxy for overall health, 60
modern versus ancient, 109
depression, 39, exercise and, 253
depression, post-partum, *77*
detoxification, natural 146, 258
diabetes, 251
bread, recommended type of, 164
cholesterol level disruptions, 194-5
circulation problems, cause of, 206
diagnosis of, 209-10
diet and, 208-9, 229-30, 241
early signs of, *203*, 210
family history and, 3, 14, 28
gestational, 79, 206-7

hunger and, 195
insulin resistance, 203-4
vitamin D and, 89
trans fat, cause of, 241
dietary guidelines, ancient 5
modern, 117, 200
diet-heart hypothesis, 168
dieting, 241
disease, model of, 2, 3, 7-8, *7,* 12
DNA, 22-35
hexagonal/pentagonal geometry and, 175
"junk" DNA, 23-4, 30, 32-3
language in, 31
memory of, 22-31
mutation, *7,* evidence against random mutation, 22-31
nutrient deficiency and, 79
symmetry and, 45
doctor
attitudes of, 37, 88-9, 157, 165, 166-7, 199-200, 249
education of, 9, 39-40, 166-7
special interest groups and, 86-88, 94
dog food, comparison to cereal etc. 113-116

E

eating:
class differential, 116-7
connection to our environment, 105
cultural experiences of, 6, 12, 74, 103
historical shifts in, 11, 15, 117, 124-5, 168, 176-7, 233
how to, according to past wisdom, 21
inadequacy of majority, 76
lack of time for, 93, 201
E. coli, as pathogen, 147
eczema, 218, 271
education, medical *see*: doctor, education
eggs, 13, 69, *116, 235, 239, 266*
free range versus industrial, 14
Egypt, 36, 58
Beer recipe, cuneiform, 143
Cave of Swimmers, *120*
fermentation, use of in dough, 142
makeup, 273-4
understanding of phi, 42-3
elastin, 282-3
endorphins, 254-5
endothelial function test, 184-6
environment, health of, 63, *206*
influence on genes, 3, 7, 23, 30-3, 62-3, *64,*
enzyme(s), *29,* 161, 179, 195, *196 fig. 8b, c, and f,* 278
activation of, 257, 270
damage to, 161, 175
weight gain and, 239-41, *240*
digestive, 149, 153, 155, 190
liver, 187
in bacteria/microbes, 143-46
in seeds, 149
in saliva, 229
increased metabolism and, 257
use as catch-phrase, 142
enzyme inhibitors, 143
Enig, Mary, 177
epigenetics, 2-4, 9, 14-8, 23-33
ancient wisdom and, 7, 283
beauty and, 47
childhood development and, *79,* 79, 97-9, 164, 200, 219
milk and, 154, 156
see also: genes, genetic
erectile dysfunction (ED), 185
Eskimo 65, 123
estrogen, 83-4, 211-2
effects on child's growth, 83
Etcoff, Nancy, 51, 55
eugenics, 57
exercise, 202, 217, 249
anti-inflammatory effect, 251
benefits from, aerobic versus anaerobic, 253-8
effect on metabolism, 240, 251
failure to lose weight from, 240-2, 248
memory improvements from, 255
overtraining, 257
eye, development, 110
missing eyes, 32-3
evolution, 83, 108, 117, 121
evidence against random mutation model, 3, 24, 29-30, 108
language encoded in DNA, 31-4
intelligence behind, 33-4

F

family history, 99, 215-6
Farmer, Fanny, 112
farmers, 66, 95, 134, local, 168
fast food, 130, 185, birth defects and, 199
fat, flavor of, 132-3
fat tissue:
  as source of stem cells, 244-8, *245*
  comparison to cancer, 250-3
  hormones and, 236-7, 244
  see also: cellulite
fats:
  bad versus good, table, *173*
  bloodstream and, 187-8
  first 'bad' fat, 171-3
  inflammation effect on, 184, 238-41
  lipid hydroperoxides (MegaTrans), 182-3
  oxidation of, 239-41
  polyunsaturated, 177, *178,* 179
  saturated, 178
  trans, 166, 173, 182, 239-41
  versus oil, *170*
  see also: omega-3
fatty acid (see fats)
fatty liver, 240, 250
fatty streak, 192
female body type, 53-5, *54*
fermentation, 142-8, 153, 155, 161
  neutralizing effect on toxins, 147-8
  nutrient preservation and, 148
fetal alcohol syndrome, 90, *91,* 207-8
fiber, in fruit 231
Fibonacci sequence, 41-2, 45
Fiennes, Ralph, *86*
Fiennes, Joe, *86*
Filipino food, in Hawaii, 72-4
flax oil, 180, 235
flour *see: wheat*
flavor, five major: 132-3
  antioxidants and flavor, 132
  development of flavor during cooking, 128-30, 184
  minerals and flavor, 130, 132
  fat and, 133
food:
  as cellular/genetic language 7, 33, 234
  class differential and food quality, *116,* 117
  complexity of, 130, *206*
  declining nutritional quality of, 95-6
  foodspeak, 104
  modern characterization of, 105, 112
  importance of source, 113
  relation to soil health, 95
Food and Drug Administration, 226, *276*
food industry 112, 247
  use of sugar, 225-7
  use of vegetable oil, 171, 274
food pyramid, 117
form-function relationship, 47, 62-4
Four Pillars Of World Cuisine, 15-16, 20, 121-65
  recipes, online at www.DrCate.com
free radicals, 181, 183-4, *197*
  arterial disease and, 184, 198
  birth defects and, 199
  erectile dysfunction and, 185-6
  saturated fat, resistance to, 178-80
free range, benefits of, 14
  see also: bioconcentration, pasture-raised
freezers, influence on height 101
French Cuisine, 124-5
French paradox, 125
fructose 226-7, *226*
  added to "100 percent" juice, 266
  in table sugar, 230
  fat-storing metabolic effects, 231, 242
fruit, 101, 133, 142. 153
  antioxidants in, 151-2
  digestion and, 153, 231
  nutrient levels in, 95-6, 118
  elevated triglycerides and, 87
  sugar and, 230-1
  recommended amount of, 231
fruit growers, influence on health research, 87,8
fruit juice, 146, 147, 212, 220, 224
  commercial sugar doping of, 226
Funny Looking Kid, FLK, 38

G

gateway 'drug', most common, 219-20
genes 16, 23-4

designer genes, 2
genetic disease, cause of 26-7
mutations in, 1, 2
nutrient/food effects on, 7, 13, 26-7, 28, 31, 32
osteoporosis and, 27
regulation of, 24, 25, 31, 32
see also: DNA, epigenetic
genetic engineering, 1, 32
genetic intelligence/memory, evidence for 'librarian' model of genetic change, 33
mouse study, 28
vitamin A and, 32
vitamin C and, 31
genetic momentum, 16
genetic wealth, 16-7, 35, 64,*64,* 99
GERD, gastro-esophageal reflux disease, 250
germinate, 145
germination, 149-50
Ghandi, 94
ginseng, 150
glucose, 202, 208, 209, 211-2, 227
relationship to starch, 229-30
see also: sugar
gluten intolerance, *see*: wheat intolerance
government, 117, 122, 157, 177
grains, 69, 110
processing of, 70
sprouting/sprouted, benefits of, 143, 149-50, 230
grain fed animals, 131, 132, 235
grass-fed animals, *66,* 133-4
Groves, Barry, PhD, 167
growth hormones, 134
group-think, in medicine 93

H

Hartman, Thom, 155
Harvard School of Public Health, findings on health of low-fat diets, 166
Hawaiians, native, 100, 165
HDL, 187-9
blood sugar effects on levels, 194
head size, low-fat diet and, 200
headaches, 216-8, 269
health:
birth order and, 76-9
class differential, 117
decline in, 15,16, 71, 85, 96-8, 115
genetic momentum/wealth and, 16-7
of Indigenous Peoples, 12, 61, *62, 63,* 66,
relationship to beauty, 17, 23, 37-9, 61, 63,
relationship to healthy environment, 63, 64, 65, 70
relationship to cultural mythology, 86-88, 94-5, 104-5, 112, 114
value to culture, 4-5, 68-9, 88, 94, 110, 115
versus health care, *206*
heart attack, *183*
cause, 167, 169, 184, 195-9, *196-7,* 208
cholesterol levels and, 187-95, 200-1
creating fear of, 168
historical trends, 170
sugar levels and, 208-9
tests to predict, 184-6, 187
heart surgery, 199
heart tests, 184-6, 187, 189, 213
heart beat, irregular, *see*: palpitations
heartburn, inflammation as cause, 269
heart disease
animal fat and,
cholesterol myths and, 21, 168-71
health 'paradox' and, 125
see also: heart attack, atherosclerosis
height, benefits of (for men), 100
herbs, antioxidants in, 151-2
heroin, 220
hexagon, bio-molecules and, 175
high blood sugar, 195, 205, 210 *see also*: blood sugar, high, glucose, and sugar
high blood pressure, 3, 195
Hilton, Nicky, *81*
Hilton, Paris, *81*
Hippocratic oath, *14*
homeopathy, applied to diet, 141
hormone receptors, *193,* 198, 203, 204
human engineering, 34, 68-70
hunter-gatherers, 108, 110-1, 123, 137m 155
Hygieia, *5, 14*

hypertension, *see* high blood pressure
hypoglycemia, 210-12

I

immigrant health, *see* Latina Paradox
immune system, 64, 122
  allergies and, 270-1
  effects of sugar cross-links on, 207
  inflammation and, 260, 270-1
  sleep and, *249*
  probiotics and, 147-8, 154
indigestion, fatty liver as cause, 250
inflammation, 206, 238-41, *240,* 260, 269-70
  aging and, 262, 270
  allergy and, 151, 261
  cause of, 151, 171, 183-4, 195, 242
  cellulite and, *252*
  exercise and, 251, 252, 254-5, 258
  intestinal, 269
  immune system and, 270-1
  joints and, 267, 270
  pregnancy and, *255*
  probiotics and, 148
  skin health and, 271-3, 274, 278-9
  weight gain and, 242, 246, 250-1
insulin, 211, 212
  exercise effects on, 245-6
  resistance to, 203-4, 208-9, 210, 241
  weight-promotion, 131
ions, flavor of, 130 *see also*: salt
ingestion versus absorption, 229
intelligence, factors affecting, 14, 38, 89, 222
iron, 65, 77, 95, 130
irritable bowel, *see*: inflammation, intestinal

J

Japanese, 146, height of, *101*
joint-building foods, 134-7, 141, *267*
  joint health, 129, 163, 251, 258, 260, 264
joint damage, 267, *264,* see *also*: arthritis
juice, hidden corn syrup in, 266-7

K

Kassirer, Jerome, MD. 200
Keys, Ancel, father of diet-heart hypothesis 167-70, *170*

L

lactose intolerance, 155-6
Latina paradox, 88
leavening, benefits of, 145
life expectancy 11, *70,* 282
linoleic acid, *172*
lipid cycle, 187-91
lipid hypothesis, *see* diet-heart hypothesis
lipoapoptosis, 240
lipoproteins, 187-8, *188,* 189-92, 192-95, *192,* 198, 205
  effect of sugar on levels, 215-6, *216*
LDL, healthy levels, *190,* 200
  effect of sugar on levels, 194, 200, 215-6
liver, nutrients in, 139, *140*
liver, role in cholesterol levels, 191, 194
liver, role in sugar levels, 210
low-fat diets, effects on collagen/skin, *277*

M

Maasai 68-9, 103
  beauty of, 104
  lifestyle, work and, 107
  milk consumed by, 119
  mythology of, 104
  toughness of connective tissue, 277
malformations, 38, 69, 90, 106
margarine, 13, 17, 74, 168-9, 171, *172,* 177
  "one molecule from plastic" 184
Marquardt, Stephen R, 40-5, 55-6
Marquardt mask, *44, 56, 52, 281*
meat:
  animal health effects on, 95-6, 133-4
  cooking principles, 125-32
  safety of undercooking, 162-3
MegaTrans, 182, 183-7, 195, *196* 198
  weight gain and, 239-41
memory loss
  from MSG, 131
  from sugar, 203
men, ED and, 185
menopause, 211
menstrual irregularities, 146

metabolism, 79, 175, 234, 256-7
microbe 143, 144-5, 147-8
  skin and, 271, 274
  sugar metabolism and, 232
milk:
  fresh v. pasteurized, 154-5, 156-62, *160*
  Maasai dependence on, 68-9
  shopping for, 161
  see also: dairy, lactose intolerance, soymilk
minerals:
  bioavailability influenced by, 145, 146, 152, 160, 161
  influence on facial development, 79
  influence on genes, 31-2
  loss during childbearing, 77
  presence in broth, 136-7
  presence in grains, 67, 69, 145, 230
  requirements for, 65
  slow cooking and, 130, 163
  traditional farming and, 95
monounsaturated fat, 133, *170,* 178, *178*
moon food, 118-20
MSG, in hydrolyzed soy and protein, 131
mutation (*see* DNA, mutation of)

N

Native Americans, 12, 106, 137, 150
nerve cell, 46, *46,* 49, 222, *222,* 255
Nurses' Health Study, 241
nutrients:
  access to, 67, 70-2, 92, 95
  influence on genes, 27-30, 79, 96, *101*
  interaction between, 132-3, 176
  loss with heating, 127, 153, 159, 163
  loss with storage, 118
  probiotics and, 144-6, 163
  release during cooking, 125, 128
  release by germination, 149
nutrient requirements, 64-67, 76
nutrition science, 13, 66-7
nuts, *174*

O

obesity, 79, 238, *see also*: overweight
olive oil, *173,* 178, 179, 274
Okinawan diet, 19, 122
omega-3 fatty acid, 11, *172,*
  anti-inflammatory effect of, 180, 280
  best dietary sources of, 141
  cancer cells and, 235
  damage by heat, 180
  in fat from pastured animals, 132
  pregnancy and, 69, 77
  traditional diets and 69, 236
omega-6 fatty acid, *172,* 235-6
Oprah, *54*
orange juice, sugar doping, 226
organ meats:
  traditional diets and, 69, 72-5, 138-9
  value of, *116,* 138-40, *140,* 141-2, 163
organically grown, 118, 119, 133-4, 149, 162
Ornish, Dean, *277*
osteoporosis, 154
  genes and, 27
overweight, 'apple shape,' *203*
  leptin and, 238
  pregnancy and, *255*
  viscous cycle, 252

P

Paleodiet, 18
palpitations, heart, 213-4, 218
pancreas, 208, 211
Parkinson's disease, 243
peptides, *127,* 129, 130
pesticides, 133, 149, 175
phosphorus, 65, 77, 140
phytates, 145, 149
phytoestrogens, 145-6
plants, 96
  antioxidants in, 152
  domestication of, 106, 219
  growth pattern of, 46-7
  fertilization of, 95
  pesticides in, 133-4
  self-defense, 142-3
  starch in, 228, 230
plastic surgery, 39
platelets, *196-7*
Pollan, Michael, 21, 219
polyunsaturated fat , 177-9, *178*
  see also: fatty acids, polyunsaturated
postpartum depression, *77*
potassium, 77, 130

bioconcentration of, 134
pre-eclampsia, 89
prediabetes, 187, 193, 208-10
pregnancy
cod liver oil and, 89
foods to avoid during, 79
preparation for, 69
smoking and, 30
soy-foods and, 146
spacing of, 76-9, 94
sugar consumption during, 208
prenatal vitamins, 86-94
Price, Weston A., 59-66, *62, 106,* 155-6
probiotic, 147-8
in milk, 158
protection from pathogens, 163, 274
vitamins derived from, 164
see also: bacteria, fermentation, microbe
processed food, 98, 112
low-cholesterol, as selling point, 169
sugar and vegetable oil in, 165, 201
protein
allergies to, 149, 156, 270, 271
collagenous proteins, 13, 264
cooking and, 126-7, *127,* 129
damage by sugar, 194, 204-5
gene products, 24, 26, 31
hydrolysed protein, 130
reducing food to, dangers of, 112-4
'sports' products and powders, 118
proto-farming, 155

Q

quality improvement programs for physicians, 286

R

radiation, DNA mutation from, 7
rats:
brain studies, 48
cereal study, 102
chocolate ensure study, 219
recipes, to read and to share: see www.DrCate.com
recommended daily allowance, RDA, set to low, 64-7, 71
refined foods, 118
shift from whole food to, 112-3
retinal health, 110, 141
riboflavin *see vitamin B_2*
Robinson, Jo, 235-6
Roosevelt, Franklin Delenor (FDR), 95

S

sacred geometry, *5*
salmon, 112, *206*
saturated fat *see fatty acids, saturated*
sausage, traditional 13
screening tests, medicalization and, 214
angiogram, 198-9
blood sugar, 209-10
endothelial function, 184-5
scurvy, 5-6
seafood, 19, 153
Second Sibling Syndrome, 84
selenium, 77
sexual development/dimorphism, 83, 85
shin splints, 8-9, 14
Singh, Simon, 46
skin:
anatomy, *263*
bacteria on, 271, 273-4
basis for preferring smooth skin, *281*
collagen and, *262,* 264, 265
dark blotches, cause of, 280
low fat diets and, *277*
oils in, 272-3
sun damage to, minimizing, 275, *276*
vitamin D and, 276-8
skin care products healthier than health foods, 274
sleep, importance of, 164, 236, 258
sleep apnea, 38, 108
smoking:
effects on children, 29-30, 79
government reluctance to reveal health effects of, 177
soda, 98, 154, 214, 224, 241
soil, fortification of, 64-5, 95-6
effect on animal health, 140
soy, difference between traditional use and modern 'health' food, 145-6
soymilk, comparison to yoohoo, 162
soy proteins, effect on thyroid, 145-6
soy sauce, brewed versus hydrolyzed, 131

spina bifida, 89, 90
statins, *see* cholesterol, drugs to reduce
stew, 128-30
stress
  degenerative effect of, 251
  effect on adrenal gland, 280
  effect on genes, 4, 33
  sugar dependence and inability to handle, 221
swelling, from inflammation, 269, 270
sucrose analgesia, 220
sugar
  as gateway drug, 219
  as pro-inflammatory compound, 242, 261-3
  addictiveness, 218-220, *219*
  atherosclerosis and, 195, 196-99
  birth defects and, 199, 207-8
  carbohydrates and, 112
  effects on child growth, 78-80, 85
  effects on cholesterol levels, 194
  effects on cell membranes, 203, *216*
  effects on circulatory system, 205-7
  effects on joints, 267
  effects on brain cells, 220-3, *222*
  in fruit, *see*: fructose
  loss of sensitivity to, 223
  metabolism into energy, 256
  most people eat more than they realize, 225-30
  pasteurization and protein damage by sugar, 158, 159, 160
  stickiness, cause of and damage due to, 194, 204-5
  stiffening effect of, 204
  see also: advanced glycation end-products, blood sugar, diabetes, hyopoglycemia
Surivial of The Prettiest, 50-1
sun, and wrinkles, 274-9, *276, 277*
sunscreen, *276,* 279
supplements, lack of potency, 92, 141

T

tallow, 171, *173*
taste buds, 130 *see also*: flavor
tea, Iraq study on effects of sugar in, 223
thrombosis, events leading to *196*
thyroid, soy protein effect on, 145-6
trans fat:
  association with MegaTrans, 182-4
  degenerative effect from, 260, *277*
  definition, 173
  delayed action by politicians, 177
  diet heart hypothesis and, 167-71
  doctors unaware of effects, 167
  damage to enzymes, 239-40, *240*
  damage to blood vessels,
  insulin resistance and, 241
  presence in "trans free" foods, 177
  presence in organic canola oil, 181
  pro-inflammatory effect, 239
  weight-gain from, 240-1, 243
triglycerides, definition, *170*
  blood levels of, 189
  diabetes and, 194
  fruit consumption and, 87
Tudge, Colin, 155
tumor necrosis factor, 255

U

ultrasound test for fatty liver, 240
unsaturated fat, *170*
UVA rays, *276,* 278-9
UVB rays, *276,* 278-9
UV-induced collagen damage, *276*

V

vegetable oil, definition, 179
  avoidance of, as way of avoiding heart surgery, 199
  birth defects and, 199
  consumption of in US, correlation with heart disease, 170
  effects of consumption on energy levels, 185
  effects of consumption on arterial walls, *196-7,* 198
  endothelial function and, 184-5
  fatty acids in, 179
  free radicals from, 181, 183-4
  hidden trans fat in, 175, 177
  interference with normal growth, 78-9, 83, 85, 98
  omega-6 in, 235
  processing of, 180-1
  trans fat, manufactured from, 168-70

ubiquitousness in processed foods, 113, 118
vegetables
antioxidants in, 151, 152
digestion of, 152
fermentation of, 143
influence of soil health on vitamin content, 95
nutrient loss in fridge, 148
vegetarians, 142
vitamin A:
bioavailability of (retinoids), 153
distinguishing between retinoids and, *144*
influence on DNA, 31-2
levels of in US populations, 71, 87, 89
reduced by childbearing, 77
sources of, 14, 141
protective effect on collagen, 280
vitamin B_2
effect of deficiency, 14
levels of in US populations, 71
vitamin B_6:
levels of in US populations, 89
set too low by RDA, 66
vitamin B_{12}
levels of in US populations, 89
loss during childbearing, 77
vitamin C:
in adrenal glands, 6
inaccurate package labeling, 95
loss of human gene for, 31
lost during storage, 148
vitamin D:
from sun, 275, 279
in liver oils, 275
levels of in US populations, 71, 89
loss during childbearing, 77
vitamin E:
consumption of supplements may increase mortality, 92
levels of in US populations, 71
vitamin K, unknown requirements for, 71
vitamins:
organ meats as source of, 139-41, *140*
probiotics and, 144
protective effect on skin, 280
synthetic versus natural, 92

W

walking, 254-5
water molecules, hexagonal geometry, 175
weight gain:
blood sugar and, 210
calories and, 234
cause of, 234
degenerative disease and, 260
invasive fat, 250-3
low fat diets as cause of, 242-3
leptin resistance and, 138
yo-yo diets and, 249-50
weight loss: *249*
carbohydrate consumption and, 242
exercise and, 248-9, 253-8
Deep Nutrition 'formula,' 236
metabolism and, 246, 257
why diets fail, 241
Weil, Andrew, 11
wheat:
benefits of leavening, 145
benefits of sprouting, 149
historical use, 143, 149-50
toasting, changes in, 204
wheat berries, 149
wheat intolerance, 148-9
whole food, value of, 130, 152
White House dinner, 116
wild animals, nutrition and, 134
wine, effects of fermentation on fruit, 143, 146

X

xanthine oxidase, 161

Y

yoghurt:
as alternative to raw milk, 161
lactose intolerance and, 155-6
probiotics and, 146
yoga, 253

Z

zinc, 77, 95
dwarfism and, 145

References 307

1 Dr. Michael Dexter, Wellcome Trust

2 Transposable Elements: Targets for Early Nutritional Effects on Epigenetic Gene Regulation. Waterland RA. Molecular and Cellular Biology, August 2003, p. 5293-5300, Vol. 23, No. 15

3 *Nutrition And Physical Degeneration*. Price W. The Price-Pottenger Foundation Inc. 1945. P 75.

4 Lifetime Risk for Diabetes Mellitus in the United States. Venkat Narayan KM Jama. 2003;290:1884-1890.

5 Guts And Grease: The Diet Of Native Americans. Fallon S. Wise Traditions.

6 A mechanistic link between chick diet and decline in seabirds? Proceedings of the Royal Society of Biological Sciences, Volume 273, Number 1585 / February 22, 2006 p445-550

7 Maternal Vitamin D Status During Pregnancy and Childhood Bone Mass at Age 9 Years: A Longitudinal Study. Javaid MK. Obstetrical & Gynecological Survey. 61(5):305-307, May 2006.

8 Epigenetic Epidemiology of the Developmental Origins Hypothesis, Waterland RA, Annual Review of Nutrition, Vol. 27: 363-388 (Volume publication date August 2007)

9 See chapter 11.

10 *The Paleo Diet: Lose Weight and Get Healthy by Eating the Food You Were Designed to Eat*. Loren Cordain. Wiley, 2002. P39

11 *In Defense of Food: An Eater's Manifesto*, Michael Pollan. Penguin Press, 2008.

12 We have between 10 and 100 trillion cells in our body, and each cell has two to three meters of DNA, totaling between 20 and 300 trillion meters. It's only 3,844,000,000 meters to the moon.

13 Pluripotency of mesenchymal stem cells derived from adult marrow. Jiang Y, Nature. 2002 Jul 4;418(6893):41-9. Epub 2002 Jun 20.

14 Environmental Health Perspectives Volume 114, Number 3, March 2006.

15 Epigenetic differences arise during the lifetime of monozygotic twins, Fraga MF. PNAS July 26, 200 5 vol. 102 no. 30 pp 10604-9

16 *Osteoporosis: Diagnostic and Therapeutic Principles*. Clifford J. Rosen, Humana Press, 1996, p51.

17 Genetics of Osteoporosis. Peacock M, Endocrine Reviews 23 (3): 303-326

18 The Ghost In Your Genes. NOVA Partial transcript accessed online at: http://www.bbc.co.uk/sn/tvradio/programmes/horizon/ghostgenes.shtml

19 Transposable Elements: Targets for Early Nutritional Effects on Epigenetic Gene Regulation. Waterland RA. Molecular and Cellular Biology, August 2003, p. 5293-5300, Vol. 23, No. 15

20 Decreased birthweights in infants after maternal in utero exposure to the Dutch famine of 1944-1945, L.H. Lumey, Paediatr Perinat Ep, 6:240-53, 1992.

21 Pregnant smokers increases grandkids' asthma risk. Vince G. NewScientist.com news sevice. 22:00 11 April 2005

22 Epigenetics: Genome, Meet Your Environment. Pray L. Volume 18. Issue 13. 14, Jul. 5, 2004

23 Accessed online at: http://bioinfo.mbb.yale.edu/mbb452a/projects/Dov-S-Greenbaum.html#_ednref63. Aug 19, 2007. Dov Greenbaum works with Dr. Mark Gernstein, the center's director.

24 Accessed online at: http://bioinfo.mbb.yale.edu/mbb452a/projects/Dov-S-Greenbaum.html#_ednref63. Aug 19, 2007. Dov Greenbaum works with Dr. Mark Gernstein, the center's director.

25 Influence of S-Adenosylmethionine Pool Size on Spontaneous Mutation, Dam Methylation, and Cell Growth of Escherichia coli. Posnick LM. Journal of Bacteriology, November 1999, p. 6756-6762, Vol. 181, No. 21

26 Zipf's law states that, if one were to create a histogram containing the total amount of words in a language and their occurrence, the arrangement in rank order would be linear on a double logarithmic scale with a slope of -z. This is the case for all natural languages

27 Hints of a language in Junk DNA, Flam F. Science 266:1320, 1994

28 Power Spectra of DNA Sequences in Phage and Tumor Suppressor Genes (TSG) Eisei Takushi Genome Informatics 13: 412–413 (2002)

29 Mantegna RN et al Physics Review Letters 73, 3169 (1994)

30 Non-coding DNA Can Regulate Gene Transcription by its Base Pair's Distribution. Sandler U. Journal of Theoretical Biology, Volume 193, Number 1, July 1998 , pp. 85-90(6)

31 The relation of maternal vitamin A deficiency to microopthalmia in pigs. Hale F. Texas S J Med 33:228, 1937.

32 The Modulation of DNA Content: Proximate Causes and Ultimate Consequences. Gregory TR, Genome Research Vol. 9, Issue 4, 317-324, April 1999

33 *Smiths Recognizable Patterns of Human Malformation*, Jones KL, 6th ed. Sept 2005.

34 Evaluation of the palate dimensions of patients with perennial allergic rhinitis. dePreietas FCN, Int. J. Pediatric Dent. Vol 11, Issue 5, Page 365. Sept 2001.

35 Dentofacial morphology of mouthbreathing children. Preto R, Braz. Cent. J. Vol. 13 No. 2. 2002.

36 Cephalometric comparisons of craniofacial and upper airway structures in young children with obstructive sleep apnea syndrome. Kawashima S, Ear Nose And Throat Journal. July 2000.

37 Sleep apnea-related cognitive deficits and intelligence: an implication of cognitive reserve theory. Achantis M, J Sleep Res. 2005 Mar;12(1):69-75.

38 Central nervous malformations in presence of clefts reflect developmental interplay. Mueller AA, Int J Oral Maxillofac Surg. 2007 Apr;36(4):289-95. Epub 2007 Jan 24.

39 Body weight, waist-to-hip ratio, breasts and hips: Role in judgments of female attractiveness and desirability for relationships. Singh D, Ethology and Sociobiology. 16, 483-507. 1995.

40 Waist-to-hip ratio and body dissatisfaction among college women and men: The moderating role of depressed symptoms and gender. Joiner T, Int. J. Eating Disor. 16, 199-203. 1994.

41 Appearance of symmetry, beauty and health in human faces. Zaidel DW, Brain and Cognition 57 (2005) 261-263.

42 Waist-to-hip ratio and body dissatisfaction among college women and men: The moderating role of depressed symptoms and gender. Joiner T, Int. J. Eating Disor. 16, 199-203. 1994.

43 Physical Attractiveness, Dangerousness, and the Canadian Criminal Code1. Esses V, Journal of Applied Social Psychology 18 (12), 1017-1031.

44 Cross-Cultural Implications of Physical Attractiveness Stereotypes in Personnel Selection. Shahani-Denning C, Presentation at 27th Annual Conference on Personnel Assessment. Available online at ipmacc.org/conf/03/shahani-denning.pdf.

45 For more details of how the mask is constructed, go online at Dr. Marquardt's www site: Beautyanalysis.com.

46 Mathematical lives of plants: why plants grow in geometrically curious patterns. Julie J. Rehmeyer | Jul 21, 2007 http://www.mywire.com/pubs/ScienceNews/2007/07/21/4250760

47 Excerpted from the July 11, 1998 Sunday Telegraph, Simon Singh's review of Ian Stewart's book Nature's Numbers.

48 *Chaotic Climate Dynamics*. Selvan AM. Luniver Press, 2007.

49 A Superstring Theory for Fractal Spacetime,Chaos and Quantumlike Mechanics in Atmospheric Flows by A.M.Selvan and Suvarna Fadnavis published with modification in Chaos,Solitons and Fractals 10(8), 1321 - 1334 (1999)

50 Language in context: emergent features of word, sentence, and narrative comprehension. Xu J, Neuroimage. 2005 Apr 15;25(3):1002-15.

51 The effect of emergent features on judgments of quantity in configural and separable displays. Peebles D, J Exp Psychol Appl. 2008 Jun;14(2):85-100.

52 Facial symmetry and judgements of apparent health Support for a "good genes" explanation of the attractiveness–symmetry relationship. Jones BC. Evolution and Human Behavior Volume 22, Issue 6, November 2001, Pages 417-429

53 An objective system for measuring facial attractiveness. Bashour M, Plast. Reconstr. Surg. 118: 757, 2006.
Chapter 3, Figure 8. "Checkerboard patterns trigger organized EEG waves," from: Lack of long-term cortical reorganization after macaque retinal lesions Nature Vol 435 May 2005, see figure 2 and text regarding cortical response to images lacking pattern. Attentive staring enables "optimization of sensory integration within the corticothalamic neural pathways," from: Thalamic bursting in rats during different awake behavioral states. Proc Natl Acad Sci U S A. 2001;98:15330–15335. That our brains respond to pattern. from: Spatial frequency modulates visual cortical response to temporal frequency variation of visual stimuli: an fMRI study Physiol. Meas. 28 547-554. That symmetrical objects trigger bloodflow to the pleasure centers, from: Sex, beauty, and the orbitofrontal cortex, International Journal of Psychophysiology Volume 63, Issue 2, February 2007, Pages 181-185. And that infants prefer and learn symmetrical images faster than asymmetrical ones from: The effect of stimulus attractiveness on visual tracking in 2- to 6- month old infants. Infant Behavior and Development, Volume 26, Number 2, April 2003 , pp. 135-150(16)

54 Waist and hip circumferences and all-cause mortality: usefulness of the waist-to-hip ratio? Bigaard J, Nature Obesity, Volume 28(6), June 2004, pp 741-747

55 Waist circumference and body composition in relation to all-cause mortality in middle-aged men and women. Bigaard J,Int J Obes (Lond). 2005 Jul;29(7):778-84.

56 The shape of things to wear: scientists identify how women's figures have changed in 50 years, By Helen McCormack, The Independent UK, Monday, 21 November 2005

57 Waist circumference and body composition in relation to all-cause mortality in middle-aged men and women. Bigaard J,Int J Obes (Lond). 2005 Jul;29(7):778-84.

58 Ancient Precision Stone Cutting. Lee L. Ancient American: Archaeology of the Americas Before Columbus. Feb 1997.

59 *Nutrition And Physical Degeneration*, Price Pottenger Foundation 1945. p5.

60 *Nutrition And Physical Degeneration*, Price Pottenger Foundation 1945. p1.

61 *Nutrition And Physical Degeneration*, Price Pottenger Foundation 1945. p1.

62 *Nutrition And Physical Degeneration*, Price Pottenger Foundation 1945. p31.

63 *Nutrition And Physical Degeneration*, Price Pottenger Foundation 1945. p275.

64 Influence of vitamin B6 intake on the content of the vitamin in human milk. West KD. Am J Clin Nutr. 1976 Sep;29(9):961-9.

65 *Nutrition And Physical Degeneration*, Price Pottenger Foundation 1945. p110

66 Wise Traditions, Vol 8, No 4, p 24.

67 *Nutrition And Physical Degeneration*, Price Pottenger Foundation 1945. p402.

68 *The Ways Of My Grandmothers*. Beverly Hungry Wolf. Quill. 1982. P186.

69 *Nutrition And Physical Degeneration*, Price Pottenger Foundation 1945. p402,3.

70 Vitamins for Fetal Development: Conception to Birth. Masterjohn C. Wise Traditions Vol 8 No 4 Winter 2007.

71 *Nutrition And Physical Degeneration*, Price Pottenger Foundation 1945. p401.

72 *Nutrition And Physical Degeneration*, Price Pottenger Foundation 1945. p402

73 Hiraoka, M. Nutritional status of vitamin A, E, C, B1, B2, B6, nicotinic acid, B12, folate, and beta-carotene in young women. J Nutr Sci Vitaminol. 2001 Feb;47(1):20-27.

74 Serum vitamin A concentrations in asthmatic children in Japan, Mizuno Y. Pediatrics International. V 48, Is. 3, pp 261-4

75 Vitamin D inadequacy has been reported in up to 36% of otherwise healthy young adults, and up to 57% of general medicine inpatients in the US, from "High prevalence of vitamin D inadequacy and implications for health" Mayo Clin Proc. 2006 Mar: 81(3):297-9

76 Nutrient intakes of infants and toddlers. Devaney B, Journal of the American Dietetic Association, 104 (1), Suppl 1, S14–S21 (2004)

77 Less than adequate vitamin E status observed in a group of preschool boys and girls living in the United States." J Nutr Biochem. 2006 Feb;17(2):132-8.

78 Vitamin K status of lactating mothers and their infants, Greer, FR. Acta Paediatr Suppl. 1999 Aug;88(430):95-103.

79 Nutritional status of vitamin A, E, C, B1, B2, B6, nicotinic acid, B12, folate, and beta-carotene in young women. Hiraoka, M. J Nutr Sci Vitaminol. 2001 Feb;47(1):20-27.

80 Consumption of calcium among African American adolescent girls. Goolsby SL. Ethn Dis. 2006 Spring;16(2):476-82.

81 Nutritional supplements in pregnancy: commercial push or evidence based? Glennville M. Curr Opin Obstet Gynecol. 2006 Dec;18(6):642-7

82 *The Contribution of Nutrition To Human And Animal Health*. 1992. Cambridge University Press. Ed: Widdowson. p263

83 Reduced brain DHA content after a single reproductive cycle in female rats fed a diet deficient in N-3 polyunsaturated fatty acids. Levant B. Biol Psychiatry. 2006 Nov 1;60(9):987-90.

84 Maternal parity and diet (n-3) polyunsaturated fatty acid concentration influence accretion of brain phospholipid docosahexaenoic acid in developing rats. Levant B. J Nutr. 2007 Jan;137(1):125-9.

85 Epigenetic regulation of metabolism in children born small for gestational age. Holness MJ. Curr Opin Clin Nutr Metab Care. 2006 Jul;9(4):482-8. Review

86 Early-life family structure and microbially induced cancer risk. Blaser MJ. PLoS Med. 2007 Jan;4(1):e7.

87 The effect of birth order and parental age on the risk of type 1 and 2 diabetes among young adults. Lammi N. Diabetologia. 2007 Dec;50(12):2433-8. Epub 2007 Oct 18.

88 Associations of birth defects with adult intellectual performance, disability and mortality: population-based cohort study. Eide MG. Pediatr Res. 2006 Jun;59(6):848-53. Epub 2006 Apr 26.

89 Nutritional factors affecting the development of a functional ruminant—a historical perspective. Warner, R. G. Pages 1–12 in Proc. Cornell Nutr. Conf. Feed Manuf., Syracuse, NY. Cornell Univ., Ithaca, NY. 1991.

90 The many faces and factors of orofacial clefts. Schutte, B. Human Molecular Genetics, 1999, Vol. 8, No. 10 1853-1859

91 Unpublished communication with PhD at UCLA Jonsson Comprehensive Cancer Center. Oct. 11, 2006.

92 Lillian Gelberg, MD. UCLA Jonsson Comprehensive Cancer Center. Unpublished communication Oct. 11, 2006.

93 Schulz, C. Vitamin A and beta-carotene supply of women with gemini or short birth intervals: A pilot study. Eur J Nutr. 2006 Nov 10.

94 From Vitamin profile of 563 gravidas during trimesters of pregnancy. (Baker H, J Am Coll Nutr. 2002 Feb;21(1):33-7.)

95 High prevalence of vitamin D insufficiency in black and white pregnant women residing in the northern United States and their neonates. Bodnar LM, J Nutr. 2007 Feb;137(2):447-52)

96 Maternal supplementation with very-long-chain n-3 fatty acids during pregnancy and lactation augments children's IQ at 4 years of age. Helland IB. Pediatrics. 2003 Jan;111(1):e39-44.

97 The fetal origins of memory: the role of dietary choline in optimal brain development. Zeises SH. J Pediatr. 2006 Nov;149(5 Suppl):S131-6. Review

98 Choline: are our university students eating enough? Gossell-Williams M. West Indian Med J. 2006 Jun;55(3):197-9.

99 Prevention of neural tube defects: results of the Medical Research Council Vitamin Study. MRC Vitamin Study Research Group. [no authors listed] Lancet. 1991 Jul 20;338(8760):131-7.

100 Nutritional supplements in pregnancy: commercial push or evidence based? Glenville M. Current Opinion in Obstetrics and Gynecology 2006, 18:642-647.

101 *Beyond Deficiency: New Views on the Function and Health Effects of Vitamins*. Annals of the New York Academy of Sciences, Vol 669, 1992. Pp 8-10.

102 *Natural Causes: Death, Lies, and Politics in America's Vitamin and Herbal Supplement Industry*. Dan Hurly. Broadway 2006.

103 Traditional Methods of Birth Control in Zaire. Waife RS. Pathfinder Papers No. 4. Chestnut Hill, MA, 1978.

104 "Le Bebe En Brousse": European Women, African Birth Spacing And Colonial Intervention In The Belgian Congo. Hunt NR. The International Journal of African Historical Studies, 21, 3 (1988) 401-32.

105 Intimate Colonialism: The Imperial Production of Reproduction in Uganda, 1907-1925.Carol Summers. Signs, Vol. 16, No. 4, Women, Family, State, and Economy in Africa (Summer, 1991), pp. 787-807

106 *Nutrition And Physical Degeneration*, Price Pottenger Foundation 1945. p398.

107 Nutritional supplements in pregnancy: commercial push or evidence based? Glenville M. Current Opinion in Obstetrics and Gynecology 2006, 18:642-647.

108 Lifetime Risk for Diabetes Mellitus in the United States. Venkat Narayan KM Jama. 2003;290:1884-1890.

109 America's Children in Brief: Key National Indicators of Well-Being, 2008, Federal interagency Forum on Child and Family Statistics.

110 Anna Stainer-Knittel: portrait of a femme vitale. Kain E. Women's Art Journal: Vol 20, No.2 pp 13-71.

111 *Mirror, Mirror...The Importance of Looks in Everyday Life*. Hatfield, E. 1986. SUNY Press

112 New Light on the "Dark Ages": The Remarkably Tall Stature of Northern European Men during the Medieval Era. Steckel RH, Social Science History 2004 28(2):211-229;

113 *The Cambridge World History of Food*, Cambridge University Press, 2000

114 *Fighting the Food Giants*, Paul A. Stitt. Natural Press, 1981, pp. 61-66

115 Accessed online at lostgirlsworld.blogspot.com/2006/12/becoming-maasai.html on July 27, 2008

116 Accessed online at: www.bluegecko.org/kenya/tribes/maasai/beliefs.htm on Sept 4, 2008

117 *Nutrition and Physical Degeneration*. Price WA. Price-Pottenger Foudation, 1945. P 226.

118 *Nutrition and Physical Degeneration*. Price WA. Price-Pottenger Foudation, 1945. P 10.

119 *Nutrition and Physical Degeneration*. Price WA. Price-Pottenger Foudation, 1945. P 228.

120 *Nutrition and Physical Degeneration*. Price WA. Price-Pottenger Foudation, 1945. P 248.

121 Archaeological Amerindian and Eskimo cranioskeletal size variation along coastal western North America: relation to climate, the reconstructed diet high in marine animal foods, and demographic stress. Ivanhoe F. International Journal of Osteoarchaeology. Volume 8, Issue 3, Pages 135 - 179

122 Craniofacial variation and population continuity during the South African Holocene. Stynder DD. American Journal of Physical Anthroplogly. Published Online: 4 Sep 2007

123 Craniofacial morphology in the Argentine center-west: Consequences of the transition to food production. Marina L. Sardi. The American Journal of Physical Anthropology. Volume 130, Issue 3, Pages 333 - 343

124 *The Cambridge World History Of Food*, Cambridge University Press, 2000. p1704.

125 Stone Age Economics, Sahlins M. Aldine Transaction, 1972. pp1-40.

126 Stone Age Economics, Sahlins M. Aldine Transaction, 1972. pp1-40.

127 The question of robusticity and the relationship between cranial size and shape in Homo sapiens. Lahr MM. Journal of Human Evolution (1996) 31, 157-191.

128 Dental carries in prehistoric South Africans. Dryer, TF. Nature, 136:302, 1935. "The indication from this area [...] bears out the experience of European anthropologists that carries is a comparatively modern disease and that no skull showing this condition can be regarded as ancient."

129 Dental Anthropology, Scott GR, Annual Review of Anthropology Vol 17:99-126 Oct 1988. "Pronounced forms of malocclusion are a relatively recent development"

130 *Bioarchaeology of Southeast Asia*, Oxenham M. Cambridge University Press 2006. "[H]unter-gatherers typically have low frequencies of carries, calculus, malocclusion and alveolar resorption, a high frequency of severe attrition [wear] and large jaw size. Agricultural populations typically have the opposite profile, low rates of severe attrition (except in cases where food contains abrasives) and high rates of carries, calculus, resorption, dental crowding and malocculsion."

131 *Nutrition and Physical Degeneration*. Price WA. Price-Pottenger Foudation, 1945. P 279.

132 Jan 20, 2001 Inaugural luncheon menu served at the US State capitol. Accessed online Oct 31, 2007 at: http://www.gwu.edu/%7Eaction/inaulu.html

133 The content of bioactive compounds in rat experimental diets based on organic, low-input, and conventional plant materials. Leifert C. 3rd QLIF Congress, Honeheim, Germany, March 20-23, 2007. Archived at http://orgprints.org/view/projects/int_conf_qlif2007.html.

134 Nutritional comparison of fresh, frozen, and canned fruits and vegetables II. Vitamin A and carotenoids, vitamin E, minerals and fiber Joy C RickmanJ Sci Food Agric (in press)

135 The Vitamin A, B, and C Content of Artificially Versus Naturally Ripened Tomatoes. House MC. The Journal of Biological Chemistry, Vol LXXXI, No. 3. Received for publication Dec 13, 1928.

136 The Vitamin A, B, and C Content of Artificially Versus Naturally Ripened Tomatoes. House MC. The Journal of Biological Chemistry, Vol LXXXI, No. 3. Received for publication Dec 13, 1928.

137 Nutritional comparison of fresh, frozen and canned fruits and vegetables. Part 1. Vitamins C and B and phenolic compounds Joy C Rickman, J Sci Food Agric 87:930–944 (2007)

138 *The Cambridge World History of Food,* Cambridge University Press 2000 p1210

139 *The Cambridge World History of Food,* Cambridge University Press 2000 p1210

140 Dietary advanced glycation endproducts (AGEs) and their health effects--PRO. Sebeková K, Mol Nutr Food Res. 2007 Sep;51(9):1079-84.

141 Methylglyoxal in food and living organisms. Nemet I, Mol Nutr Food Res. 2006 Dec;50(12):1105-17. Review.

142 Multidimensional scaling of ferrous sulfate and basic tastes. Stevens D, Physiology & behavior, 2006, vol. 87, no2, pp. 272-279

143 Neural Circuits for Taste: Excitation, Inhibition, and Synaptic Plasticity in the Rostral Gustatory Zone of the Nucleus of the Solitary Tract. Bradley RM. Annals of the New York Academy of Sciences 855 (1), 467–474.

144 *Excitotoxins: The Taste That Kills,* Russel Blaylock, Health Press 1996

145 Body Composition of White Tailed Deer, Robbins C, 1974. 38:871-876. J Anim Sci

146 University of New Hampshire Cooperative Extension. Accessed online Aug 19, 2008 at: http://extension.unh.edu/news/feedeer.htm

147 *The Journals of Samuel Hearne,* S Hearne 1768, "On the twenty-second of July, we met several strangers, whom we joined in pursuit of the caribou, which were at this time so plentiful that we got everyday a sufficient number for our support, and indeed too frequently killed several merely for the tongues, marrow and fat."

148 *The Narrative of Cabeza De Vaca.* Cabeza de Vaca, Álvar Núñez. Translation of La Relacion by Rolena Adorno and Patrick Charles Pautz. University of Nebraska Press 2003.

149 CD36 involvement in orosensory detection of dietary lipids, spontaneous fat preference, and digestive secretions. Laugerette F. J. Clin. Invest. 115:3177-3184 (2005)

150 Evidence for Human Orosensory (Taste?) Sensitivity to Free Fatty Acids. Chale-Rush A, Chem Senses, June 1, 2007; 32(5): 423 - 431.

151 Multiple routes of chemosensitivity to free fatty acids in humans. Chale-Rush A, Am J Physiol Gastrointest Liver Physiol 292: G1206-G1212, 2007

152 *Seeds of Deception, Exposing Industry and Government Lies About the Safety of the Genetically Engineered Foods You're Eating,* Smith J. Yes! Books, 2003. pp77-105.

153 Nutraceuticals As Therapeutic Agents In Osteoarthritis: The Role of Glucosamine, Chondroitin Sulfate, and Collagen Hydrolysate. Deal CL, Rheumatic Disease Clinics of North America. Volume 25, Issue 2, 1 May 1999, Pages 379-395

154 Nutraceuticals As Therapeutic Agents In Osteoarthritis: The Role of Glucosamine, Chondroitin Sulfate, and Collagen Hydrolysate. Deal CL, Rheumatic Disease Clinics of North America. Volume 25, Issue 2, 1 May 1999, Pages 379-395

155 The Heparin-Binding (Fibroblast) Growth Factor Family of Proteins. Burgess W. Annual Review of Biochemistry,Vol. 58: 575-602, July 1989

156 As posted on The Stone Foundation For Arthritis Help And Research, accessed 10-10-07 at: www.stoneclinic.com/jjanews.htm

157 Determinants and Implications of Bone Grease Rendering: A Pacific Northwest Example. Prince P. North American Archaeologist Volume 28, Number 1 / 2007

158 A New Approach to Identifying Bone Marrow and Grease Exploitation: Why the "Indeterminate" Fragments should not be Ignored. Outram AK. Journal of Archaeological Science (2001) 28, 401-410.

159 Freezing for two weeks at -4 degrees F will kill parasites

160 *Let's Cook It Right,* Adelle Davis, Signet Classics 1970 p87,

161 USDA Agricultural Resource Service Nutrient Data Library. Accessed online at www.nal.usda.gov/fnic/foodcomp/search/ Dec 23, 2005.

162 Paraphrased by H.E. Jacob in *Six Thousand Years of Bread: It's Holy and Unholy History.* Skyhorse Publishing, 2007, p26.

163 *The Cambridge World History of Food.* Cambridge Unviersity Press 2000 p1474.

164 *Wind, Water, Work: Ancient and Medieval Milling Technology,* Adam Lucas. Brill Academic Publishers, 2005.

165 The gut flora as a forgotten organ. Shanahan F. EMBO reports 7, 7, 688–693 (2006)

166 Nutrition and colonic health: the critical role of the microbiota. O'keefe SJ. Curr Opin Gastroenterol. 2008 Jan;24(1):51-58.

167 Serum or plasma cartilage oligomeric matrix protein concentration as a diagnostic marker in pseudoachondroplasia: differential diagnosis of a family A Cevik Tufan et. al. Eur J Hum Genet 15: 1023-1028.

168 *The Cambridge World History of Food.* Cambridge Press 2000. p1473.

169 Effects of soy protein and soybean isoflavones on thyroid function in healthy adults and hypothyroid patients: a review of the relevant literature. Messina M, Thyroid, 2006 Mar; 16(3):249-58.

170 Infant feeding with soy formula milk: effects on puberty progression, reproductive function and testicular cell numbers in marmoset monkeys in adulthood. Tan KA. Hum Reprod. 2006 Apr;21(4):896-904.

171 Food Values of Portions Commonly Used, Pennington J, HarperPerrenial 1989

172 Quorum sensing: cell-to-cell communication in bacteria. Waters CM, Bassler BL. Annu Rev Cell Dev Biol 21: 319-346 2005

173 The gut flora as a forgotten organ. Shanahan F. EMBO reports 7, 7, 688–693 (2006)

174 Probiotics in human disease. Isolauri E. Am J Clin Nutr. 2001 Jun;73(6):1142S-1146S. Review.

175 Commensal bacteria (normal microflora), mucosal immunity and chronic inflammatory and autoimmune diseases. Sokol D. Immunol Lett. 2004 May 15;93(2-3):97-108. Review.

176 Probiotics and their fermented food products are beneficial for health. Parvez S. J Appl Microbiol. 2006 Jun;100(6):1171-85. Review

177 Nutritional comparison of fresh, frozen, and canned fruits and vegetables, Executive Summary of the Department of Food Science and Technology, University of California Davis, Davis, CA. 95616, Rickman J. Accessed online at: www.mealtime.org/uploadedFiles/Mealtime/Content/ucdavisstudyexecutivesummary.pdf -

178 Whole wheat and white wheat flour—the mycobiota and potential mycotoxins. Weidenbörner M, Food Microbiology Volume 17, Issue 1, February 2000, Pages 103-107

179 The Impact of Processing on the Nutritional Quality of Food Proteins. Meade S, Journal of AOAC International, 2005, vol. 88, no3, pp. 904-922

180 *Let's Have Healthy Children*, Adelle Davis Signet 1972 p95.

181 Bioavailability and bioconversion of carotenoids. Castenmiller JJM Annual Review of Nutrition Vol. 18: 19-38 July 1998

182 The apparent incidence of hip fracture in Europe: A study of national register sources. Johnel O, Ostoporosis International, Volume 2, Number 6 / November, 1992

183 The Milk Book: The Milk of Human Kindness is Not Pasteurized. William Campbell Douglass II, MD. Rhino Publishing 2005.

184 Continuous Thermal Processing of Foods: Pasteurization and Uht. Heppell NJ. Springer 2000 P194

185 Dr. North and the Kansas City Newspaper War: Public Health Advocacy Collides with Main Street Respectability. Kovarik B. Paper presented at the Annual Meeting of the Association for Education in Journalism and Mass Communication (72nd, Washington, DC, August 10-13, 1989) accessed online Dec 27, 2007 at www.radford.edu/wkovarik/papers/aej98.html

186 *The Milk Book: The Milk of Human Kindness is Not Pasteurized.* William Campbell Douglass II, MD. Rhino Publishing 2005.

187 *The Milk Book: The Milk of Human Kindness is Not Pasteurized.* William Campbell Douglass II, MD. Rhino Publishing 2005. p11.

188 Modifications in milk proteins induced by heat treatment and homogenization and their influence on susceptibility to proteolysis. Garcia-Risco MR. International Dairy Journal 12 (2002) 679-688.

189 Soluble, dialyzable and ionic calcium in raw and processed skim milk, whole milk and spinach. Reykdal O. Journal of Food Science 56 3, pp. 864–866. 1991

190 Calcium bioavailability in human milk, cow milk and infant formulas—comparison between dialysis and solubility methods Roig MJ. Food Chemistry Vol 65, Issue 3, P353-357.

191 Carbonylation of milk powder proteins as a consequence of processing conditions François Fenaille. Proteomics Vol 5 Issue 12 pp3097-3104

192 Modifications in milk proteins induced by heat treatment and homogenization and their influence on susceptibility to proteolysis. Garcia-Risco MR. International Dairy Journal 12 (2002) 679-688.

193 *Chemistry And Safety of Acrylamide In Food*, Friedman M. p141. Springer 2005

194 *Dietary Fat Requirements in Health and Development*, Thomas H Applewhite, American Oil Chemists Society 1988 p30

195 Types of Dietary Fat and Risk of Coronary Heart Disease: A Critical Review. HU F, Journal of the American College of Nutrition, Vol 2-, 1, 5-19 (2001)

196 In *Food Choices and Coronary Heart Disease: A Population Based Cohort Study of Rural Swedish Men with 12 Years of Follow-up*" (Int. J. Environ. Res. Public Health 2009, 6, 2626-2638) the authors assert "The diet-heart hypothesis from the 1950s stating that saturated fats lead to heart disease via blood lipid derangement is under re-evaluation." Barry Groves, PhD, cites over 1,000 articles in his book *Trick and Treat: How Healthy Eating is Making Us Ill* published by Hammersmith Press in 2008. Gary Taubes' 640 page *Good Calories, Bad Calories* (Knopf, 2007) is similarly well-referenced.

197 Health Revolutionary: The Life and Work of Ancel Keys, accessed online at http://209.85.141.104/search?q=cache:PVHCLllMKzQJ:www.asph.org/movies/keys.pdf+%22i'll+show+those+guys%22+keys&hl=en&ct=clnk&cd=1&gl=us&client=firefox-a

198 Hydrogenated fats in the diet and lipids in the serum of man. Anderson JT. J Nutr. 75 (4):338, 1961

199 Hydrogenated fats in the diet and lipids in the serum of man. Anderson JT. J Nutr. 75 (4):338, 1961

200 Health Revolutionary: The Life and Work of Ancel Keys, accessed online at http://209.85.141.104/search?q=cache:PVHCLlIMKzQJ:www.asph.org/movies/keys.pdf+%22i'll+show+those+guys%22+keys&hl=en&ct=clnk&cd=1&gl=us&client=firefox-a

201 Tracing citations in consensus articles and other policy setting research statements leads us back to Keys and his junk science. Case in point, the 2004 National Cholesterol Education Program (NCEP) coordinating committee issued an update to the third Adult Treatment Panel (ATP III) Consensus panel statement

202 *Know Your Fats, The Complete Primer for Understanding the Nutrition of Fats, Oils, and Cholesterol*, Mary G Enig PhD Bethesda Press 2000 p94.

203 *The Cholesterol Myths*, Uffe Ravnskov MD, PhD. New Trends Publishing 2000, p 30.

204 Myths And Truths About Beef. Fallon S. Wise Traditions in Food, Farming and the Healing Arts. Spring 2000.

205 *Trans Fatty Acids in the Food Supply: A Comprehensive Report Covering 60 Years of Research*, 2nd Edition, Enig, Mary G, PhD, Enig Associates, Inc, Silver Spring, MD, 1995, 4-8

206 Heart Disease and Stroke Statistics- 2003 Update. American Heart Association

207 The Rise and Fall of Ischemic Heart Disease, Stallones RA, Sci Am. 1980 Nov;243(5):53-9.

208 Sex matters: secular and geographical trends in sex differences in coronary heart disease mortality Lawlor DA, BMJ 2001;323:541-545 (8 September)

209 The Lowdown On Oleo. Kapica C. Chicago Wellness Magazine. Sept-Oct 2007.

210 See Chapter 11

211 The ABCs of vitamin E and ß-carotene absorption, Traber MG, American Journal of Clinical Nutrition, Vol. 80, No. 1, 3-4, July 2004

212 Absorption, metabolism, and transport of carotenoids. Parker RS. FASEB J. 1996 Apr;10(5):542-51.

213 Human plasma transport of vitamin D after its endogenous synthesis. Haddad JG, Matsuoka LY, Hollis BW, Hu YZ, Wortsman J

214 Physicochemical and physiological mechanisms for the effects of food on drug absorption: The role of lipids and pH Journal of Pharmaceutical Sciences Volume 86, Issue 3, Pages 269 - 282

215 Plasma lipoproteins as carriers of phylloquinone (vitamin K1) in humans. Am J Clin Nutr. 1998 Jun;67(6):1226-31

216 Vitamin E: absorption, plasma transport and cell uptake. Hacquebard M, Carpentier YA. Curr Opin Clin Nutr Metab Care. 2005 Mar;8(2):133-8.

217 PUFAs reduce the formation of post-prandial triglycerides that carry lipid soluble nutrients from your last meal.

218 "...it is now generally recognized that the replacement of saturated fats by vegetable oils containing high levels of polyunsaturated fatty acids (PUFAs) may also render individuals susceptible to cardiovascular lesions." In Vivo Absorption, Metabolism, and Urinary Excretion of alpha, beta-Unsaturated Aldehydes in Experimental Animals: Relevance to the Development of Cardiovascular Diseases by the Dietary Ingestion of Thermally Stressed Polyunsaturate-rich Culinary Oils. Grootveld M. J. Clin. Invest. Volume 101, Number 6, March 1998, 1210-1218

219 Dietary oxidized fatty acids: an atherogenic risk? Meera Penumetchaa M. Journal of Lipid Research, Vol. 41, 1473-1480, September 2000

220 Determination of total trans fats and oils by infrared spectroscopy for regulatory compliance, Mossoba M. Anal Bioanal Chem (2007) 389:87–92

221 Lipoxygenase-Catalyzed Oxygenation of Storage Lipids is Implicated in Lipid Mobilization During Germination,I Feussner, Proceedings of the National Academy of Sciences, Vol 92, 11849-11853

222 Formation of modified fatty acids and oxyphytosterols during refining of low erucic acid rapeseed oil. (AKA Canola oil). Lambelet P. J Agric Food Chem. 2003 Jul 16;51(15):4284-90.

223 Formation of modified fatty acids and oxyphytosterols during refining of low erucic acid rapeseed oil. (AKA Canola oil). J Agric Food Chem. 2003 Jul 16;51(15):4284-90.

224 Impaired endothelial function following a meal rich in used cooking fat. Williams M. J Am Coll Cardiol, 1999; 33:1050-1055

225 A local restaurant owner explained one of the benefits of the new "reduced trans" cooking oils is that you can stretch their useful life from one week to two. By then, he said, the stuff turns so black and rancid, you've got no choice but to change it out. Bon appetit!

226 Two consecutive high-fat meals affect endothelial-dependent vasodilation, oxidative stress and cellular microparticles in healthy men. Tushuizen ME J Thromb Haemost. 2006 May;4(5):1003-10.

227.Non enzymatic glycation of apolipoprotein A-I. Effects on its self-association and lipid binding properties. Calvo C. Biochem Biophys Res Commun. 1988 Jun 30;153(3):1060-7

228 Lipoprotein Lipase Mediates the Uptake of Glycated LDL in Fibroblasts, Endothelial Cells, and Macrophages. Robert Zimmermann

229 Glycation of very low density lipoprotein from rat plasma impairs its catabolism. Mamo JC. Diabetologia. 1990 Jun;33(6):339-45.

230 Modification of low density lipoprotein by advanced glycation end products contributes to the dyslipidemia of diabetes and renal insufficiency. Bucala R. Proc Natl Acad Sci U S A. 1994 Sep 27;91(20):9441-5.

231 Glycation of very low density lipoprotein from rat plasma impairs its catabolism. Mamo JC. Diabetologia. 1990 Jun;33(6):339-45. The study concludes: "Glycation [sugar sticking to stuff] of VLDL appears to interfere with the lipolysis [the unloading] of its triglyceride. This may explain the delayed clearance of glycated VLDL triglyceride in vivo."

232 Thermally oxidized dietary fats increase the susceptibility of rat LDL to lipid peroxidation but not their uptake by macrophages. Eder K, J Nutr. 2003 Sep;133(9):2830-7

233 Myeloperoxidase and Plaque Vulnerability. Hazen SL. Arteriosclerosis, Thrombosis, and Vascular Biology. 2004;24:1143.

234 Oxidation-reduction controls fetal hypoplastic lung growth. Fisher JC. J Surg Res. 2002 Aug;106(2):287-91.

235 Intake of high levels of vitamin A and polyunsaturated fatty acids during different developmental periods modifies the expression of morphogenesis genes in European sea bass (Dicentrarchus labrax). Villeneuve LA. Br J Nutr. 2006 Apr;95(4):677-87.

236 Neural tube defects and maternal biomarkers of folate, homocysteine, and glutathione metabolism. Zhao W Birth Defects Res A Clin Mol Teratol. 2006 Apr;76(4):230-6.

237 Congenital heart defects and maternal biomarkers of oxidative stress. Hobbs CA Am J Clin Nutr. 2005 Sep;82(3):598-604

238 A reduction state potentiates the glucocorticoid response through receptor protein stabilization. Kitugawa H. Genes Cells. 2007 Nov;12(11):1281-7.

239 Trends in Serum Lipids and Lipoproteins of Adults, 1960-2002. Carrol MD. Vol 294 No 14, oct 12, 2005.

240 *On The Take: How Medicine's Complicity With Big Business Can Endanger Your Health.* Jerome P. Kassirer. Oxford University Press. 2005.

241 *Overdosed America: The Broken Promise of American Medicine,* John Abramson, Harper Collins, 2004.

242 Adverse Birth Outcomes Among Mothers With Low Serum Cholesterol. Edison RJ. Pediatrics Vol. 120 No. 4 October 2007, pp. 723-733

243 Cane sugar: 160 pounds per capita per year. High fructose corn syrup: 44 pounds per capita per year.

244 Maternal obesity and risk for birth defects. Watkins ML Pediatrics Vol. 111 No. 5 May 2003, pp. 1152-1158

245 Fasting Glucose in Acute Myocardial Infarction. Incremental value for long-term mortality and relationship with left ventricular systolic function. Aronson D. Diabetes Care 30:960-966, 2007

246 IGT and IFG. Time for revision? K. Borch-Johnsen Diabetic Medicine. Volume 19 Issue 9 Page 707-707, September 2002

247 The Modern Nutritional Diseases. Ottoboni F. 2002. "Epidemiologic studies among human populations showed that atherosclerotic cardiovascular diseases occurred at higher rates in affluent societies and among the higher socioeconomic classes. These studies associated the high disease rates with "luxurious food" consumption, excessive caloric intake, sweets, sedentary lifestyle, and stress."

248 America's Eating Habits: Changes and Consequences. Frazao E (ed) Agriculture Information Bulletin No. (AIB750) 484 pp, May 1999 Chapter 7: Trends in the US food supply: 1970-97.

249 Restricted daily consumption of a highly palatable food (chocolate Ensure®) alters striatal enkephalin gene expression, Kelley AE, European Journal of Neuroscience 18 (9) , 2592–2598. The authors conclude that "repeated consumption of a highly rewarding, energy-dense food induces neuroadaptations in cognitive-motivational circuits." Numerous other similar studies exist to support the idea that animals addicted to sugar have the same chemical changes in their brains as if they were addicted to opiates.

250 Routine Sucrose Analgesia During the First Week of Life in Neonates Younger Than 31 Weeks' Postconceptional Age. Johnston CC. PEDIATRICS Vol. 110 No. 3 September 2002, pp. 523-528.

251 Routine Sucrose Analgesia During the First Week of Life in Neonates Younger Than 31 Weeks' Postconceptional Age. Johnston CC. PEDIATRICS Vol. 110 No. 3 September 2002, pp. 523-528

252 Routine Sucrose Analgesia During the First Week of Life in Neonates Younger Than 31 Weeks' Postconceptional Age. Johnston CC. PEDIATRICS Vol. 110 No. 3 September 2002, pp. 523-528

253 Central insulin resistance as a trigger for sporadic Alzheimer-like pathology: an experimental approach. Salkovic-Petrisic M, Hoyer S.J Neural Transm Suppl. 2007;(72):217-33. Review

254 Aging of the brain. Mech Ageing Dev. Anderton BH. 2002 Apr;123(7):811-7. Review

255 Taste Preference for Sweetness in Urban and Rural Populations in Iraq. Jamel HA. J Dent Res 75(11): 1879-1884, November, 1996

256 Pediasure brand nutritional supplement. Label information downloaded from www.pediasure.com/pedia_info.aspx. accessed Aug 22, 2007.

257 Observations on the Economic Adulteration of High Value Food Products. Fairchild GF. Journal of Food Distribution Research Vol 32 No. 2. July 2003. 38-45

258 Jaenisch, R. Epigenetic regulation of gene expression: how the genome integrates intrinsic and environmental signals. Nature Genetics. 33, 245-254 (2003)

259 Orexins in the Brain-Gut Axis. Kirchgessner AL, Endocrine Reviews 23 (1): 1-15

260 Adipose tissue as an endocrine organ. Prins JB. Best Practice & Research Clinical Endocrinology and Metabolism Vol.16 No. 4, pp639-651, 2002.

261 Reduction in Adiposity Affects the Extent of Afferent Projections to Growth Hormone-Releasing Hormone and Somatostatin Neurons and the Degree of Colocalization of Neuropeptides in Growth Hormone-Releasing Hormone and Somatostatin Cells of the Ovine Hypothalamus. Javed Iqbal J. Endocrinology Vol. 146, No. 11 4776-4785

262 Peroxisome Proliferator-Activated Receptor {gamma} and Adipose Tissue—Understanding Obesity-Related Changes in Regulation of Lipid and Glucose Metabolism. Sharma AM. The Journal of Clinical Endocrinology & Metabolism Vol. 92, No. 2 386-395

263 Leptin-induced Growth Stimulation of Breast Cancer Cells Involves Recruitment of Histone Acetyltransferases and Mediator Complex to CYCLIN D1 Promoter via Activation of Stat3, Saxena NK. J. Biol. Chem., Vol. 282, Issue 18, 13316-13325, May 4, 2007

264 Effect of dietary trans fatty acids on the delta 5, delta 6 and delta 9 desaturases of rat liver microsomes in vivo. Mahfouz M. Acta Biol Med Ger. 1981;40(12):1699-1705."This study shows that the dietary trans fatty acids are differentially incorporated into the liver microsomal lipids and act as inhibitors for delta 9 and delta 6 desaturases. The delta 6 desaturase is considered as the key enzyme in the conversion of the essential fatty acids to arachidonic acid and prostaglandins. This indicates that the presence of trans fatty acids in the diet may induce some effects on the EFA metabolism through their action on the desaturases."

265 A defect in the activity of delta 6 and delta 5 desaturases may be a factor predisposing to the development of insulin resistance syndrome. Das UN. Prostaglandins, Leukotrienes and Essential Fatty Acids. Volume 72, Issue 5, May 2005, Pages 343-350

266 Liver mitochondrial dysfunction and oxidative stress in the pathogenesis of experimental nonalcoholic fatty liver disease. Oliveira CP, Braz J Med Biol Res. 2006 Feb;39(2):189-94. Epub 2006 Feb 2.

267 The significance of differences in fatty acid metabolism between obese and non-obese patients with non-alcoholic fatty liver disease. Nakamuta M, Int J Mol Med. 2008 Nov;22(5):663-7.

268 Insulin resistance, inflammation, and non-alcoholic fatty liver disease. Tilg H, Trends Endocrinol Metab. 2008 Oct 15. [Epub ahead of print]

269 Apoptosis in skeletal muscle myotubes is induced by ceramide and is positively related to insulin resistance. Turpin SM, Am J Physiol Endocrinol Metab 291: E1341–E1350, 2006.

270 Minireview: weapons of lean body mass destruction: the role of ectopic lipids in the metabolic syndrome. Unger RH, Endocrinology. 2003 Dec;144(12):5159-65.

271 *Prostaglandins*, Chuck S. Bronson. Nova Publishers, 2006. p51.

272 Dietary fat intake and risk of type 2 diabetes in women. Salmeron J. American Journal of Clinical Nutrition, Vol. 73, No. 6, 1019-1026, June 2001

273 Regulation of adipose cell number in man. Prins JB. Clin Sci (Lond) 1997; 92: 3-11

274 The Cellular Plasticity of Human Adipocytes, Tholpady SS, Annals of Plastic Surgery, Vol 54 No6, June 2005. p651-6

275 Transdifferentiation potential of human mesenchymal stem cells derived from bone marrow. Song L, The FASEB Journal, Vol. 18 June 2004 pp980-2

276 Reversible transdifferentiation of secretory epithelial cells into adipocytes in the mammary gland. Morron M, PNAS November 30, 2004 vol. 101 no. 48 16801–16806

277 Identification of cartilage progenitor cells in the adult ear perichondrium: utilization for cartilage reconstruction. Togo T, Laboratory Investigation (2006) 86, 445 – 457

278 The Cellular Plasticity of Human Adipocytes. Tholpady S, Ann Plast Surg 2005; 54: 651– 656

279 "The Health Report," ABC Radio International, Transcript July 9, 2007. Presented by Norman Swain.

280 Transdifferentiation potential of human mesenchymal stem cells derived from bone marrow. Song L. FASEB Vol 18, June 2004, 980-2.

281 Changes in nerve cells of the nucleus basalis of Meynert in Alzheimer's disease and their relationship to ageing and to the accumulation of lipofuscin pigment. Mann DM. Mech Ageing Dev. 1984 Apr-May;25(1-2):189-204

282 Mechanisms of Disease: Is osteoporosis the obesity of bone? Rosen CJ. Nature Clinical Practice Rheumatology (2006) 2, 35-43

283 Endocrinology of adipose tissue – an update. Fischer-Pozovsky P, Hormone Metabolism Research 2007 May;36(5):314-21.

284 Exercise and the Treatment of Clinical Depression in Adults: Recent Findings and Future Directions. Brosse A. Sports Medicine. 32(12):741-760, 2002.

285 Beta-endorphin decreases fatigue and increases glucose uptake independently in normal and dystrophic mice. Kahn S, Muscle Nerve. 2005 Apr;31(4):481-6.

286 The differential contribution of tumour necrosis factor to thermal and mechanical hyperalgesia during chronic inflammation. Inglis JJ. Arthritis Res Ther. 2005;7(4):R807-16. Epub 2005 Apr 12.

287 TNF-related weak inducer of apoptosis (TWEAK) is a potent skeletal muscle-wasting cytokine. FASEB J. 2007 Jun;21(8):1857-69.

288 Aerobic Exercise Training Increases Brain Volume in Aging Humans. Colcombe J. The Journals of Gerontology Series A: Biological Sciences and Medical Sciences 61:1166-1170 (2006)

289 Running increases cell proliferation and neurogenesis in the adult mouse dentate gyrus. Gage FH. Nat Neurosci. 1999 Mar;2(3):266-70.

290 Six sessions of sprint interval training increases muscle oxidative potential and cycle endurance capacity in humans. Burgomaster KA. J Appl Physiol 98: 1985-1990, 2005.

291 Six sessions of sprint interval training increases muscle oxidative potential and cycle endurance capacity in humans. Burgomaster KA. J Appl Physiol 98: 1985-1990, 2005.

292 Plasma ghrelin is altered after maximal exercise in elite male rowers. Jürimäe J, Exp Biol Med (Maywood). 2007 Jul;232(7):904-9.

293 Update on food allergy, Sampson, H. Journal of Allergy and Clinical Immunology , Volume 113, Issue 5, Pages 805 - 819

294 Hypermobility and sports injuries in junior netball players. Smith R, British Journal of Sports Medicine 2005; 39:628-631

295 The hypermobility syndrome: musculoskeletal complaints in 100 consecutive cases of generalized joint hypermobility. Finsterbush A, Clin Orthop 1982;168:124–7.

296 Does generalised ligamentous laxity increase seasonal incidence of injuries in male first division club rugby players? Stewart DR, Br J Sports Med. 2004 Aug;38(4):457-60.

297 See how AGEs cross-link collagen in Chapter 10.

298 Metabolic fate of exogenous chondroitin sulfate in the experimental animal. Palmieri L, Arzneimittelforschung. 1990 Mar;40(3):319-23.

299 Silbert JE. Proteoglycans and glycosaminoglycans. In: Goldsmith LA, ed. *Biochemistry and Physiology of the Skin*. New York, NY: Oxford University; 1983:448-461

300 Anti-inflammatory activity of chondroitin sulfate. Ronca F, Osteoarthritis Cartilage. 1998 May;6 Suppl A:14-21.

301 Cellulite and Its Treatment. Rawlings A, International Journal of Cosmetic Science, 2006, 28, 175–190

302 Modern Acne Treatment, Zouboilis C, Aktuelle Dermatologie, 2003, vol. 29, no1-2, pp. 49-57

303 Flesh Eating Bacteria: A Legacy of War and Call For Peace. Shanahan C. The Pacific Journal Vol 1 Issue 1, 2007.

304 Kinetics of UV Light–induced Cyclobutane Pyrimidine Dimers in Human Skin In Vivo: An Immunohistochemical Analysis of both Epidermis and Dermis. Katiyar S, Photochemistry and Photobiology, Volume 72 Issue 6, Pages 788 - 793

305 The vitamin D content of fortified milk and infant formula, Holick MF. NEJM, Volume 326:1178-1181, April 30, 1992

Vitamin D intoxication associated with an over-the-counter supplement. Koutikia P,: N Engl J Med. 2001 Jul 5;345(1):66-7.

307 Vitamin D: the underappreciated D-lightful hormone that is important for skeletal and cellular health. Holick M, Current Opinion in Endocrinology & Diabetes. 9(1):87-98, February 2002.

308 With the exception of Northern American Native Peoples. The exception may be due to the fact that they only migrated far north recently, or that they ate so much vitamin D rich animal tissue their skin never needed to lose the melanin to enable UV to penetrate enough to make their own. "The evolution of human skin coloration." Jablonski, Nina G., and George Chaplin. Journal of Human Evolution 39: 57-106. 2000.

309 Skin aging induced by ultraviolet exposure and tobacco smoking: evidence from epidemiological and molecular studies. Lei Y, Photodermatol Photoimmunol Photomed 2001; 17: 178–183

310 Molecular basis of sun-induced premature skin ageing and retinoid antagonism. Fisher GJ, Nature Volume 379(6563), 25 January 1996, pp 335-339

311 Eicosapentaenoic acid inhibits UV-induced MMP-1expression in human dermal fibroblasts. Hyeon HK, Journal of Lipid Research Vol 46, 2005, pp 1712-20.

312 Influence of glucosamine on matrix metalloproteinase expression and activity in lipopolysaccharide-stimulated equine chondrocytes. Byron CR. American Journal of Veterinary Research. June 2003, Vol. 64, No. 6, Pages 666-671

313 The Lung: Development, Aging and The Environment, Ed: Plopper C, Elsevier Publishing 2003. p259

314 *Overdosed America: The Broken Promise of American Medicine*, John Abrams, Harper Collins, 2004.

315 *On The Take: How Medicine's Complicity With Big Business Can Endanger Your Health*, Jerome Kassirer, Oxford University Press, USA, 2005.

316 Current Molecular Medicine 2005, 5, 309-322

CPSIA information can be obtained at www.ICGtesting.com
Printed in the USA
LVOW081115300412

279684LV00002B/1/P